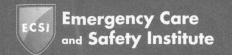
ECSI Emergency Care and Safety Institute

AAOS

First Aid, CPR, and AED
Fifth Edition

Alton Thygerson, Ed.D.
Medical Writer

Benjamin Gulli, MD
Medical Editor

Jon R. Krohmer, MD, FACEP
Medical Editor

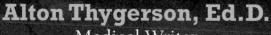
American College of Emergency Physicians®
ADVANCING EMERGENCY CARE ——

D0608329

JONES AND BARTLETT PUBLISHERS
Sudbury, Massachusetts
BOSTON   TORONTO   LONDON   SINGAPORE

Jones and Bartlett Publishers

World Headquarters
40 Tall Pine Drive
Sudbury, MA 01776
info@jbpub.com
www.ECSInstitute.org

Jones and Bartlett Publishers Canada
6339 Ormindale Way
Mississauga, Ontario L5V 1J2
Canada

Jones and Bartlett Publishers International
Barb House, Barb Mews
London W6 7PA
United Kingdom

Jones and Bartlett's books and products are available through most bookstores and online booksellers. To contact Jones and Bartlett Publishers directly, call 800-832-0034, fax 978-443-8000, or visit our website www.jbpub.com.

Substantial discounts on bulk quantities of Jones and Bartlett's publications are available to corporations, professional associations, and other qualified organizations. For details and specific discount information, contact the special sales department at Jones and Bartlett via the above contact information or send an email to specialsales@jbpub.com.

American Academy of Orthopaedic Surgeons

Production Credits
Chief Executive Officer: Clayton E. Jones
Chief Operating Officer: Donald W. Jones, Jr.
President, Higher Education and Professional Publishing: Robert W. Holland, Jr.
V.P., Sales and Marketing: William J. Kane
V.P., Production and Design: Anne Spencer
V.P., Manufacturing and Inventory Control: Therese Connell
Publisher: Lawrence Newell
Publisher, Public Safety Group: Kimberly Brophy
Editor: Jennifer S. Kling

Production Editor: Jenny L. McIsaac
Photo Research Manager/Photographer: Kimberly Potvin
Director of Marketing: Alisha Weisman
Interior Design: Anne Spencer
Cover Design: Kristin E. Ohlin
Cover Image: © Brad Wrobleski/Masterfile
Composition: Shepherd, Inc.
Text Printing and Binding: Courier Kendallville
Cover Printing: Courier Kendallville

The first aid, CPR, and AED procedures in this book are based on the most current recommendations of responsible medical sources. The American Academy of Orthopaedic Surgeons and the Publisher, however, make no guarantee as to, and assume no responsibility for, the correctness, sufficiency, or completeness of such information or recommendations. Other or additional safety measures may be required under particular circumstances.

Reviewed by the American College of Emergency Physicians

The American College of Emergency Physicians (ACEP) makes every effort to ensure that its product and program reviewers are knowledgeable content experts and recognized authorities in their fields. Readers are nevertheless advised that the statements and opinions expressed in this publication are provided as guidelines and should not be construed as College policy unless specifically referred to as such. The College disclaims any liability or responsibility for the consequences of any actions taken in reliance on those statements or opinions. The materials contained herein are not intended to establish policy, procedure, or a standard of care. To contact ACEP write to: PO Box 619911, Dallas, TX 75261-9911; call toll-free 800-798-1822, touch 6, or 972-550-0911.

Library of Congress Catologing-in-Publication Data

Thygerson, Alton L.
First aid, CPR, and AED / Alton Thygerson, Benjamin Gulli, Jon Krohmer ; American Academy of Orthopaedic Surgeons, American College of Emergency Physicians. — 5th ed.
    p. ; cm.
    Includes index.
    ISBN-13: 978-0-7637-4209-6 (pbk.)
    ISBN-10: 0-7637-4209-0 (pbk.)
    1. First aid in illness and injury. 2. CPR (First aid) 3. Automated external defibrillation.   I. Gulli, Benjamin. II. Krohmer, Jon R.
III. American Academy of Orthopaedic Surgeons. IV. American College of Emergency Physicians. V. Title.
    [DNLM: 1. First Aid. 2. Cardiopulmonary Resuscitation. 3. Electric Countershock.   WA 292 T549fi 2007]
RD86.7.T473 2007
616.02'52--dc22

                        2006008738

6048

Additional photographic and illustration credits appear on page 420, which constitutes a continuation of the copyright page.

Printed in the United States of America
10 09 08 07 06   10 9 8 7 6 5 4 3 2

brief contents

contents

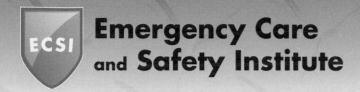
Emergency Care and Safety Institute

welcome

Welcome to the Emergency Care and Safety Institute

Welcome to the Emergency Care and Safety Institute (ECSI), brought to you by the American Academy of Orthopaedic Surgeons (AAOS) and the American College of Emergency Physicians (ACEP).

The ECSI is an educational organization created for the purpose of delivering the highest quality training to laypersons and professionals in the areas of First Aid, CPR, AED, Bloodborne Pathogens, and related safety and health fields.

Two of the most respected names in injury, illness, and emergency medical care—AAOS and ACEP—have approved the content of our training materials.

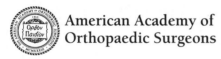
American Academy of Orthopaedic Surgeons

About the AAOS

The AAOS provides education and practice management services for orthopaedic surgeons and allied health professionals. The AAOS also serves as an advocate for improved patient care and informs the public about the science of orthopaedics. Founded in 1933, the not-for-profit AAOS has grown from a small organization serving less than 500 members to the world's largest medical association of musculoskeletal specialists. The AAOS now serves about 24,000 members internationally.

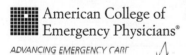
American College of Emergency Physicians®

ADVANCING EMERGENCY CARE

About ACEP

ACEP was founded in 1968 and is the world's oldest and largest emergency medicine specialty organization. Today it represents more than 23,000 members and is the emergency medicine specialty society recognized as the acknowledged leader in emergency medicine.

ECSI Course Catalog

Individuals seeking training in ECSI subjects can choose from among various online and offline course offerings. The following courses are available through the ECSI:

First Aid, CPR, and AED Standard

CPR and AED

Professional Rescuer CPR

First Aid

Wilderness First Aid

Bloodborne Pathogens

First Responder

First Aid and CPR Online

First Aid Online

Adult CPR Online

Adult and Pediatric CPR Online

Professional Rescuer CPR Online

AED Online

Adult CPR and AED Online

Bloodborne Pathogens Online

The ECSI offers a wide range of textbooks, instructor and student support materials, and interactive technology, including online courses. Every ECSI textbook is the center of an integrated teaching and learning system that offers instructor, student, and technology resources to better support instructors and prepare students. The instructor supplements provide practical hands-on, time-saving tools like PowerPoint presentations, DVDs, and web-based distance learning resources. The student supplements are designed to help students retain the most important information and to assist them in preparing for exams. And, a key component to the teaching and learning systems are technology resources that provide interactive exercises and simulations to help students become great emergency responders.

Documents attesting to the ECSI's recognitions of satisfactory course completion will be issued to those who successfully meet the course objectives and criteria for passing the course. Written acknowledgement of a participant's successful course completion is provided in the form of a Course Completion Card, issued by the ECSI.

Visit www.ECSInstitute.org today!

resource preview

This textbook is the core of the First Aid, CPR, and AED program with features that will reinforce and expand on the essential information.

Features include:

Chapter at a Glance
Guides students through the topics covered in the chapter.

Skill Drills Provide step-by-step explanations and visual summaries of important skills for first aiders.

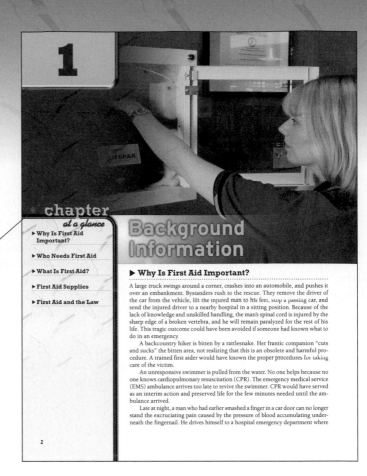

1

chapter
at a glance

▶ Why Is First Aid Important?

▶ Who Needs First Aid

▶ What Is First Aid?

▶ First Aid Supplies

▶ First Aid and the Law

Background Information

▶ Why Is First Aid Important?

A large truck swings around a corner, crashes into an automobile, and pushes it over an embankment. Bystanders rush to the rescue. They remove the driver of the car from the vehicle, lift the injured man to his feet, stop a passing car, and send the injured driver to a nearby hospital in a sitting position. Because of the lack of knowledge and unskilled handling, the man's spinal cord is injured by the sharp edge of a broken vertebra, and he will remain paralyzed for the rest of his life. This tragic outcome could have been avoided if someone had known what to do in an emergency.

A backcountry hiker is bitten by a rattlesnake. Her frantic companion "cuts and sucks" the bitten area, not realizing that this is an obsolete and harmful procedure. A trained first aider would have known the proper procedures for taking care of the victim.

An unresponsive swimmer is pulled from the water. No one helps because no one knows cardiopulmonary resuscitation (CPR). The emergency medical service (EMS) ambulance arrives too late to revive the swimmer. CPR would have served as an interim action and preserved life for the few minutes needed until the ambulance arrived.

Late at night, a man who had earlier smashed a finger in a car door can no longer stand the excruciating pain caused by the pressure of blood accumulating underneath the fingernail. He drives himself to a hospital emergency department where

2

skill drill

2-1   How to Remove Gloves

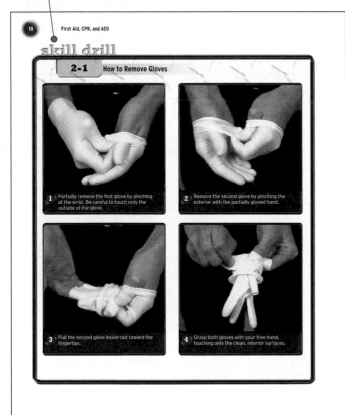

1. Partially remove the first glove by pinching at the wrist. Be careful to touch only the outside of the glove.

2. Remove the second glove by pinching the exterior with the partially gloved hand.

3. Pull the second glove inside-out toward the fingertips.

4. Grasp both gloves with your free hand, touching only the clean, interior surfaces.

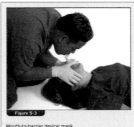

Figure 5-3
Mouth-to-barrier device: mask.

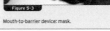

Figure 5-4
Proper hand position for infant CPR.

Mouth-to-Barrier Device

A barrier device is placed in the victim's mouth or over the victim's mouth and nose as a precaution against infection. There are several different types of barrier devices (for example, face shields and face masks), and all are easy to use with little modification to the mouth-to-mouth method **Figure 5-3**.

Mouth-to-Nose Method

If you cannot open the victim's mouth, the teeth are clenched shut, the mouth is severely injured, or you cannot make a good seal with the victim's mouth (for example, because there are no teeth), use the mouth-to-nose method. With the head tilted back, push up on the victim's chin to close the mouth. Make a seal with your mouth over the victim's nose and provide rescue breaths.

Mouth-to-Stoma Method

Some diseases of the vocal cords result in surgical removal of the larynx. People who have this surgery breathe through a small, permanent opening in the neck called a

stoma. To perform mouth-to-stoma breathing, close the victim's mouth and nose and breathe through the opening in the neck.

Chest Compressions

Chest compressions move a small but critical amount of blood to the heart and brain. Perform chest compressions with two hands for an adult, one or two hands for a child, and two fingers for an infant. Effective compressions require rescuers to push hard and fast. The chest of an adult should be compressed 1.5 to 2 inches, and the chest of a child or infant should be compressed one third to one half the depth of the chest. The chest should be allowed to return to its normal depth after each compression. The desired position for adult and child chest compressions is in the center of the chest between the nipples; for infants, it is just below the nipple line **Figure 5-4**. The victim should be on a hard, flat surface (for example, the floor) and on his or her back.

Caution Boxes
Emphasize crucial actions that first aiders should or should not take while administering treatment.

FYI Boxes Include valuable information related to the injuries or illnesses discussed in that section, including prevention tips and risk factors.

FYI

Avoiding Stomach Distention

Rescue breaths can cause stomach distention. Minimize this problem by limiting the breaths to the amount needed to make the chest rise. Avoid overinflating the victim's lungs by just taking a normal breath yourself before breathing into the victim. Gastric distention can cause regurgitation of stomach contents and complicate care.

CAUTION

First aiders DO NOT:
Check for a pulse or other signs of circulation (for example, movement).
Give rescue breaths without chest compressions.
Use a jaw thrust to open the airway—only health care providers use this maneuver.

Decision Tables Provide a concise summary of what first aiders should look for and what treatment steps they should take.

Flowcharts Pose a central question and organize treatment options by injury or illness type.

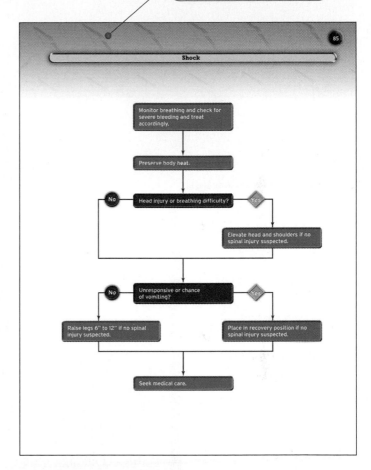

▶ Shock

What to Look For	What to Do
• Agitation • Anxiety • Restlessness • Feeling of impending doom • Altered mental status • Weak, rapid, or absent pulse • Clammy (pale, cool, moist) skin • Paleness, with cyanosis about the lips • Shallow, rapid breathing • Shortness of breath • Nausea or vomiting	1. Wear medical exam gloves. 2. Monitor breathing and provide care if needed. 3. Control all obvious bleeding. 4. Place the victim on his or her back. (Those having a heart attack or those with lung disease breathe easier in a half-sitting position). 5. Raise the victim's legs 6 to 12 inches. Do not move the victim if there are suspected fractures or head, spine, or torso injuries. 6. Splint any bone or joint injuries. 7. Place blankets under and over the victim. 8. Handle the victim gently. 9. Seek medical care by calling 9-1-1 if signs of shock are present.

▶ Anaphylaxis

What to Look For	What to Do
Skin • Flushing, itching, or burning, especially over the face and upper chest • Hives, which can spread over large areas of the body • Swelling, especially of the face, tongue, and lips • Bluish lips (cyanosis) **Circulatory system** • Weak pulse (you might be barely able to feel it) • Dizziness • Fainting and unresponsiveness **Respiratory system** • Sneezing or itching in the nostrils • Tightness in the chest, with a persistent dry cough • Breathing difficulty • Secretions of fluid and mucus into the throat and lungs • Wheezing (forced expirations during breathing) • Breathing stops	1. Monitor breathing, and if necessary, give CPR. 2. Call 9-1-1 immediately. 3. If the victim has his or her own prescribed epinephrine, help the victim use it. If you are assisting with or using an auto-injector, follow the container's instructions. 4. Give an antihistamine (such as Benadryl)—it is not life saving because it takes too long to work (20 minutes), but can prevent further reactions. 5. Keep a responsive victim sitting up to help breathing. Place an unresponsive victim on his or her side (recovery position).

prep kit

▶ Ready for Review

○ A heart attack occurs when heart muscle tissue dies because the blood supply is severely reduced or stopped.

○ The four links in the chain of survival are early access, early CPR, early defibrillation, and early advanced care.

○ CPR consists of breathing oxygen into a victim's lungs and moving blood to the heart and brain by giving chest compressions.

○ The signs of a severe airway obstruction include difficult breathing, weak and ineffective cough, inability to speak or breathe, and signs of cyanosis.

▶ Vital Vocabulary

<u>airway obstruction</u> A blockage, often the result of a foreign body, in which air flow to the lungs is reduced or completely blocked.

<u>cardiac arrest</u> Stoppage of the heartbeat.

<u>chain of survival</u> A four-step concept to help improve survival from cardiac arrest: early access, early CPR, early defibrillation, and early advanced care.

<u>chest compressions</u> Depressing the chest and allowing it to return to its normal position as part of CPR.

<u>CPR</u> Cardiopulmonary resuscitation; the act of providing rescue breaths and chest compressions for a victim in cardiac arrest.

<u>heart attack</u> Death of a part of the heart muscle.

<u>rescue breaths</u> Breathing for a person who is not breathing.

▶ Assessment in Action

You are at a local health club when you overhear someone in the weight room nearby shouting for help. You enter the room and see a person lying motionless on the floor. You quickly confirm that he is unresponsive.
Directions: Circle Yes if you agree with the statement, circle No if you disagree.

Yes No 1. The next thing to do is to start chest compressions.

Yes No 2. The ratio of chest compressions to rescue breaths is 15 to 2.

Yes No 3. Compression depth for an adult is one third the depth of the chest.

Yes No 4. Open the airway using the head tilt–chin lift method.

Yes No 5. Continue CPR until an AED becomes available or EMS personnel arrive.

Answers: 1. No; 2. No; 3. No; 4. Yes; 5. Yes

▶ Check Your Knowledge

Directions: Circle Yes if you agree with the statement, circle No if you disagree.

Yes No 1. Take 5 to 10 seconds when checking for breathing.

Yes No 2. After you determine that an adult victim is unresponsive, the next step is to call 9-1-1.

Yes No 3. Tilting the head back and lifting the chin helps move the tongue and open the airway.

Yes No 4. If you determine that a victim is not breathing, begin chest compressions.

Yes No 5. Do not start chest compressions until you have checked for a pulse.

Yes No 6. For all victims (adult, child, infant) needing CPR, give 30 compressions followed by two breaths.

Yes No 7. Use two fingers when performing CPR on an infant.

Yes No 8. A sign of choking is that the victim is unable to speak or cough.

Yes No 9. To give abdominal thrusts to a responsive choking victim, place your fist below the victim's navel.

Yes No 10. When giving abdominal thrusts to a responsive choking victim, repeat the thrusts until the object is removed or the victim becomes unresponsive.

Answers: 1. Yes; 2. Yes; 3. Yes; 4. No; 5. No; 6. Yes; 7. Yes; 8. Yes; 9. No; 10. Yes

Prep Kit End-of-chapter activities reinforce important concepts and improve students' comprehension.
Key Terms List of the key terms and definitions from the chapter.
Assessment in Action Brief case study followed by critical thinking questions that allow students to apply what they've learned.
Check Your Knowledge Questions Quiz students on the chapter's core concepts.

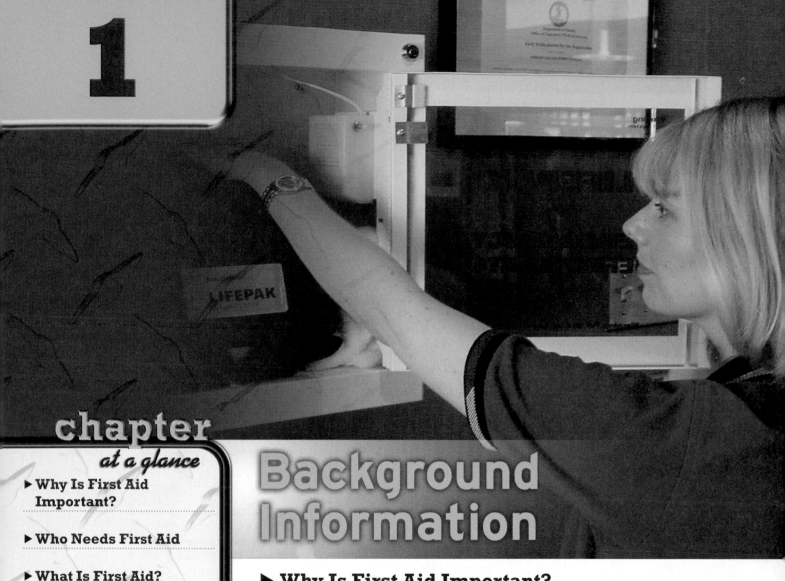

chapter
at a glance

Background Information

▶ Why Is First Aid Important?

A large truck swings around a corner, crashes into an automobile, and pushes it over an embankment. Bystanders rush to the rescue. They remove the driver of the car from the vehicle, lift the injured man to his feet, stop a passing car, and send the injured driver to a nearby hospital in a sitting position. Because of the lack of knowledge and unskilled handling, the man's spinal cord is injured by the sharp edge of a broken vertebra, and he will remain paralyzed for the rest of his life. This tragic outcome could have been avoided if someone had known what to do in an emergency.

A backcountry hiker is bitten by a rattlesnake. Her frantic companion "cuts and sucks" the bitten area, not realizing that this is an obsolete and harmful procedure. A trained first aider would have known the proper procedures for taking care of the victim.

An unresponsive swimmer is pulled from the water. No one helps because no one knows cardiopulmonary resuscitation (CPR). The emergency medical service (EMS) ambulance arrives too late to revive the swimmer. CPR would have served as an interim action and preserved life for the few minutes needed until the ambulance arrived.

Late at night, a man who had earlier smashed a finger in a car door can no longer stand the excruciating pain caused by the pressure of blood accumulating underneath the fingernail. He drives himself to a hospital emergency department where a blood clot is relieved. He later receives a bill for more than $100. If he had known the proper first aid procedure, he could have relieved the pain sooner and saved money.

These cases clearly point out the need for first aid training. *It is better to know it and not need it than to need it and not know it.* Everyone should be able to perform first aid, because most people will eventually find themselves in a situation requiring it for another person or for themselves. First aiders do not diagnose (this is what medical doctors do), but they can suspect what the problem is and then give first aid.

▶ Who Needs First Aid?

Although heart disease and cancer continue to be critical health problems in the United States, injuries—both unintentional and intentional—constitute a major threat to public health. This threat has been called the neglected epidemic. **Table 1-1** shows the role of injury as a cause of death by age group and ranking compared with other causes of death.

Death statistics do not always reflect the extent or severity of the injury problem. Most people who are injured do not die of their injuries. The extent of nonfatal injuries is reflected in nonfatal injury data. The "injury pyramid" illustrates the relationship between death and nonfatal injury **Figure 1-1** . Deaths from injury are only the tip of the iceberg.

Table 1-2 shows the leading causes of nonfatal, unintentional injury by age group in the United States. Each year, one in four people experiences a nonfatal injury serious enough to need medical care or to restrict activity for at least 1 day. More sports-related nonfatal injuries are treated in hospital emergency departments than any other type of unintentional injury.

A delay of as little as 4 minutes when a person's heart stops can mean death. Therefore, what a bystander does can mean the difference between life and death. Fortunately, most injuries do not require lifesaving efforts. During their entire lifetimes, most people will see only one or two situations involving life-threatening conditions. Most of the victims you see will have injuries requiring only first aid.

Table 1-1 Leading Causes of Death

Rank	<1	1-4	5-9	10-14	15-24	25-34	35-44	45-54	55-64	65+	All Ages
1	Congenital Anomalies 5,621	Unintentional Injury 1,717	Unintentional Injury 1,096	Unintentional Injury 1,522	Unintentional Injury 15,272	Unintentional Injury 12,541	Unintentional Injury 16,766	Malignant Neoplasms 49,843	Malignant Neoplasms 95,692	Heart Disease 563,390	Heart Disease 685,089
2	Short Gestation 4,849	Congenital Anomalies 541	Malignant Neoplasms 516	Malignant Neoplasms 560	Homicide 5,368	Suicide 5,065	Malignant Neoplasms 15,509	Heart Disease 37,732	Heart Disease 65,060	Malignant Neoplasms 388,911	Malignant Neoplasms 556,902
3	SIDS 2,162	Malignant Neoplasms 392	Congenital Anomalies 180	Suicide 244	Suicide 3,988	Homicide 4,516	Heart Disease 13,600	Unintentional Injury 15,837	Chronic Low. Respiratory Disease 12,077	Cerebro-vascular 138,134	Cerebro-vascular 157,689
4	Maternal Pregnancy Comp. 1,710	Homicide 376	Homicide 122	Congenital Anomalies 206	Malignant Neoplasms 1,651	Malignant Neoplasms 3,741	Suicide 6,602	Liver Disease 7,466	Diabetes Mellitus 10,731	Chronic Low Respiratory Disease 109,139	Chronic Low Respiratory Disease 126,382
5	Placenta Cord Membranes 1,099	Heart Disease 186	Heart Disease 104	Homicide 202	Heart Disease 1,133	Heart Disease 3,250	HIV 5,340	Suicide 6,481	Cerebro-vascular 9,946	Alzheimer's Disease 62,814	Unintentional Injury 109,277
6	Unintentional Injury 945	Influenza & Pneumonia 163	Influenza & Pneumonia 75	Heart Disease 160	Congenital Anomalies 451	HIV 1,588	Homicide 3,110	Cerebro-vascular 6,127	Unintentional Injury 9,170	Influenza & Pneumonia 57,070	Diabetes Mellitus 74,219
7	Respiratory Distress 831	Septicemia 85	Septicemia 39	Chronic Low Respiratory Disease 81	Influenza & Pneumonia 244	Diabetes Mellitus 657	Liver Disease 3,020	Diabetes Mellitus 5,658	Liver Disease 6,428	Diabetes Mellitus 54,919	Influenza & Pneumonia 65,163
8	Bacterial Sepsis 772	Perinatal Period 79	Benign Neoplasms 38	Influenza & Pneumonia 72	Cerebro-vascular 221	Cerebro-vascular 583	Cerebro-vascular 2,460	HIV 4,442	Suicide 3,843	Nephritis 35,254	Alzheimer's Disease 63,457
9	Neonatal Hemorrhage 649	Chronic Low Respiratory Disease 55	Chronic Low Respiratory Disease 37	Benign Neoplasms 41	Chronic Low Respiratory Disease 191	Congenital Anomalies 426	Diabetes Mellitus 2,049	Chronic Low Respiratory Disease 3,537	Nephritis 3,806	Unintentional Injury 34,355	Nephritis 42,453
10	Circulatory System Disease 591	Benign Neoplasms 51	Cerebro-vascular 29	Cerebro-vascular 40	HIV 178	Influenza & Pneumonia 373	Influenza & Pneumonia 992	Viral Hepatitis 2,259	Septicemia 3,651	Septicemia 26,445	Septicemia 34,069

Source: Produced by Office of Statistics and Programming, National Center for Injury Prevention and Control, US Centers for Disease Control and Prevention. Data source: National Center for Health Statistics (NCHS) Vital Statistics Systems. Available at http://webapp.cdc.gov/sasweb/ncipc/leadcaus10.htm.

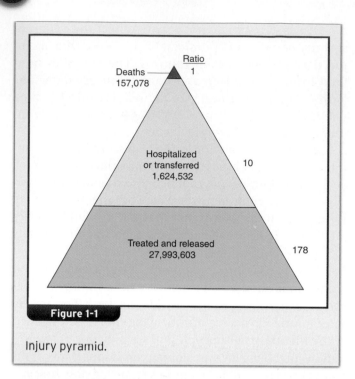

Figure 1-1

Injury pyramid.

Each year, the injuries of millions of Americans go unreported. For many of them, the injury causes temporary pain and inconvenience; for others, however, the injury leads to disability, chronic pain, and a profound change in lifestyle. Given the size of the injury problem and sudden illness, everyone should be prepared to deal with an emergency.

Value to Self

Although many people learn first aid to help others, the training primarily helps oneself. It enables a person to give proper immediate care to one's own injuries and sudden illnesses. If victims are too seriously injured to help themselves, they could be able to direct others in proper care. First aid training also helps develop safety awareness. Discussing injuries promotes injury prevention by showing how injuries occur.

Table 1-2   Ten Leading Causes of Unintentional Injury

Rank	<1	1-4	5-9	10-14	15-24	25-34	35-44	45-54	55-64	65+	All Ages
1	Unintentional Fall 126,281	Unintentional Fall 888,335	Unintentional Fall 676,704	Unintentional Fall 668,589	Unintentional Struck by/Against 980,050	Unintentional Fall 762,703	Unintentional Fall 816,521	Unintentional Fall 791,813	Unintentional Fall 607,041	Unintentional Fall 1,850,649	Unintentional Fall 8,058,498
2	Unintentional Struck by/Against 30,760	Unintentional Struck by/Against 368,104	Unintentional Struck by/Against 404,124	Unintentional Struck by/Against 593,752	Unintentional MV-Occupant 914,024	Unintentional Overexertion 673,076	Unintentional Overexertion 645,508	Unintentional Overexertion 423,692	Unintentional Struck by/Against 200,708	Unintentional Struck by/Against 214,235	Unintentional Struck by/Against 4,430,171
3	Unintentional Other Bite/Sting 12,753	Unintentional Other Bite/Sting 145,001	Unintentional Cut/Pierce 115,886	Unintentional Overexertion 272,797	Unintentional Fall 869,363	Unintentional Struck by/Against 669,346	Unintentional Struck by/Against 575,089	Unintentional Struck by/Against 393,861	Unintentional Overexertion 200,451	Unintentional MV-Occupant 185,779	Unintentional Overexertion 3,279,383
4	Unintentional Fire/Burn 11,372	Unintentional Foreign Body 113,084	Unintentional Pedal Cyclist 101,891	Unintentional Cut/Pierce 155,040	Unintentional Overexertion 739,741	Unintentional MV-Occupant 612,446	Unintentional MV-Occupant 501,564	Unintentional MV-Occupant 353,728	Unintentional MV-Occupant 197,296	Unintentional Overexertion 167,395	Unintentional MV-Occupant 3,000,866
5	Unintentional Foreign Body 9,767	Unintentional Cut/Pierce 86,787	Unintentional Other Bite/Sting 93,317	Unintentional Pedal Cyclist 140,063	Unintentional Cut/Pierce 498,856	Unintentional Cut/Pierce 440,900	Unintentional Cut/Pierce 398,151	Unintentional Cut/Pierce 296,883	Unintentional Cut/Pierce 164,110	Inintentional Cut/Pierce 122,162	Unintentional Cut/Pierce 2,285,191
6	Unintentional Other Specified 7,979	Unintentional Overexertion 76,876	Unintentional MV-Occupant 74,399	Unintentional MV-Occupant 99,353	Unintentional Other Bite/Sting 194,493	Unintentional Other Bite/Sting 173,843	Unintentional Other Specified 176,427	Unintentional Other Specified 149,760	Unintentional Other Bite/Sting 68,451	Unintentional Other Bite/Sting 74,395	Unintentional Other Bite/Sting 1,103,257
7	Unintentional Inhalation/Suffocation 7,801	Unintentional Fire/Burn 57,728	Unintentional Overexertion 73,980	Unintentional Unknown/Unspecified 95,311	Unintentional Other Specified 158,451	Unintentional Other Specified 142,385	Unintentional Other Bite/Sting 153,531	Unintentional Other Bite/Sting 117,166	Unintentional Other Specified 59,121	Unintentional Poisoning 61,888	Unintentional Other Specified 820,676
8	Unintentional MV-Occupant 6,992	Unintentional Other Specified 49,446	Unintentional Foreign Body 58,303	Unintentional Other Transport 70,429	Unintentional Unknown/Unspecified 142,089	Unintentional Other Transport 102,175	Unintentional Poisoning 118,140	Unintentional Poisoning 92,787	Unintentional Poisoning 39,802	Unintentional Other Transport 47,822	Unintentional Other Transport 623,846
9	Unintentional Cut/Pierce 6,152	Unintentional Poisoning 47,402	Unintentional Dog Bite 52,568	Unintentional Other Bite/Sting 70,286	Unintentional Other Transport 136,800	Unintentional Foreign Body 99,096	Unintentional Foreign Body 86,079	Unintentional Other Transport 67,640	Unintentional Other Transport 33,856	Unintentional Unknown/Unspecified 40,910	Unintentional Foreign Body 609,493
10	Unintentional Poisoning 5,814	Unintentional Unknown/Unspecified 47,078	Unintentional Other Transport 49,071	Unintentional Dog Bite 39,265	Unintentional Poisoning 100,145	Unintentional Poisoning 90,372	Unintentional Other Transport 82,760	Unintentional Foreign Body 62,703	Unintentional Foreign Body 32,348	Unintentional Other Specified 37,148	Unintentional Unknown/Unspecified 589,698

Source: Office of Statistics and Programming, National Center for Injury Prevention and Control, CDC.

Value to Others

People with first aid training are more likely to give proper assistance to injured family members. Although the main beneficiaries are the trained individual and family, the benefits of knowing appropriate first aid techniques extend further, usually to coworkers, acquaintances, and strangers.

Value in Remote Areas

Should injuries or sudden illness require medical care, time, distance, and availability are major considerations. EMS can reach most victims who are severely injured or suddenly ill within 10 to 20 minutes. However, some victims are long distances from medical care. Although most people associate wilderness settings involving outdoor recreational activities (for example, hiking, camping, hunting, and snowmobiling) with long distances and lack of medical care, other settings also demand that people be prepared to give first aid for an extended time. The following are some examples:

- Urban areas after a disaster that destroys or overwhelms the EMS
- Remote occupations (for example, farming, ranching, commercial fishing, and forestry)
- Remote communities
- Developing countries

First aid needed in remote locations is similar to that needed in urban settings, but extra skills are sometimes required. See chapter 24 for information on delivering first aid in remote locations.

▶ What Is First Aid?

First aid is the immediate care given to an injured or suddenly ill person. First aid does not take the place of proper medical care. It consists only of giving temporary help until competent medical care, if needed, is obtained or until the chance for recovery without medical care is assured. Most injuries and illnesses do not require medical care.

Properly applied, first aid might mean the difference between life and death, between rapid recovery and a long hospitalization, or between a temporary and a permanent disability. First aid involves more than doing things for others; it also includes treatments that people can do for themselves.

Recognizing a serious medical emergency and knowing how to get help could be crucial in saving a life. Recognition of an emergency can be delayed because neither the victim nor bystanders know basic symptoms (for example, a heart attack victim might wait hours after the

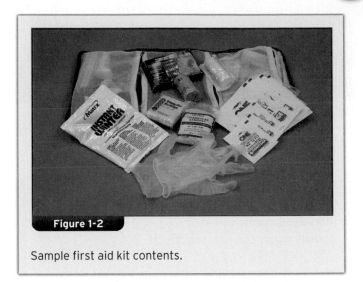

Figure 1-2

Sample first aid kit contents.

onset of symptoms before seeking help). Moreover, most people do not know first aid; even if they do, they might panic in an emergency.

▶ First Aid Supplies

The supplies in a first aid kit should be customized to include those items likely to be used on a regular basis Figure 1-2 . A kit for the home is often different than one for the workplace. A home kit may contain personal medications and a smaller number of items. A workplace kit will need more items (such as bandages) and will not include personal medications. Table 1-3 lists the basic items that should be stocked in a workplace first aid kit.

Although a first aid kit may have some medications, such as antihistamines and topical ointments, there might be local requirements that restrict the use of these items by first aiders without prior written approval. For example, teachers, activity leaders, and bus drivers in certain areas might not be able to administer these items to children without specific written permission signed by a child's parent or guardian.

▶ First Aid and the Law

Legal and ethical issues concern all first aiders. For example, is a first aider required to stop and give care at an automobile crash? Can a child with a broken arm be treated even when the parents cannot be contacted for their consent? These and many other legal and ethical questions confront first aiders.

A first aider can be sued. Do not become overly concerned about being sued—it rarely happens. Ways to minimize the risk of a suit include:

- Obtaining the victim's consent before touching him.

Table 1-3	Sample Workplace First Aid Kit *	
Equipment		**Minimum Quantity**
Adhesive strip bandages (1″ × 3″)		20
Triangular bandages (muslin, 36″ × 40″ × 36″– 40″ × 52″– 56″)		4
Sterile eye pads (2⅛″ × 2⅝″)		2
Sterile gauze pads (4″ × 4″)		6
Sterile nonstick pads (3″ × 4″)		6
Sterile trauma pads (5″ × 9″)		2
Sterile trauma pads (8″ × 10″)		1
Sterile conforming roller gauze (2″ width)		3 rolls
Sterile conforming roller gauze (4½″ width)		3 rolls
Waterproof tape (1″ × 5 yards)		1 roll
Porous adhesive tape (2″ × 5 yards)		1 roll
Elastic roller bandages (4″ and 6″)		1 each
Antiseptic skin wipes, individually wrapped		10
Antibiotic ointment, individual packets		6
Medical exam gloves (various sizes)		2 pairs per size
Mouth-to-barrier device, either a face mask with a one-way valve or a disposable face shield		1
Disposable instant cold packs		2
Sealable plastic bags (quart size)		2
Padded malleable splint (SAM splint, 4″ × 36″)		1
Emergency blanket		1
Scissors		1
Tweezers		1
Biohazard waste bag (3½ gallon capacity)		2
List of local emergency telephone numbers		1
Miniature flashlight and batteries		1 flashlight, 4 batteries

*This list does not include over-the-counter ointments, topical medications, or internal medications.

- Following this book's guidelines and not exceeding your training level.
- Explaining any first aid you are about to give.
- Once starting to care for a victim, stay with that person. You are legally bound to remain with the victim until care is turned over to an equally or better trained person.

Consent

A first aider must have the victim's **consent** (permission) before giving first aid. Touching another person without his or her permission or consent is unlawful (known as **battery**) and could be grounds for a lawsuit. Likewise, giving first aid without the victim's consent is unlawful.

Expressed Consent

Consent must be obtained from every alert, mentally competent (able to make a rational decision) person of legal age. Tell the victim that you have first aid training and explain what you will be doing. The victim may give permission verbally or with a nod of the head.

Implied Consent

Implied consent involves an unresponsive victim with a life-threatening condition. It is assumed or implied that an unresponsive victim would consent to lifesaving interventions. An alert victim who does not resist the administrations of a first aider is also assumed to have given consent.

Children and Mentally Incompetent Adults

Consent must be obtained from the parent or guardian of a child victim, as legally defined by the state. The same is true for an adult who is mentally incompetent. When life-threatening situations exist and a parent or legal guardian is not available for consent, first aid should be given based on implied consent. Do not withhold first aid from a minor just to obtain consent from a parent or guardian.

Psychiatric emergencies present difficult problems of consent. Under most conditions, a police officer is the only person with the authority to restrain and transport a person against that person's will. A first aider should not intervene unless directed to do so by a police officer or unless it is obvious that the victim is about to do life-threatening harm to himself or herself or to others.

Refusing Help

Although it seldom happens, a person might refuse assistance for countless reasons, such as religious grounds, avoidance of possible pain, or the desire to be examined by a physician rather than by a first aider. Whatever the reason for refusing medical care, or even if no reason is given, the alert and mentally competent adult can reject help.

Generally, the wisest approach is to inform the victim of his or her medical condition, what you propose to do, and why the help is necessary. If the victim understands the consequences and still refuses treatment, there is little else you can do. Call the EMS, and, while awaiting arrival:

- Try again to persuade the victim to accept care and encourage others at the scene to persuade the victim. A victim could have a change of mind after a short time.
- Make certain you have witnesses. A victim could refuse consent and then deny having done so.

- Consider calling for law enforcement assistance. In most locations, the police can place a person in protective custody and require him or her to go to a hospital.

Abandonment

<u>Abandonment</u> means leaving a victim after starting to give help without ensuring continued care at the same level or higher. Once you have responded to an emergency, you must not leave a victim who needs continuing first aid until another competent and trained person takes responsibility for the victim. This might seem obvious, but there have been cases in which critically ill or injured victims were left unattended and then died. Thus, a first aider must stay with the victim until another equally or better trained person takes over.

Negligence

<u>Negligence</u> means not following the accepted standards of care, resulting in further injury to the victim. Negligence involves:

1. Having a duty to act (required to give first aid)
2. Breaching that duty (either by giving no care or by giving substandard care)
3. Causing injury and damages
4. Exceeding your level of training

Duty to Act

No one is required to give first aid unless a legal <u>duty to act</u> exists. For example, you do not have to help a stranger unless you have a legal obligation to that person, or you were involved in the events that led to the victim's injuries regardless of who was at fault. The decision to help in an emergency is usually an ethical (moral) one. Duty to act could apply in the following situations:

- *When employment requires it.* If your employer designates you as the individual responsible for providing first aid to meet Occupational Safety and Health Administration (also known as OSHA) requirements and you are called to an injury scene, you have a duty to act. Examples of occupations that involve a legal obligation to give first aid include law enforcement officers, park rangers, athletic trainers, lifeguards, flight attendants, and firefighters.
- *When on duty (and sometimes when off duty).* Some states require certain individuals who are licensed by the state to give emergency care regardless of their on- or off-duty status. In other words, these individuals are considered to be always on duty. Other states require them to act when on duty but not generally when they are off duty, unless they are in uniform or have other visible insignia and

appear to be on duty—in which case these individuals must respond.
- *When a preexisting responsibility exists.* You might have a preexisting relationship with other persons that makes you responsible for them, which means that you must give first aid should they need it. For example, a parent has a preexisting responsibility for a child, and a driver for a passenger.

Duty to act means following guidelines for standards of care. Standards of care ensure quality care and protection for injured or suddenly ill victims. The elements that make up standards of care include the following:

- *The type of rescuer.* A first aider should provide the level and type of care expected of a reasonable person with the same amount of training and in similar circumstances. Different standards of care apply to physicians, nurses, emergency medical technicians (EMTs), and first aiders.
- *Published guidelines.* Emergency care-related organizations and societies publish recommended first aid procedures. For example, the American Heart Association publishes guidelines for giving CPR, and the Wilderness Medical Society publishes guidelines for assisting victims who are in remote locations.

Breach of Duty

A <u>breach of duty</u> happens when a first aider fails to provide the type of care that would be given by a person having the same or similar training. There are two ways to breach one's duty: acts of omission and acts of commission. An <u>act of omission</u> is the failure to do what a reasonably prudent person with the same or similar training would do in the same or similar circumstances. An <u>act of commission</u> is doing something that a reasonably prudent person would not do under the same or similar circumstances. Forgetting to put on a dressing is an act of omission; cutting a snake-bite site is an act of commission.

Injury and Damages Inflicted

In addition to physical damage, injury and damage can include physical pain and suffering, mental anguish, medical expenses, and sometimes loss of earnings and earning capacity.

Confidentiality

First aiders might learn confidential information. It is important that you be extremely cautious about revealing information you learn while caring for someone. The law recognizes that people have the right to privacy. Do not discuss what you know with anyone other than those who have a medical need to know. Some state laws, however, require the reporting of certain incidents, such as rape, abuse, and gunshot wounds.

Good Samaritan Laws

Starting in the late 1950s, a number of states (beginning with California in 1959) enacted laws designed to protect physicians and other medical personnel from legal actions that might arise from emergency treatment they provided while not in the line of duty. These laws, known as <u>Good Samaritan laws</u>, encourage people to assist others in distress by granting them immunity against lawsuits. Although the laws vary from state to state, Good Samaritan immunity generally applies only when the rescuer is (1) acting during an emergency; (2) acting in good faith, which means he or she has good intentions; (3) acting without compensation; and (4) not guilty of malicious misconduct or gross negligence toward the victim (deviating from rational first aid guidelines).

Although Good Samaritan laws primarily cover health care providers, many states have expanded them to include laypersons serving as first aiders. In fact, some states have several Good Samaritan laws that cover different types of people in various situations. Many legal experts believe Good Samaritan laws have given first aiders a false sense of security. These laws will not protect first aiders who have caused further injury to a victim. Good Samaritan laws are not a protection for poorly given first aid or for exceeding the scope of your training. Fear of lawsuits has made some people hesitant of becoming involved in emergency situations. First aiders, however, are rarely sued.

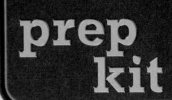

▶ Ready for Review

- Everyone should be able to perform first aid because most people will eventually find themselves in a situation requiring it for another person or for themselves.
- First aid is the immediate care given to an injured or suddenly ill person. First aid does not take the place of proper medical care.
- The supplies in a first aid kit should be customized to include those items likely to be used on a regular basis.
- Legal and ethical issues concern all first aiders.
- A first aider must have the victim's consent (permission) before giving first aid.
- First aiders might learn confidential information. It is important that you be extremely cautious about revealing information you learn while caring for someone.
- Varying from state to state, Good Samaritan laws encourage people to assist others in distress by granting them immunity against lawsuits.

▶ Vital Vocabulary

abandonment Failure to continue first aid until relieved by someone with the same or a higher level of training.

act of commission Doing something that a reasonably prudent person would not do under the same or similar circumstances.

act of omission Failure to do what a reasonably prudent person with the same or similar training would do in the same or similar circumstances.

battery Touching a person or providing first aid without consent.

breach of duty When a first aider fails to provide the type of care that would be given by a person having the same or similar training.

consent An agreement by a patient or victim to accept treatment offered as explained by medical personnel or first aiders.

duty to act An individual's responsibility to provide victim care.

first aid Immediate care given to an injured or suddenly ill person.

Good Samaritan laws Laws that encourage individuals to voluntarily help an injured or suddenly ill person by minimizing the liability for errors made while rendering emergency care in good faith.

implied consent An assumed consent given by an unconscious adult when emergency lifesaving treatment is required.

negligence Deviation from the accepted standard of care that results in further injury to the victim.

▶ Assessment in Action

You are driving slowly looking for a house number in an unfamiliar residential area. You are trying to find your friend's new home. While looking for the house, you see an elderly woman lying motionless at the bottom of a flight of porch stairs. You see no one else in the neighborhood, and you are alone. You quickly, but safely, stop your vehicle in front of the victim's house. As you approach the victim, you notice that her skin appears bluish.

Directions: Circle Yes if you agree with the statement, circle No if you disagree.

Yes   No   **1.** Do you have to stop to help her?

Yes   No   **2.** You have implied consent to help this person.

Yes   No   **3.** If she does not respond to your tapping on her shoulders and shouting, "Are you OK?" you can leave her and assume that someone else who is more competent or is a family member will arrive shortly to help her.

Yes   No   **4.** You decide to help. Without examining the victim you quickly straighten her legs, which suddenly causes a bone to protrude through the skin. Would this increase the likelihood of being sued?

Answers: **1.** No; **2.** Yes; **3.** No; **4.** Yes

prep kit

▶ Check Your Knowledge

Directions: Circle Yes if you agree with the statement, circle No if you disagree.

Yes   No   **1.** Because an ambulance can arrive within minutes in most locations, most people do not need to learn first aid.

Yes   No   **2.** Correct first aid can mean the difference between life and death.

Yes   No   **3.** During your lifetime, you are likely to encounter many life-threatening emergencies.

Yes   No   **4.** All injured victims need medical care.

Yes   No   **5.** Before giving first aid to an alert, competent adult, you must get consent (permission) from the victim.

Yes   No   **6.** If you ask an injured adult if you can help, and she says "No," you can ignore her and proceed to provide care.

Yes   No   **7.** People who are designated as first aiders by their employers must give first aid to injured employees while on the job.

Yes   No   **8.** First aiders who help injured victims are rarely sued.

Yes   No   **9.** Good Samaritan laws provide a degree of protection for first aiders who act in good faith and without compensation.

Yes   No   **10.** You are required to provide first aid to any injured or suddenly ill person you encounter.

Answers: **1.** No; **2.** Yes; **3.** No; **4.** No; **5.** Yes; **6.** No; **7.** Yes; **8.** Yes; **9.** Yes; **10.** No

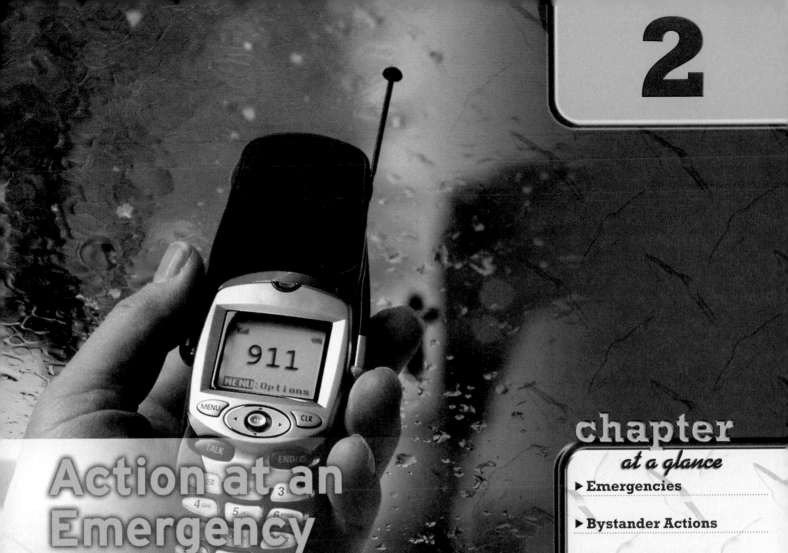

Action at an Emergency

Emergencies

Emergencies have distinctive characteristics. They are:

- Dangerous—people's lives, well-being, or property are threatened.
- Unusual and rare events—the average person will probably encounter fewer than a half a dozen serious emergencies in a lifetime.
- Different from one another—each presents a different set of problems.
- Unforeseen—they happen suddenly and without warning.
- Urgent—if the emergency is not dealt with immediately, the situation will escalate.

► Bystander Actions

The bystander is a vital link between the <u>emergency medical services (EMS)</u> and the victim. Typically it is a bystander who recognizes a situation as an emergency and acts to help the victim. If a bystander is to intervene in an emergency, he or she must make not just one but a series of decisions and actions quickly and reliably. These include:

1. Recognizing the emergency.
2. Deciding to help.
3. Calling 9-1-1, if EMS is needed.
4. Checking the victim.
5. Giving first aid.

Compared with health care providers, ordinary bystanders are significantly less likely to offer help in emergencies that occur in public places. Some reasons for this include:

- Lack of knowledge
- Confusion about what is an emergency
- Characteristics of the emergency (for example, unpleasant physical appearance of the victim, the presence of other bystanders)

Lack of Knowledge and Helping Behavior

The average layperson is unaware of many aspects of emergency care and has difficulty recognizing common medical emergencies and deciding to call 9-1-1 for help. Also, a person who does not feel competent to deal with an emergency is not likely to offer even minimal help. The person who does not feel competent can escape this uncomfortable feeling by failing to acknowledge the situation as an emergency. The implication is that bystanders who are uncertain of their ability to deal with a seriously injured victim are more likely to assume that the victim is not seriously injured.

Confusion About What Is an Emergency

Sometimes, laypersons have a great deal of difficulty deciding when an emergency exists. For example, motor vehicle crashes can be easier to recognize as emergencies than heart attacks. This can lead to delays in calling 9-1-1 and to inappropriate decisions, such as transporting victims with life-threatening problems by private vehicles rather than contacting EMS.

Other Factors That Influence Whether a Bystander Helps

In addition to lack of knowledge and confusion, bystanders encounter other barriers that can slow or prevent action in an emergency. Many people are put off by unpleasant physical characteristics such as blood, vomitus, or alcohol on the breath. Reluctance to help might reflect an unwillingness to approach or touch a bloody victim. Public attention on human immunodeficiency virus (HIV) and acquired immunodeficiency syndrome (AIDS) can make this problem more difficult. Another factor involved in helping behavior is the bystander's time of arrival. A bystander who sees the emergency happen is more likely to help than a bystander who arrives after the event.

Quality of Help Provided by Bystanders

First aid and other assistance given by bystanders can be inadequate or potentially dangerous. Failure to keep an open airway and the decision to transport the victim in a private vehicle rather than by the EMS are two examples. Many people, trained decades ago or remembering a home remedy, might use outdated and unproven first aid procedures for various injuries or sudden illnesses. A few examples include:

- Putting butter on a burn
- Treating a nosebleed by tilting the head back
- Using hydrogen peroxide to clean a wound
- Sticking an object between the teeth of a seizure victim to prevent the victim from biting his or her tongue
- Giving syrup of ipecac for a swallowed poison

▶ What Should Be Done?

As stated at the beginning of this chapter, victims would benefit if bystanders could quickly and reliably do the following:

1. Recognize the emergency.
2. Decide to help.
3. Call 9-1-1, if EMS is needed.
4. Check the victim.
5. Give first aid.

Recognize the Emergency

To help in an emergency, the bystander first has to notice that something is wrong. Noticing that something is wrong is related to four factors:

- *Severity.* Severe, catastrophic emergencies such as a traffic collision involving an overturned car or several vehicles attract attention.
- *Physical distance.* The closer a bystander is to an emergency situation, the more likely he or she will notice it.
- *Relationship.* Knowing the victim increases the likelihood of noticing an emergency. For example, you would notice your child's injuries before you might notice the same injuries in a stranger.
- *Time exposed.* Evidence indicates that the longer a bystander is aware of the situation, the more likely he or she will notice it as an emergency.

Decide to Help

At some time, everyone will have to decide whether to help another person. Unless the decision to act in an emergency is considered well in advance of an actual emergency, the many obstacles that make it difficult or unpleasant for a bystander to help a stranger are almost certain to impede action. One important strategy that people use to avoid action is to refuse (consciously or unconsciously) to acknowledge the emergency. Many emergencies do not look like the ones portrayed on television, and the uncertainty of the real event can make it easier for the bystander to avoid acknowledging the emergency.

Making a quick decision to get involved at the time of an emergency is more likely to occur if the bystander has previously considered the possibility of helping others. Thus, the most important time to make the decision to help is before you ever encounter an emergency. Deciding to help is an attitude about emergencies and about one's ability to deal with emergencies. It is an attitude that takes time to develop and is affected by a number of factors. Developing such a helping attitude means that you must:

- Appreciate the importance of bystander help to an injured or suddenly ill person.
- Feel confident enough about helping someone who is seriously injured or suddenly ill to offer help even if someone else is present.
- Be willing to take the time to help.
- Be able to put the potential risks of helping in perspective.
- Feel comfortable about taking charge at an emergency scene.
- Feel comfortable about seeing or touching a victim who is bleeding or vomiting or who appears dead.

Deciding Not to Help

A bystander could always find excuses for not helping in emergency situations. The following are reasons that people do not aid others:

- *It could be harmful.* Bystanders have lost their lives or been severely injured while attempting to rescue others. The fear of being sued or contracting a disease such as HIV or tuberculosis (TB) can also act as a deterrent. And some would-be rescuers have been attacked by dogs protecting their disabled owners.
- *Helping doesn't matter.* Some bystanders might feel that the victim is getting what he or she deserves. Rewards, if any, are not significant for rescuers, possibly consisting of a newspaper write-up or a small cash prize. Often the rescuer gets nothing more than a hurried, "Thanks," and in some cases, rescuers are never known.
- *Obstacles can prevent helping.* Many bystanders do not know how to help. They cannot swim, do not know how to control bleeding or perform cardiopulmonary resuscitation (CPR), or do not have other necessary rescue and first aid skills. Ironically, the more bystanders there are, the less likely it is that one of them will respond. Some would-be rescuers are adversely affected by the sight of blood, vomit, and other unpleasant conditions sometimes found at emergency scenes.

Call 9-1-1, if EMS Is Needed

Wrong decisions about calling 9-1-1 can be made. Examples include a delay in calling 9-1-1 until callers are absolutely sure that an emergency exists, or deciding to bypass the EMS and transport the victim to medical care in a private vehicle. Such actions can endanger a victim. Fortunately, most injuries and sudden illnesses do not require medical care—only first aid.

FYI

Actual Versus Perceived EMS Response Time
Patients' perceptions of ambulance response times are inaccurate. They tend to overestimate response time while underestimating scene time and time to medical care.
Source: Harvey AH, Gerard WC, Rice GF, Finch H: Actual vs. perceived EMS response time. *Prehosp Emerg Care* 3(1):11-14.

Check the Victim

You must decide if life-threatening conditions exist and what kind of help a victim needs. See chapter 4, *Finding Out What's Wrong*, for details.

Give First Aid

Often the most critical life support measures are effective only if started immediately by the nearest available person. That person usually will be a layperson—a bystander.

▶ Seeking Medical Care

Knowing when to call 9-1-1 for help from EMS is important. To know when to call, you must be able to tell the difference between a minor injury or illness and a life-threatening one. For example, upper abdominal pain can be indigestion, ulcers, or an early sign of a heart attack. Wheezing could be related to a person's asthma, for which the person can use his or her prescribed inhaler for quick relief, or it can be as serious as a severe allergic reaction from a bee sting.

Not every cut needs stitches, nor does every burn require medical care. It is, however, always best to err on the side of caution. According to the American College of Emergency Physicians (ACEP), if the answer to any of the following questions is "yes," or if you are unsure, call 9-1-1 for help.

- Is the victim's condition life threatening?
- Could the condition get worse and become life threatening on the way to the hospital?
- Does the victim need the skills or equipment of the EMS?
- Could the distance or traffic conditions cause a delay in getting the victim to the hospital?

ACEP also recommends immediate transport to the hospital emergency department, by the EMS or by private vehicle, for the following conditions that are warning signs of more serious conditions:

- Chest pain lasting 2 minutes or more
- Uncontrolled bleeding (see below for wounds needing immediate medical care)
- Any sudden or severe pain
- Coughing or vomiting blood
- Difficulty breathing, shortness of breath
- Sudden dizziness, weakness, fainting
- Changes in vision
- Severe or persistent vomiting or diarrhea
- Change in mental status (for example, confusion, difficulty arousing)
- Suicidal or homicidal feelings
- Wounds needing immediate medical care include (see chapter 9 for additional wounds needing medical care) those in which:
  - Bleeding from a cut does not slow during the first 15 minutes of steady direct pressure.
  - Signs of shock occur.
  - Breathing is difficult because of a cut to the neck or chest.
  - A deep cut to the abdomen causes moderate to severe pain.
  - There is a cut to the eyeball.
  - A cut amputates or partially amputates an extremity.

When a serious situation occurs, call 9-1-1 *first*. Do *not* call your doctor, the hospital, a friend, relatives, or neighbors for help before you call 9-1-1. Calling anyone else first only wastes time. Calling 9-1-1 has several advantages over driving to the hospital emergency department by private vehicle:

- Many victims should not be moved except by trained personnel.
- The EMTs who arrive with the ambulance know what to do. In addition, they are in radio contact with hospital physicians.
- Care provided by EMTs at the scene and on the way to the hospital can increase a victim's chances of survival and rate of recovery. The condition could

get worse and become life threatening on the way to the hospital.

- An EMS ambulance usually can get a victim to the hospital quicker.

If the situation is not an emergency, call your doctor. However, if you have *any* doubt about whether the situation is an emergency, call 9-1-1. Later chapters identify when to call 9-1-1 for specific problems.

▶ How to Call EMS

In most communities, to receive emergency assistance of any kind, call 9-1-1 **Figure 2-1** . Check to see if this is true in your community. Emergency telephone numbers are usually listed on the inside front cover of telephone directories. Keep these numbers near or on every telephone. Dial 0 (the operator) if you do not know the emergency number. A community 9-1-1 number has some benefits:

- There is only one number to remember.
- Calls are received by specially trained personnel.
- Response time is reduced.

When you call EMS, speak slowly and clearly. Be ready to give the dispatcher the following information:

1. *The victim's location.* Give the address, names of intersecting roads, and other landmarks, if possible. This information is the most important thing you can give. Also, tell the specific location of the victim. (For example, "in the basement" or "in the backyard.")
2. *The phone number you are calling from and your name.* This allows dispatchers to detect false reports, thus minimizing their frequency, and it al-

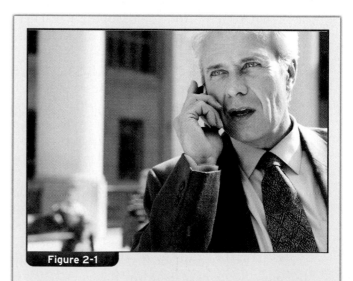

Figure 2-1

For help, phone 9-1-1 or the local emergency number.

lows a dispatch center without the enhanced 9-1-1 system to call back if disconnected or for additional information if needed.

3. *What happened.* State the nature of the emergency. (For example, "My husband fell off a ladder and is not moving.")

4. *Number of persons needing help and any special conditions.* (For example, "There was a car crash involving two cars. Three people are trapped.")

5. *Victim's condition* (for example, "My husband's head is bleeding.") and any first aid you have tried (such as pressing on the site of the bleeding).

Do *not* hang up the phone unless the dispatcher instructs you to do so. Enhanced 9-1-1 systems can track a call, but some communities lack this technology. Also, the EMS dispatcher could tell you how to best care for the victim. If you send someone else to call, have the person report back to you so you can be sure the call was made. Other tips include:

- Teach children what 9-1-1 is for and how and when to call. Refer to "nine-one-one," not "nine-eleven," because children might expect to find an eleven on the dial or on the push buttons.
- Do not hang up without explanation if you call 9-1-1 by mistake, or the dispatcher will have to call back to see if you need help.
- If your area does not have a 9-1-1 system, add EMS, fire, and police numbers to a list by your phones. During an emergency, you might not have the time or presence of mind to find a directory listing.

▶ Rescuer Reactions

The sight of blood and the cries of victims can be upsetting to people attempting to rescue and help an injured person. Seeing a grotesque amputation, being splattered with vomit or blood, or smelling disagreeable odors from urine and feces can be unnerving. More than one rescuer has felt nauseated and weak, vomited, or fainted when helping injured victims. Even the toughest of physicians and emergency medical technicians (EMTs) have difficult moments when exposed to certain situations.

It is essential that first aiders stay alert and working at an injury scene. A first aider who collapses while aiding an injured person detracts attention from the original victim, whose condition is usually more serious. All the knowledge and skills a rescuer has are useless if he or she collapses or has to leave the scene because of weakness or fainting.

Some emergency care providers seem to have ice in their veins. They always appear calm and unaffected by even the worst injuries. These people might seem callous, but the proper psychological term is *desensitized*. A specialty within psychology deals with desensitization and suggests ways of overcoming anxieties caused by unpleasant sights and sounds. Desensitization is a deconditioning or a counterconditioning process that can be effective in eliminating fears and anxieties. The idea is to weaken an undesirable response such as fainting by strengthening an incompatible response. When responses are incompatible (calmness versus anxiety), the occurrence of either one prevents the occurrence of the other. By desensitizing, you learn to associate relaxation with situations that elicit anxiety so that eventually you do not experience anxiety. But you first need to learn how to invoke relaxation before gradually exposing yourself to anxiety-producing situations such as the sight of blood.

A simple way to desensitize (calm) yourself while helping another person is to change your thought patterns from the unpleasant to the pleasant by singing a favorite song to yourself (not out loud, of course, for the obvious reason of how you might appear to the victim or observers). You can begin a process of gradual exposure to unpleasant scenes by viewing television programs, videos, DVDs, or pictures of injuries in medical journals. You might eventually consider volunteering at a hospital emergency department where you can see injuries.

In a number of cases, a first aider who fainted had failed to eat breakfast. It is strongly recommended that everyone maintain an adequate blood glucose level through proper eating habits, especially eating breakfast.

Postcare Reactions

After giving first aid for severe injuries, a person might feel an emotional letdown, which is frequently overlooked. A stressful event can be psychologically overwhelming and can result in a condition known as **posttraumatic stress disorder (PTSD)**. Its symptoms include depression and flashbacks of the event.

Discussing your feelings, fears, and reactions within 24 to 72 hours of helping at an emergency helps prevent later emotional problems. You could discuss your feelings with a trusted friend, a mental health professional, or a member of the clergy. Bringing out your feelings quickly can relieve personal anxieties and stress.

▶ Scene Size-Up

If you are at the scene of an emergency situation, do a 10-second **scene size-up** Figure 2-2 , looking for three things: (1) hazards that could be dangerous to you, the victim(s), or bystanders; (2) the cause of the injury or illness; and (3) the number of victims. As you approach an emergency scene, scan the area for immediate dangers to

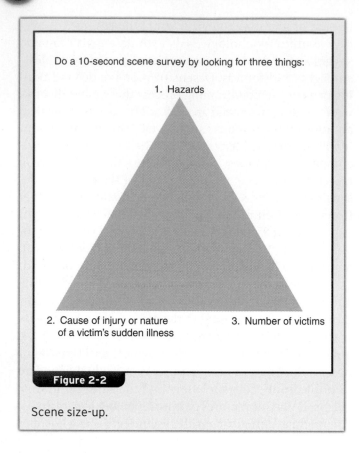

Do a 10-second scene survey by looking for three things:

1. Hazards

2. Cause of injury or nature of a victim's sudden illness

3. Number of victims

Figure 2-2

Scene size-up.

▶ Disease Precautions

First aiders must understand the risks from infectious diseases, which can range in severity from mild to life threatening. First aiders should know how to reduce the risk of contamination to themselves and to others. Precautionary measures help protect against infection from viruses and bacteria.

An **infectious disease** can be transmitted from one person to another. Also known as **communicable diseases**, their transmission can be minimized with proper precautions. Because there are so many different infectious diseases to be concerned about, the Centers for Disease Control and Prevention (CDC) developed a set of **universal precautions**, which advise you to assume that all blood and certain body fluids pose a risk for transmission of infectious diseases. These protective measures are designed to prevent first aiders from coming into direct contact with infectious agents. The term universal is meant to remind you to apply precautions in *all* situations in which you have contact with a victim. Because it is difficult to tell whether an individual is free from a communicable disease, you should always take the necessary precautions.

Following **body substance isolation (BSI)** techniques provides additional protection. Use BSI under the assumption that *all* body fluids are potentially infectious. Infectious diseases can spread through:

- Blood or fluid splash
- Surface contamination
- Lack of or improper handwashing

yourself or to the victim. For example, if a car crash is obstructing traffic, you have to consider whether you can safely go to that vehicle to help the victim. Or you might notice that gasoline is dripping from the gas tank and that the battery has shorted out and is sparking. Other conditions include hazardous conditions such as chemical spills, toxic fumes, explosives, gas leaks, or live electric wires. Other locations might have a danger of an avalanche, landslides, fires, flash floods, or attack dogs. If the scene is dangerous, stay away and call 9-1-1. You are not being cowardly, merely realistic. Never attempt a rescue that you have not been specifically trained to do. You cannot help another if you also become a victim. For details about hazards at an emergency scene, refer to chapter 23.

The second thing is to try to determine the cause of the injury. For example, if the emergency department physician knows that a victim was thrown against a steering wheel, he or she will check for liver, spleen, and cardiac injuries. Be sure to tell EMS personnel about your findings, so that they can identify the extent of any injuries. Finally, determine how many people are involved. There could be more than one victim, so look around and ask about others involved.

FYI

What Is the Risk of HIV Transmission from Contacting Blood?

In professional football, there are almost four bleeding injuries per game, yet researchers estimate that the risk of HIV transmission in an NFL game is less than one in one million.

Source: Brown LS, et al: Bleeding injuries in professional football: estimating the risk for HIV transmission. *Ann Intern Med* 122:271-274.

Handwashing

Handwashing is one of the simplest, yet most effective ways to control disease transmission. Even if you are wearing gloves, you should wash your hands before, if possible, and definitely after every victim contact. The longer the germs remain with you, the greater their chance of infecting you.

The proper procedure for washing your hands is as follows:

1. Use soap and warm water, if possible.
2. Rub your hands together for 15 to 20 seconds to work up a lather. Wash all surfaces well, including wrists, palms, backs of hands, and fingers. Clean the dirt from under your fingernails.
3. Rinse the soap from your hands.
4. Dry your hands completely with a clean towel if possible (this helps remove the germs). However, if towels are not available, it is okay to allow your hands to air dry.

If soap and water are not available, use an alcohol-based hand sanitizer to clean your hands **Figure 2-3** . Apply the gel to one hand and rub hands together, covering all surfaces of hands and fingers, until the hands are dry. If your mucous membranes (for example, your eyes, nose, or mouth) are splashed by a bloody fluid, immediately flush the area with clean water.

Personal Protective Equipment

Personal protective equipment (PPE) includes medical exam gloves, mouth-to-barrier devices, eye protection, and gowns. PPE provides a barrier between the first aider and infectious diseases.

Medical Exam Gloves

Medical exam gloves should always be worn when there is any possibility of exposure to blood or body fluids. The Food and Drug Administration (FDA), the CDC, and the Occupational Safety and Health Administration (OSHA) have stated that both vinyl and latex gloves provide adequate protection. Research indicates that latex has fewer micropores (very small holes) and, thus, offers the most protection. However, latex tends to break down faster (within several years) while the gloves are in a first aid kit waiting to be used. All first aid kits should contain several pairs of gloves. Because some rescuers have allergic reactions to latex, latex-free gloves should also be available.

It is important to use the proper technique when removing used gloves so you do not contaminate yourself. When removing used gloves, do not touch their outside surface **Skill Drill 2-1** . The proper method of removing gloves is:

1. Begin by partially removing one glove. With the other gloved hand, pinch the first glove at the wrist—being certain to touch only the outside of the first glove—and start to roll it back off the hand, inside out. Leave the exterior of the fingers on that first gloved hand exposed (**Step ❶**).
2. Use the still-gloved fingers of the first hand to pinch the wrist of the second glove and begin to pull it off, rolling it inside-out toward the fingertips as you did with the first glove (**Step ❷**).
3. Continue pulling the second glove off until you can pull the second hand free (**Step ❸**).
4. With your now-ungloved second hand, grasp the exposed inside of the first glove and pull it free of your first hand and over the now-loose second glove. Be sure that you touch only clean, interior surfaces with your ungloved hand (**Step ❹**).

Figure 2-3

Use a waterless handwashing solution if there is no running water available.

FYI

Latex Allergies: A Growing Risk

Allergies to latex, or natural rubber, can be disabling and even life threatening, producing reactions ranging from mild dermatitis to wheezing, urticaria (skin eruptions with intense itching), and anaphylaxis (life-threatening anaphylactic shock). With the emphasis on protection against HIV and other bloodborne pathogens, latex products are becoming very common, increasing the opportunities for and likelihood of exposure to latex. Alternatives to latex examination gloves are products made of nitrile, neoprene, or vinyl. Latex allergy can be a serious barrier to pursuing a career in health care. For those in the health care field who are severely allergic and react even to latex particles in the air, the only option might be to abandon the field of health care.

Source: Kolsun J: Latex allergies: a growing risk. *Emerg Med* 30:66,71.

skill drill

2-1   How to Remove Gloves

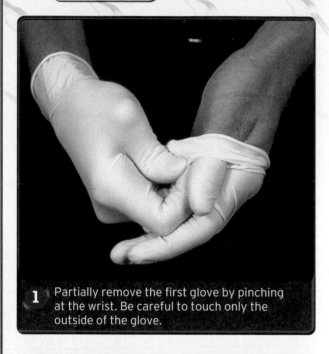

1 Partially remove the first glove by pinching at the wrist. Be careful to touch only the outside of the glove.

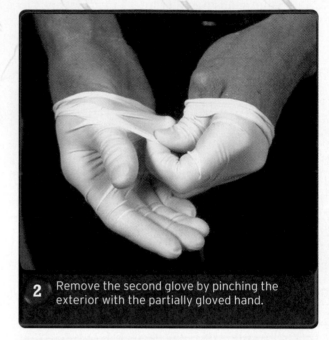

2 Remove the second glove by pinching the exterior with the partially gloved hand.

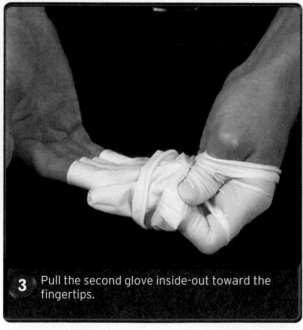

3 Pull the second glove inside-out toward the fingertips.

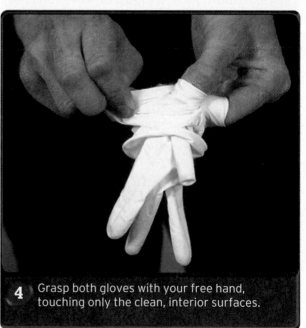

4 Grasp both gloves with your free hand, touching only the clean, interior surfaces.

FYI

Do Gloves Really Protect?

A study tested the effectiveness of vinyl and latex gloves as barriers to hand contamination. Gloves were checked according to the American Society for Testing and Materials, and leaks occurred with 43% of vinyl gloves and 9% of latex gloves. The researchers concluded that latex gloves and, to a lesser extent, vinyl gloves provide substantial protection during hand contact with moist body substances, functioning as a barrier even when leaks are present. Because leaks are not always detected by the wearer, handwashing should routinely follow the use of disposable gloves.

Source: Olsen RJ, et al: Examination gloves as barriers to hand contamination in clinical practice. *JAMA* 270:350-353.

If the gloves are cut or torn, replace them. You might consider putting on a second pair of gloves over the first if there is major, significant external bleeding or body fluid.

Mouth-to-Barrier Devices

Mouth-to-barrier devices are recommended for rescue breathing and CPR **Figure 2-4**. Although there are no documented cases of disease transmission to rescuers as a result of performing unprotected mouth-to-mouth resuscitation on a victim with an infection, you should use a barrier device such as a pocket mask when providing rescue breaths.

Other Personal Protective Equipment

Other PPE includes eye protection and gowns and aprons. OSHA requires these to be available in some workplaces, especially for health care workers. These are not required for first aiders and usually will not be available.

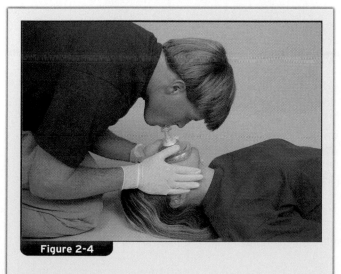

Figure 2-4

Pocket face mask, one-way valve.

Cleaning Up After an Emergency

When cleaning up blood or other body fluids, protect yourself and others against disease transmission by following these steps:

1. Wear heavier gloves than lightweight latex or vinyl.
2. If you have been trained in the correct procedures, use absorbent barriers to soak up blood or other infectious materials.
3. Clean the spill area using soap and water. After cleaning, disinfect with a bleach and water solution at a 1:10 dilution. Isopropyl alcohol can also be used to disinfect. These solutions can corrode or discolor certain fabrics, leathers, vinyl, or other synthetic materials.
4. Discard contaminated materials in an appropriate waste disposal container.

If you have been exposed to blood or body fluids:

1. Use soap and water to wash the parts of your body that have been contaminated.
2. If the exposure happened at work, report the incident to your supervisor. Otherwise, contact your personal physician. Early action can prevent the development of certain infections.

The best protection against disease is using the safeguards described here. By following these guidelines, first aiders can decrease their chances of contracting bloodborne illnesses.

Some Diseases of Special Concern

Bloodborne Diseases

Some diseases are carried by an infected person's blood (**bloodborne diseases**). **HIV (human immunodeficiency virus)** is the virus that can cause acquired immunodeficiency syndrome (AIDS). The virus is transmitted by direct contact with infected blood, semen, or vaginal secretions; there is no scientific documentation that the virus is transmitted by contact with sweat, saliva, tears, sputum, urine, feces, vomitus, or nasal secretions, unless these fluids contain visible signs of blood. There is currently no vaccine available to prevent HIV infection.

Hepatitis B virus (HBV) is also spread by direct contact with infected blood. The term hepatitis refers to an inflammation (and often infection) of the liver. A vaccine is available for HBV and is recommended for all infants and for adults who might have contact with carriers of the disease or with blood. **Hepatitis C virus (HCV)** can cause liver disease or cancer. It cannot be cured, and there is no vaccine.

Airborne Diseases

Airborne diseases are transmitted through the air by coughing or sneezing. **Tuberculosis**, a chronic bacterial disease that usually affects the lungs, is becoming a common problem, and is hard to distinguish from other diseases. Victims who present the highest risk often have a cough. Tuberculosis is more common in people who have lived in a homeless shelter, or in a developing country.

SARS (severe acute respiratory syndrome) is a potentially life-threatening viral infection. It is thought to be transmitted by close person-to-person contact. If a surgical mask is available, wear it or wrap a handkerchief over your nose and mouth.

FYI

On-the-Job Protection

Individuals infected with HBV or HIV might not show symptoms and might not even know they are infectious. For that reason, all human blood and body fluids should be considered potentially infectious, and precautions should be taken to avoid contact. BSI procedures recommend you assume that *all* body fluids are a possible risk. EMS personnel routinely follow BSI procedures, even if blood or body fluids are not visible.

OSHA requires any company with employees who are expected to give first aid in an emergency to follow universal precautions. OSHA applies the "Good Samaritan" definition to an employee who assists another with a nosebleed or a cut. Such acts, however, are not considered occupational exposure unless the employee who provides the assistance is a member of a first aid team or is designated or expected to provide first aid as part of his or her job. In essence, OSHA's requirement excludes unassigned employees who perform unanticipated first aid.

Whenever there is a chance that you could be exposed to bloodborne pathogens, your employer must provide appropriate PPE, which might include eye protection, gloves, gowns, and masks. The PPE must be accessible, and your employer must provide training to help you choose the right PPE for your work.

EMS personnel follow BSI procedures, and OSHA requires designated work-site first aiders to follow universal precautions—but what procedures should a typical first aider follow? It makes sense for first aiders to follow BSI procedures and assume that *all* blood and body fluids are infectious and follow appropriate protective measures.

FYI

Emergency Medical Service

If you or someone you know is ever sick or injured and needs emergency help, remember, there are lots of people who are specially trained to help you!

Emergency medical technicians: Emergency medical technicians, sometimes called EMTs, have different amounts of training, depending on their jobs. Sometimes EMTs are dispatchers who answer calls for help and send ambulances and rescue vehicles to the scene of the emergency. Other EMTs drive the ambulance, assist with rescues, and perform basic emergency medical care.

Paramedics: Paramedics are EMTs with the highest level of training. They are able to perform many medical procedures at the scene of the emergency or in the ambulance on the way to the hospital. Using a radio to communicate, paramedics often get instructions from a doctor at the emergency room or at the base station (the paramedic's headquarters).

Emergency nurses: If you were a patient in the emergency department, an emergency nurse would probably be the first person you'd see. One of the nurse's jobs is to ask you questions about your problem and help decide when you can see the doctor. Emergency nurses are specially trained to help treat emergency patients.

Emergency physicians: Emergency physicians are doctors who are specially trained to take care of a certain type of patient: emergency patients. Doctors who are specially trained are often called specialists. Emergency physicians specialize in helping people who are injured or who become sick very suddenly, such as someone who is having a heart attack or has a very high fever.

Others: Police officers and firefighters are some of the other people who might help you, especially if you have to be rescued.

Source: American College of Emergency Physicians.

▶ Death and Dying

There are few incidents that involve more emotional stress than the life-and-death situations that you might face. Seeing death and dying are the unfortunate parts of providing emergency care.

The Dying Victim

A dying person presents a difficult situation. To assist such a victim:

- Avoid negative statements about the victim's condition. Even an unresponsive person can hear what is being said.
- Assure the victim that you will locate and inform his or her family of what has happened. Attempt to have family members present—they can provide great comfort to the victim.
- Allow some hope. Don't tell the victim that he or she is dying. Instead, say something like, "I won't give up on you, so don't give up on yourself."
- Do not volunteer information about the victim or others who might also be injured. However, if the victim asks a question about a family member, tell the truth. Provide simple, honest, clear information if it is requested and repeat it as often as necessary.
- Use a gentle tone of voice.
- Use a reassuring touch, if appropriate.
- Let the person know that everything that can be done to help will be done.

The Stages of Grieving

People who lose a loved one go through a **grieving process**. This process generally involves five stages, but not all people move through the process in the same way or at the same pace.

1. *Denial* ("Not me.") The person cannot believe what is happening. This stage serves as a buffer for the person experiencing the situation. This reaction is normal.
2. *Anger* ("Why me?") First aiders and bystanders could be the target of the anger. Do not take the anger or insults personally. Be tolerant, use good listening skills, and be empathetic.
3. *Bargaining* ("OK, but first let me . . .") In the victim's mind, an agreement will postpone an unpleasant event (such as the death).
4. *Depression* ("OK, but I haven't . . .") This stage is characterized by sadness and despair. The person is usually silent and retreats into his or her own world.
5. *Acceptance* ("OK, I am not afraid.") This does not mean a person is happy about the situation. The family often requires more support during this stage than the victim does.

With an understanding of these five stages, you can better understand the reactions of those who are grieving and also your reactions to stressful situations.

Dealing With Survivors

Deal with the family members of a dead or dying victim as follows:

- Do not pronounce death; leave the confirmation of death to a physician.
- Allow survivors to grieve in whatever way seems right to them (anger, rage, crying).
- Provide simple, honest, clear information as it is requested, and repeat it as often as necessary. The survivors should not be told everything at once.
- Offer as much support and comfort as possible by your presence and by your words. Do not leave an individual survivor alone, but respect that person's right to privacy.
- Use a gentle tone of voice.
- Use a reassuring touch, if appropriate.

prep kit

▶ Ready for Review

- Emergencies are dangerous, unusual, rare, unforeseen, and must be dealt with before the situation becomes worse.
- A bystander is a vital link between EMS and the victim.
- Victims would benefit if bystanders could quickly and reliably do the following:
  - Recognize the emergency.
  - Decide to help.
  - Call 9-1-1, if EMS is needed.
  - Check the victim.
  - Give first aid.
- Knowing when to call 9-1-1 is important. To do so, you must be able to tell the difference between a minor injury or illness and a life-threatening one.
- In most communities, call 9-1-1 to receive emergency assistance.
- The sight of blood and the cries of victims can be upsetting, but it is essential that first aiders remain alert and working at an injury scene.
- If you are at the scene of an emergency situation, do a 10-second scene size-up looking for hazards, the cause of the injury or illness, and the number of victims.
- First aiders should take BSI precautions to protect against infectious diseases.
- There are few incidents that involve emotional stress like the life-and-death situations that you might face.

▶ Vital Vocabulary

airborne diseases Infections transmitted through the air, such as tuberculosis.

bloodborne diseases Infections transmitted through the blood, such as HIV or HBV.

body substance isolation (BSI) Procedures that treat all bodily fluids as potentially infectious.

communicable diseases Diseases that can be spread from person to person, or from animal to person.

emergency medical services (EMS) A system that represents the combined efforts of several professionals and agencies to provide emergency medical care.

grieving process Feelings and emotions after a stressful situation that cause personal pain. People go through several stages of grieving.

hepatitis B virus (HBV) A viral infection of the liver for which a vaccine is available.

hepatitis C virus (HCV) A viral infection of the liver for which no vaccine is available.

human immunodeficiency virus (HIV) The virus that can cause acquired immunodeficiency syndrome (AIDS).

infectious disease A disease that is caused by an infection.

personal protection equipment (PPE) Equipment, such as medical exam gloves, used to block the entry of an organism into the body.

posttraumatic stress disorder A delayed stress reaction to a prior emergency event.

SARS (severe acute respiratory syndrome) A potentially life-threatening viral infection that usually starts with flu-like symptoms.

scene size-up Steps taken when approaching an emergency scene. Steps include checking for hazards, noting the cause of the injury of illness, and determining the number of victims.

tuberculosis A bacterial disease usually affecting the lungs.

universal precautions Protective measures that have traditionally been developed by the Centers for Disease Control and Prevention (CDC) for use in dealing with objects, blood, body fluids, or other potential exposure risks of communicable disease.

▶ Assessment in Action

You are rushing to an important appointment and are running five minutes late. It's beginning to rain and the rush hour is about to begin. Suddenly, you see a motorcyclist skid off the highway and into a ditch. You have a cellular telephone in your car.

Directions: Circle Yes if you agree with the statement, circle No if you disagree.

Yes   No   **1.** As you approach the victim, you should not be concerned about any other possible victims.

Yes   No   **2.** This crash scene could be dangerous.

Yes   No   **3.** In most communities, 9-1-1 can be used to contact the EMS.

Yes   No   **4.** Expect to give your name when you call 9-1-1.

Yes   No   **5.** If you do not know the exact address of the emergency, be prepared to give a description of the location as best as you can.

Answers: **1.** No; **2.** Yes; **3.** Yes; **4.** Yes; **5.** Yes

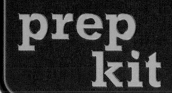

▶ Check Your Knowledge

Directions: Circle Yes if you agree with the statement, circle No if you disagree.

Yes   No   **1.** A scene survey should be done before giving first aid to an injured victim.

Yes   No   **2.** For a severely injured victim, call the victim's doctor before calling for an ambulance.

Yes   No   **3.** Dial 0 (for the telephone operator) if you do not know the emergency telephone number.

Yes   No   **4.** First aiders should assume that blood and all body fluids are infectious.

Yes   No   **5.** If you are exposed to blood while on the job, report it to your supervisor, and if off the job, to your personal physician.

Yes   No   **6.** First aid kits should contain medical exam gloves.

Yes   No   **7.** Wash your hands with soap and water after giving first aid.

Yes   No   **8.** Vaccinations are available for both HBV and HCV.

Yes   No   **9.** Medical exam gloves can be made of almost any material as long as they fit the hand well.

Yes   No   **10.** Tuberculosis is a bloodborne disease.

Answers: **1.** Yes; **2.** No; **3.** Yes; **4.** Yes; **5.** Yes; **6.** Yes; **7.** Yes; **8.** No; **9.** No; **10.** No

3

The Human Body

The Human Body

To adequately assess a victim's condition and to give effective first aid, a first aider must be familiar with the basic structure and functions of the human body. This knowledge provides a solid cornerstone for building the essentials of quality victim assessment and emergency first aid. By using the proper medical terms, you will be able to communicate more effectively with medical care providers.

In injuries and illnesses, most life-threatening conditions affect the respiratory, circulatory, and nervous systems. These three body systems include the most important and sensitive organs: the lungs, the heart, the brain, and the spinal cord. The other body systems are also important, and thorough assessment of the victim can locate injury and/or sudden illnesses affecting them as well. The major body systems described in this chapter are the respiratory, circulatory, nervous, skeletal, and muscular systems. The skin is also described. The other body systems—the endocrine, gastrointestinal, and genitourinary systems—are not discussed.

▶ The Respiratory System

The body can store food to last several weeks and water to last several days, but it can store enough oxygen for only a few minutes. Ordinarily, this does not matter because we have only to inhale air to get the oxygen we need. If the body's oxygen supply is cut off, as in drowning, choking, or smothering, death will result in about 4 to 6 minutes unless the oxygen intake is restored. Oxygen from air is made

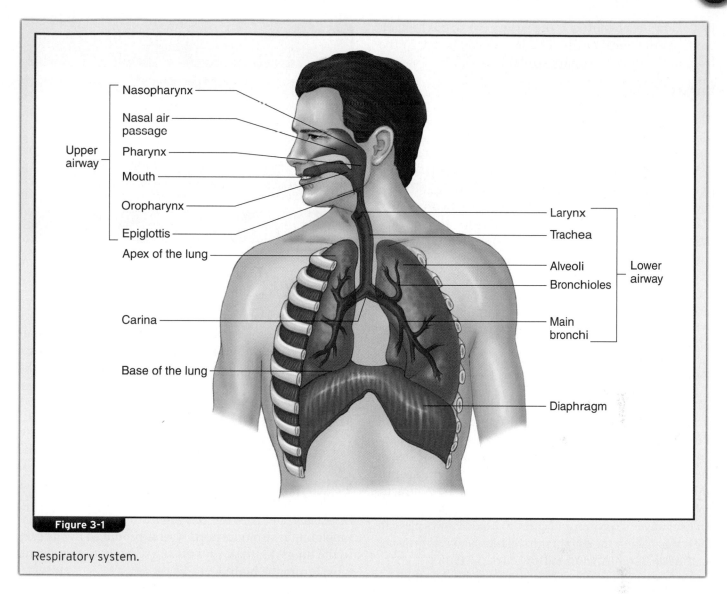

Figure 3-1

Respiratory system.

available to the blood through the <u>respiratory system</u> and then to the body cells by the circulatory system.

Nose

Air normally enters the body during inhalation through the nostrils. It is warmed, moistened, and filtered as it flows over the damp, mucous membrane (sticky lining) of the nose. When a person breathes through the mouth instead of the nose, there is less filtration and warming. After passing through the nasal passages, air enters the nasal portion of the pharynx (throat).

Pharynx and Trachea

From the back of the nose or the mouth, the air enters the throat or pharynx **Figure 3-1** . The pharynx is a common passageway for food and air. At its lower end, the pharynx divides into two passageways, one for food and the other for air. Muscular control in the back of

the throat routes food to the <u>esophagus</u> (food tube), which leads to the stomach; air is routed from the pharynx to the <u>trachea</u> (windpipe), which leads to the lungs. The trachea and the esophagus are separated by a small flap of tissue, the epiglottis, which diverts food away from the trachea. Usually this diversion works automatically to keep food out of the trachea and to prevent air from entering the esophagus. If the muscles of the pharynx and larynx are not coordinated, food or other liquid can enter the trachea instead of the esophagus.

However, normal swallowing controls do not operate if a person is unresponsive. That is why a first aider should never pour liquid into the mouth of an unresponsive person in an attempt to revive him or her. The liquid could flow down into the windpipe and suffocate the victim. Foreign objects, such as false teeth or a piece of food, might also lodge in the throat or windpipe and cut off the passage of air. In the upper 2 inches of the trachea, just below the epiglottis, is the <u>larynx</u> (voice box), which contains the vocal cords. The larynx can be felt in the front of the throat (<u>Adam's apple</u>).

Lungs

The trachea branches into two main tubes (bronchial tubes or bronchi), one for each lung. Each bronchus divides and subdivides somewhat like the branches of a tree. The smallest bronchi end in thousands of tiny pouches (<u>alveoli</u>, or air sacs), just as the twigs of a tree end in leaves. Each air sac is enclosed in a network of capillaries. The walls that separate the air sacs and the capillaries are very thin. Through those walls, oxygen combines with the hemoglobin in red blood cells to form oxyhemoglobin, which is carried to all parts of the body. Carbon dioxide and certain other waste gases in the blood move across the capillary walls into the air sacs and are exhaled from the body. The lungs occupy most of the chest cavity.

Mechanics of Breathing

The passage of air into and out of the lungs is called respiration. Breathing in is called inhalation; breathing out is exhalation. Respiration is a mechanical process brought about by alternately increasing and decreasing the size of the chest cavity. When the <u>diaphragm</u> (the dome-shaped muscle dividing the chest from the <u>abdomen</u>) contracts, the chest expands, drawing air into the lungs (inhalation). An exchange of oxygen and carbon dioxide takes place in the lungs. When the diaphragm relaxes, it exerts pressure on the lungs, causing air to flow out (exhalation).

Infants and children differ from adults. Their respiratory structures are smaller and more easily obstructed than those of adults. Infants' and children's tongues take up proportionally more space in the mouth than do the tongues of adults. The trachea is more flexible in infants and children. The primary cause of cardiac arrest in infants and children is an uncorrected respiratory problem. The average rate of breathing in an adult at rest is 12 to 20 complete respirations per minute **Table 3-1**.

Normal rates for children are from 15 to 30 times per minute; infant rates are between 25 and 50 times per minute. Normally the rate slows when a person is lying down and speeds up during vigorous exercise. The rate of breathing is controlled by a nerve center in the brain. Signs of inadequate breathing include a rate of breathing outside the normal range, cool or clammy skin that is pale or cyanotic (blue-gray), and nasal flaring, especially in children.

When a person performs hard muscular work, the lungs cannot get rid of carbon dioxide or take in oxygen fast enough at the normal rate. As carbon dioxide increases in the blood and tissues, the brain sends impulses along its nerves to cause deeper and more rapid respirations. At the same time, the heart rate increases. This faster heart rate increases the supply of oxygen available to the body as the heart pumps more blood through the lungs.

Table 3-1	Normal Respiration Rate Ranges
	Breaths per Minute*
Adults	12 to 20
Children	15 to 30
Infants	25 to 50

*To obtain the breathing rate in a person, count the number of breaths in a 30-second period and multiply by 2. A person's awareness that respirations are being counted can influence the respiratory rate, so avoid letting the person know you are counting respirations.

▶ The Circulatory System

The <u>circulatory system</u> **Figure 3-2** is made up of the blood, the heart, and the blood vessels. Blood is the great delivery system for cells throughout the body. It carries nutrients and other products from the digestive tract in its plasma, and it carries oxygen from the lungs in its hemoglobin. It also transports wastes produced by the cells to the lungs, kidneys, and other excretory organs for removal from the body.

Heart

The human circulatory system is a completely closed circuit of tubelike vessels through which blood flows. The <u>heart</u> **Figure 3-3**, by contracting and relaxing, pumps blood through the vessels. It is a powerful, hollow, muscular organ about as big as a man's clenched fist, shaped like a pear, and located in the left center of the chest, behind the sternum (breastbone). The heart is divided by a wall in the middle. Right and left compartments are divided into two chambers, the atrium above and the ventricle below. Check valves are located between each atrium and its corresponding ventricle and at the exit of the major arteries leading out of each ventricle. The opening and shutting of these valves at just the right time in the heartbeat keeps the blood from backing up.

At each beat, or contraction, the heart pumps blood rich in carbon dioxide and low in oxygen from the right ventricle to the lungs and returns oxygen-rich blood to

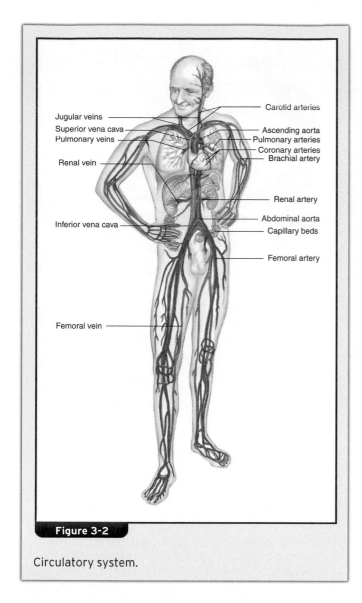

Figure 3-2

Circulatory system.

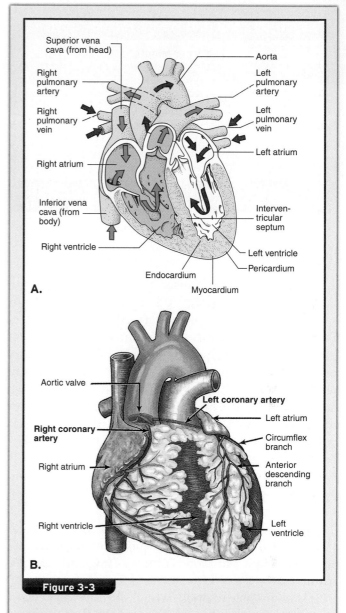

A.

B.

Figure 3-3

The heart. **A.** Circulation (internal view). **B.** The two main coronary arteries supply the heart with blood.

the left atrium of the heart from the lungs. The left ventricle pushes blood rich in oxygen freshly obtained to the rest of the body and returns oxygen-poor blood to the right atrium. At each relaxation of the heart, blood flows into the left atrium from the lungs and into the right atrium from the rest of the body ⬤ Table 3-2 .

Table 3-2   Normal Heart Rates

	Beats per Minute*
Adults	60 to 100
Children	80 to 100
Toddlers	100 to 120
Newborns	120 to 140

*To obtain a heart rate in most people, count the number of beats in a 30-second period and multiply by 2.

Blood Vessels

The <u>arteries</u> are elastic, muscular tubes that carry blood away from the heart **Figure 3-4**. They begin at the heart as two large tubes: the pulmonary artery, which carries blood to the lungs for the carbon dioxide—oxygen exchange, and the <u>aorta</u>, which carries blood to all the other parts of the body. The aorta divides and subdivides until it ends in networks of extremely fine vessels (<u>capillaries</u>) smaller than hairs. Through the thin walls of the capillaries, oxygen and food pass out of the bloodstream into the stationary cells of the body, while the body cells discharge their waste products into the bloodstream. In the capillaries of the lungs, carbon dioxide is released and oxygen is absorbed. Capillaries, having reached their limit of subdivision, begin to join together again into veins. The <u>veins</u> become larger and larger and finally form major trunks that empty blood returning from the body into the right atrium and blood from the lungs into the left atrium.

It is impossible to prick normal skin anywhere without puncturing capillaries. Because the flow of blood through the capillaries is relatively slow and under little pressure, blood merely oozes from a punctured capillary and usually has time to clot, promptly plugging the leak.

Each time the heart contracts, the surge of blood can be felt as a **pulse** at any point where an artery lies close to the surface of the body, near the skin surface and over a bone. When an artery is cut, blood spurts out. There is no pulse in a vein because the pulse is lost by the time the blood has passed through the capillaries. Hence, blood from a cut vein flows out in a steady stream. It has much less pressure behind it than blood from a cut artery.

Major locations for feeling pulses include the following:

- <u>Carotid artery</u>: The major artery of the neck, which supplies the head with blood. Pulsations can be palpated (felt) on either side of the neck (do not try to feel both at the same time). Health care

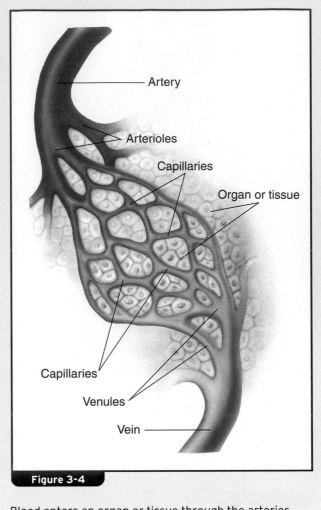

Figure 3-4

Blood enters an organ or tissue through the arteries and leaves through the veins. This process provides adequate blood flow to the tissue to meet the cells' needs.

providers use the carotid to check an unresponsive person's pulse.

- <u>Femoral artery</u>: The major artery of the thigh supplying the lower extremities with blood. Pulsations can be palpated in the groin area (the crease between the abdomen and thigh).
- <u>Radial artery</u>: The major artery of the lower arm. Pulsations can be palpated at the palm side of the wrist on the thumb side. Use the radial location to check an alert person's pulse.
- <u>Brachial artery</u>: An artery of the upper arm. Pulsations can be palpated on the inside of the arm between the elbow and the armpit. Health care providers use the brachial location to determine a pulse in an infant.

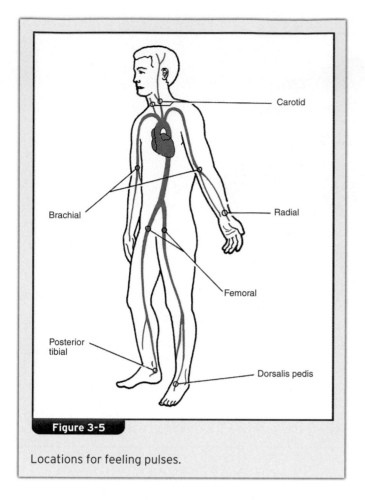

Figure 3-5

Locations for feeling pulses.

- **Posterior tibial artery**: Located behind the inside ankle knob. Pulsations can be palpated behind the posterior surface of the medial malleolus.
- **Dorsalis pedis artery**: Pulsations can be palpated on the top surface of the foot **Figure 3-5** (20% of the population have no pulsations here).

Blood Pressure

Blood pressure is a measure of the pressure exerted by the blood on the walls of the flexible arteries. Blood pressure might be high or low according to the resistance offered by the walls to the passage of blood. This difference in resistance could have several causes. For example, if blood does not fill the system, as following hemorrhage, the pressure will be low (hypotension). High blood pressure (hypertension) might be present when the arterial walls have become hard and cannot expand readily.

Blood

<u>Blood</u> has liquid and solid portions. The liquid portion is called plasma. The solid portion, which is transported by the plasma, includes disklike red blood cells; slightly larger, irregularly shaped white blood cells; and an immense number of smaller bodies called <u>platelets</u>.

<u>Plasma</u>, the liquid part of the blood, is about 90% water, in which minerals, sugar, and other materials are dissolved. Plasma carries food materials picked up from the digestive tract and transports them to the body cells. It also carries waste materials produced by cells to the kidneys, digestive tract, sweat glands, and lungs for elimination (excretion) in urine, feces, sweat, and expired breath.

The <u>red blood cells</u>, which give blood its color, carry oxygen to the organs. The <u>white blood cells</u> are part of the body's defense against infection. These cells can go wherever they are needed in the body to fight infection, for example, to a wound in the skin or other tissue that is diseased or injured. Pus, a sign of wound infection, gets its yellowish white color from the innumerable white blood cells that are fighting the invading bacteria.

Platelets are essential for the formation of blood clots. If blood plasma did not clot at the site of a wound, the slightest cut or abrasion would produce death from bleeding. Clots plug the openings through which blood escapes from punctured blood vessels. Bleeding from a large blood vessel could be too rapid to permit the formation of a clot. Hemorrhage is the term for profuse bleeding. **Perfusion** refers to the circulation of blood through an organ or a structure. Hypoperfusion is the inadequate circulation of blood through an organ or a structure. The average-size man has about 6 quarts (12 pints) of blood.

Inadequate circulation is known as shock (hypoperfusion). Shock is a state of profound depression of the vital processes of the body characterized by the following signs and symptoms: pale or cyanotic (bluish), cool, clammy skin; rapid pulse; rapid breathing; restlessness, anxiety, or mental dullness; nausea and vomiting; reduction in total blood volume; low or decreasing blood pressure; and subnormal body temperature.

▶ The Nervous System

The <u>nervous system</u> is a complex collection of nerve cells (neurons) that coordinate the work of all parts of the human body and keep the individual in touch with the outside world. Neurons receive stimuli from the environment and transmit impulses to nerve centers in the brain and spinal cord. Then, by a complicated process of thinking (reasoning) plus reflex and automatic reactions, they produce nerve impulses that regulate and coordinate all bodily movements and functions and govern behavior and consciousness.

Once neurons have been destroyed, the body cannot regenerate them. Some limited nerve repair is possible, however, as long as the vital cell body is intact. If a nerve

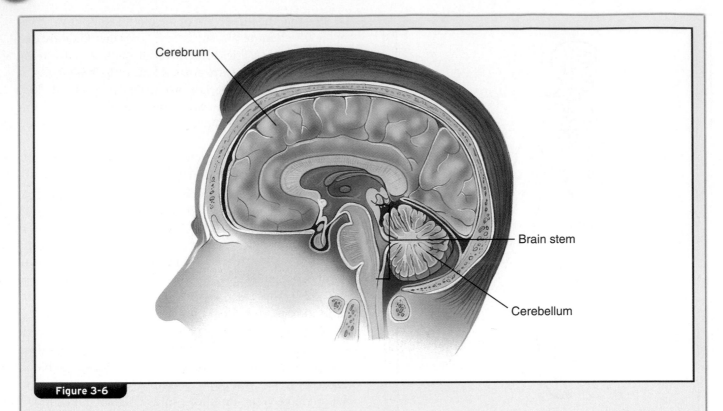

The brain lies well protected within the skull. Its principal subdivisions are the cerebrum, the cerebellum, and the brain stem.

fiber is cut or injured, the section attached to the cell body remains alive, but the part beyond the injury withers away.

The nervous system can be classified in different ways. From a structural standpoint, there are the **central nervous system (CNS)**, which includes the brain and the spinal cord, and the peripheral nervous system, a network of nerve cells that originates in the brain and spinal cord and extends to all parts of the body, including the muscles, the surface of the skin, and the special sense organs, such as the eyes and the ears. The peripheral nervous system is further subdivided into the voluntary and the autonomic (involuntary) nervous systems.

Central Nervous System

The CNS consists of the brain **Figure 3-6** , which is enclosed within the skull, and the spinal cord, which is housed in a semiflexible bony column of vertebrae. The CNS serves as the controlling organ of the body. The brain enables us to think, judge, and act. The spinal cord is a major communication pathway between the brain and the rest of the body.

Brain

The **brain**, which is the headquarters of the human nervous system, is probably the most highly specialized or-

gan in the body. It weighs about 3 pounds in the average adult, is richly supplied with blood vessels, and requires considerable oxygen to perform effectively.

The brain has three main subdivisions: the **cerebrum** (large brain), which occupies nearly all (75%) of the cranial cavity; the **cerebellum** (small brain); and the **brain stem**. The cerebrum is divided into two hemispheres by a deep cleft. The outer surface of the cerebrum, the cerebral cortex, is about one eighth-inch thick, composed mainly of cell bodies of nerve cells, and often referred to as gray matter.

Certain sections of the cerebrum are localized to control specific body functions such as sensation, thought, and associative memory, which allows us to store, recall, and make use of past experiences. The sight center of the brain is located at the back of the cerebrum, which is called the occipital lobe. The temporal lobes, at the sides of the head, deal with smell and hearing. The cerebellum is located at the back of the **cranium** (skull) and below the cerebrum. Its main function is to coordinate muscular activity and balance. The third major area of the brain is the brain stem, which extends from the base of the cerebrum to the foramen magnum (a large opening at the base of the skull). The brain stem controls automatic functions such as breathing and heart rate.

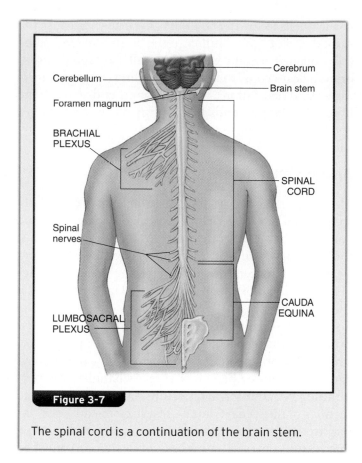

Cerebellum

Cerebrum

Brain stem

Foramen magnum

BRACHIAL PLEXUS

SPINAL CORD

Spinal nerves

CAUDA EQUINA

LUMBOSACRAL PLEXUS

Figure 3-7

The spinal cord is a continuation of the brain stem.

Because the spinal cord lies close to the bony walls of the vertebra, especially in the cervical (neck) and thoracic (chest) regions, it is particularly vulnerable to injury. Damage to the cord is almost always irreversible. An injury to the lumbar (lower back) spine causes paralysis and loss of sensation in the legs; an injury to the cervical cord causes paralysis and loss of sensation in the arms and the legs.

Peripheral Nervous System

At each vertebral level and on each side of the spinal cord, a spinal nerve exits the spinal cord through an opening in the bony canal. These nerves make up the peripheral nervous system. The peripheral nervous system consists of the sensory and motor nerves. The sensory nerves carry sensations such as smell, touch, heat, and sound from the body to the brain and the spinal cord. The motor nerves carry information from the brain and the spinal cord to the muscles of the body.

If a nerve is cut or seriously damaged, disrupting the connection between the brain and the body, the body part will not be able to work. For example, if the motor nerve going to the right leg is cut, the leg will be unable to move. This can be a permanent loss. Injuries to the nerves in the spinal cord can be very serious.

Fortunately, the CNS is well protected against injury. The brain is enclosed in the cranial cavity of the skull. The spinal cord is contained in the hollow space of the vertebrae. The brain and the spinal cord are also protected by three layers of tissue known as the meninges. The space between the layers of the meninges is filled with CSF, which also helps protects the brain and spinal cord from injury.

Autonomic Nervous System

The autonomic nervous system consists of a group of nerves that control heart rate, digestion, sweating, and other automatic body processes. These processes are not controlled by the conscious mind, but they can be influenced by the CNS to a limited extent.

▶ The Skeletal System

The human body is shaped by its bony framework. Without its bones, the body would collapse. The adult skeleton **Figure 3-8** has 206 bones. <u>Bones</u> are composed of living cells surrounded by hard deposits of calcium. The bone cells are well supplied by blood vessels and nerves. The calcium deposits give bones their strength and rigidity. Broken bones are repaired by bone-building cells lying in the bone and its covering sheath, the periosteum. New bone is formed at the site of the break, much as two pieces of steel are welded together.

Small cavities in the brain contain the <u>cerebrospinal fluid (CSF)</u>, a clear, watery solution similar to blood plasma. Circulating throughout the brain and the spinal cord, CSF serves as a protective cushion and exchanges food and waste materials. The total quantity of CSF in the brain–spinal cord system is 100 to 150 mL, although up to several liters can be produced daily. It is constantly being produced and reabsorbed.

Knowledge of nerve structure and function enables physicians to locate diseased brain sections. Because nerves from one side of the body eventually connect with the opposite side of the brain, a person whose left arm is paralyzed after a stroke will have suffered damage to the right side of the brain.

Spinal Cord

The <u>spinal cord</u> **Figure 3-7** is a soft column of nerve tissue continuous with the lower part of the brain that is enclosed in the bony vertebral column. The spinal cord exits the brain through the foramen magnum, which is a hole in the base of the skull. Thirty-one pairs of spinal nerves branch from the spinal cord. These nerves are large trunks that are similar to telephone cables because they house many nerve fibers. Some fibers carry impulses into the spinal cord; others carry impulses away from it. Spinal nerves at different levels of the cord regulate activities of various parts of the body.

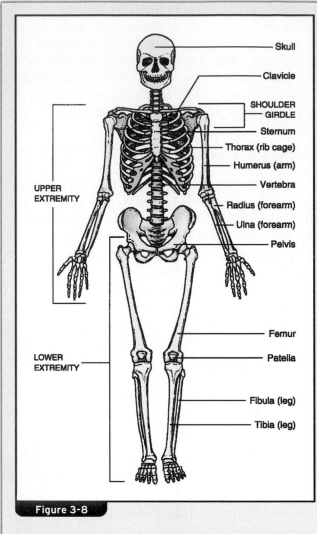

	Skull
	Clavicle
	SHOULDER GIRDLE
	Sternum
	Thorax (rib cage)
	Humerus (arm)
	Vertebra
	Radius (forearm)
	Ulna (forearm)
	Pelvis
	Femur
	Patella
	Fibula (leg)
	Tibia (leg)

UPPER EXTREMITY

LOWER EXTREMITY

Figure 3-8

The 206 bones from the skeleton give us our form, protect our vital organs, and allow us to move.

Skull

The skull rests at the top of the spinal column. It contains the brain, certain special-purpose glands (such as the pituitary and the pineal), and the centers of special senses—sight, hearing, taste, and smell. The skull has two parts, the brain case (cranium) and the face **Figure 3-9**. Blood vessels and nerve trunks pass to and from the brain through openings in the skull, mostly at the base. The largest opening is the foramen magnum, where the spinal cord exits the skull and joins the brain. The brain, which fits snugly in the cranium, is covered by the meninges. The very narrow spaces between the meninges are filled with CSF.

Although the skull is very tough, a blow can fracture it. Even if there is no fracture, a sudden impact can tear or bruise the brain and cause it to swell, just as any soft tissue swells following an injury or a bruise. Because the skull does not "give," injury to the brain is magnified by the contained pressure within the skull. Unresponsiveness or even death could result from swelling (edema), a tearing wound (laceration), bleeding, or other damage to the brain. The face extends from the eyebrows to the chin and forms the eyes, nose, cheeks, mouth, and lower jaw (mandible).

Spinal Column

The spinal column **Figure 3-10** is made up of irregularly shaped bones called vertebrae (singular is vertebra). Lying one on top of the other to form a strong, flexible column, the vertebrae are bound firmly together by strong ligaments. Between every two vertebrae is an intervertebral disk, a pad of tough elastic cartilage that acts as a shock absorber.

The spinal column can be damaged by disease or by injury. A crushed or displaced vertebra can squeeze, stretch, tear, or sever the spinal cord. Moving the disabled part by the injured person or careless handling by well-meaning but uninformed persons can further displace sections of the spinal column, resulting in additional injury to the cord and possibly permanent paralysis. For that reason, a person with a back or neck injury must be handled with extreme care.

Thorax

The thorax (rib cage) is made up of ribs and the sternum (breastbone). The sternum is a flat, narrow bone in the middle of the front wall of the chest. The collar bones and certain ribs are attached to the sternum. The 24 ribs are semiflexible arches of bone. There are 12 on each side of the chest. The back ends of the 12 pairs of ribs are attached to the 12 thoracic vertebrae. Strong ligaments bind the back ends of the ribs to the backbone but allow slight gliding or tilting movements. The front ends of the top 10 pairs of ribs are attached to the sternum by cartilage. The front ends of the last two pairs (pairs 11 and 12) hang free, giving them the name floating ribs.

Fractures of the sternum or the ribs usually result from crushing or squeezing the chest. A fall, blow, or penetration of the chest wall by an object can have the same effect. The chief danger from such injuries is that the lungs or heart might be punctured by the sharp ends of the broken bones. The lowest portion of the sternum is the xiphoid process.

Pelvis

The two hipbones and the sacrum form the pelvic girdle (pelvis). Muscles help attach the pelvic bones, the trunk,

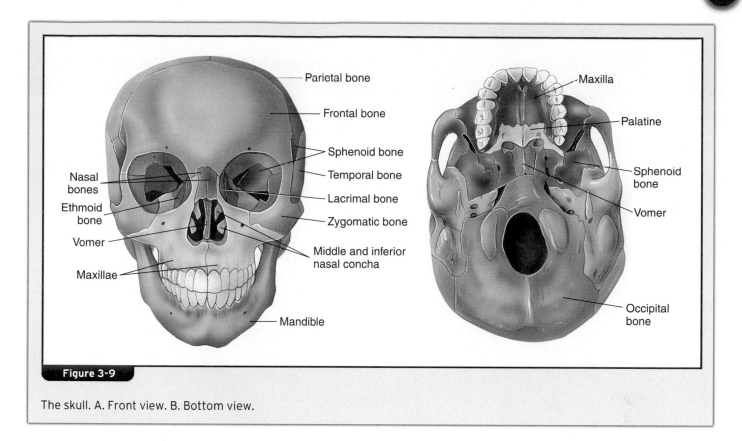

Figure 3-9

The skull. A. Front view. B. Bottom view.

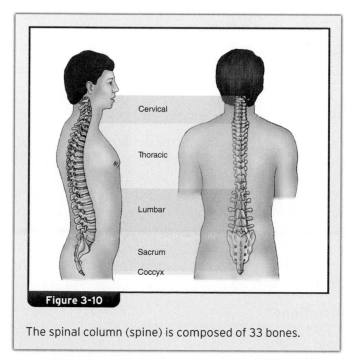

Figure 3-10

The spinal column (spine) is composed of 33 bones.

the thighs, and the legs. The pelvis forms the floor of the abdominal cavity. The lower part of the cavity, sometimes called the pelvic cavity, holds the bladder, rectum, and internal parts of the reproductive organs. The floor of the pelvic cavity helps to support the intestines.

Leg Bones

Upper Leg (Thigh)

At the outer side of each hipbone is a deep socket into which the round head of the thighbone (**femur**) fits, forming a ball-and-socket joint. The lower end of the femur is flat and has two knobs. These knobs articulate with the shinbone (tibia) at the knee joint. Although the femur is the longest and strongest bone in the skeleton, it is a common fracture site. A fractured femur is always serious because it is difficult to align the broken or splintered ends to create a strong union. Because of the force required to break the femur, laceration of the surrounding tissues, pain, and blood loss could be extensive.

Knee

The knee joint is the largest joint in the body and is a strong hinge joint **Figure 3-11**. The joint is protected and stabilized in the front by the kneecap (patella). The **patella** is a small, triangular-shaped bone in front of and between the femur and the tibia and within the tendon of the large muscle (the quadraceps) of the front of the thigh. Because the patella usually receives the force of falls or blows to the knee, it is frequently bruised or dislocated and sometimes fractured.

Lower Leg

The lower leg refers to the portion of the lower extremity between the knee and the ankle. Its two bones are the

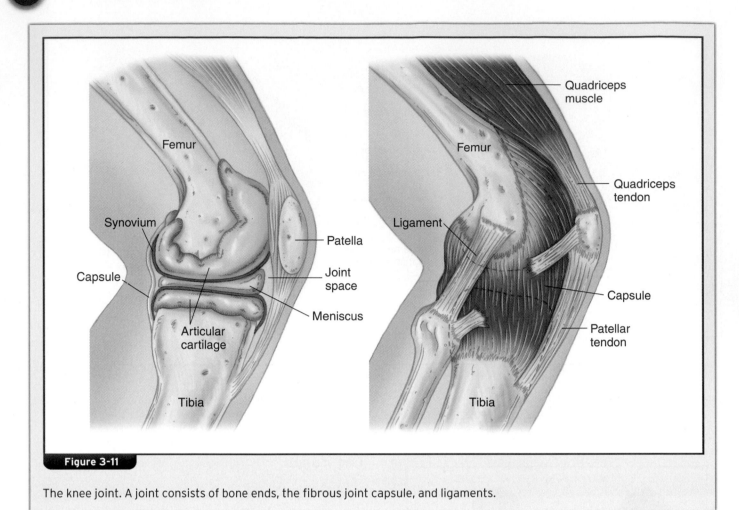

Figure 3-11

The knee joint. A joint consists of bone ends, the fibrous joint capsule, and ligaments.

tibia and the fibula **Figure 3-12**. The tibia (shin bone) is at the front and inner side of the leg. It is palpable throughout its length. Its broad upper surface receives the end of the femur to form the knee joint. The lower end, much smaller than the upper end, forms the inner rounded knob of the ankle (medial malleolus). The fibula, which is not a part of the true knee joint, is attached at the top to the tibia. Its lower end forms the outside ankle knob (lateral malleolus). The fibula is more often fractured alone than is the tibia.

Ankles, Feet, and Toes

The ends of the tibia and fibula form the socket of the ankle joint. Both ankle knobs are easily palpated. The seven ankle bones (tarsals) are bound firmly together by tough ligaments. The heel bone (calcaneus) transmits the weight of the body to the ground and forms a base for the muscles of the calf of the leg when walking **Figure 3-13**. The sole and the instep of the foot are formed by the five long metatarsals. These articulate with the tarsals and with the front row of toe bones (phalanges).

Shoulder

The collar bone (clavicle) and the shoulder blade (scapula) form the shoulder girdle. Each clavicle—a long, slightly double-curved bone—is attached to the sternum at its inner end and to the scapula at its outer end. Each clavicle can be palpated throughout its length. Fractures are common because the clavicle lies close to the surface and must absorb blows. Each scapula—a large, flat, triangular bone—is located over the upper ribs at the back of the thorax.

Arm Bones

Upper Arm

The bone of the upper arm, the humerus, is the arm's largest bone. Its upper end (the head) is round; its lower end is flat. The round head fits into a shallow cup in the shoulder blade, forming a ball-and-socket joint. This is the most freely movable joint in the body and is easily dislocated. Dislocations can tear the capsule of the joint (synovial membrane) and cause damage. Improper ma-

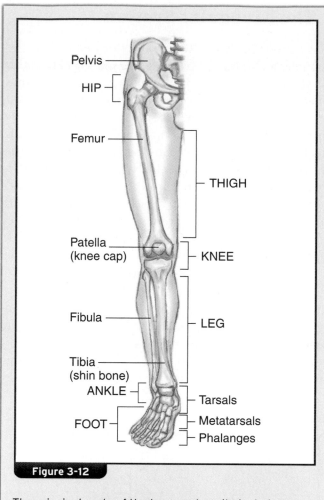

Figure 3-12

The principal parts of the lower extremity include the thigh, leg, and foot. The principal parts of the leg include the tibia and fibula.

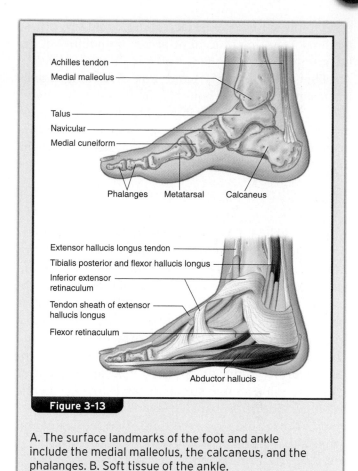

Figure 3-13

A. The surface landmarks of the foot and ankle include the medial malleolus, the calcaneus, and the phalanges. B. Soft tissue of the ankle.

nipulation during attempts to reduce or set the dislocation could add to the damage. Therefore, it is important to treat dislocations of the shoulder with gentle care.

Forearm

The two bones of the forearm (radius and ulna) lie side by side. The larger of the two, the <u>ulna</u>, is on the little finger side, and part of it forms the elbow. The flat, curved lower end of the humerus fits into a big notch at the upper end of the ulna to form the elbow joint. This hinge joint permits movement in one direction only. The <u>radius</u>, shorter and smaller than the ulna, is on the thumb side of the forearm **Figure 3-14** .

Wrist, Hand, and Fingers

The wrist is composed of eight small, irregularly shaped bones (carpals) united by ligaments. Tendons extending from the muscles of the forearm to the bones of the hand and fingers pass down the front and the back of the wrist

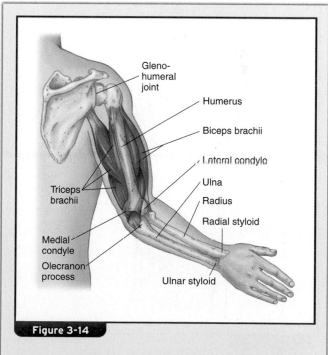

Figure 3-14

The principal bones in the arm and forearm include the humerus, the radius, and the ulna.

close to the surface. Wrist lacerations could sever these tendons, resulting in total or partial immobility of the fingers.

The palm of the hand has five long bones (metacarpals). The 14 bones of the fingers (phalanges) give the hand its great flexibility. The thumb is the most important digit. A good thumb and one or two fingers make a far more useful hand than four fingers minus the thumb **Figure 3-15** .

Joints

A <u>joint</u> is where two or more bones meet or join. Some joints, such as those in the cranium, allow little, if any, movement of the bones. Other joints, such as the hip and the shoulder, allow a wide range of motion. In a typical joint, a layer of cartilage (gristle), which is softer than bone, acts as a pad or buffer. The bones of such a joint are held in place by firmly attached ligaments, which are bands of very dense, tough, but flexible connective tissue. Joints are enclosed in a capsule, a layer of thin, tough material, strengthened by the ligaments. The inner side of the capsule (synovial membrane) secretes a thick fluid (synovial fluid) that lubricates and protects the joint.

▶ The Muscular System

Body movement is due to work performed by muscles. Examples are walking, breathing, the beating of the heart, and the movements of the stomach and the intestines. What enables muscle tissue to perform work is its ability to contract—that is, to become shorter and thicker—when stimulated by a nerve impulse. The cells of a muscle, usually long and threadlike, are called fibers. Each muscle has countless bundles of closely packed, overlapping fibers bound together by connective tissue. The three kinds of muscles are skeletal muscle (voluntary), smooth muscle (involuntary), and cardiac muscle (heart). They differ in appearance and in the specific jobs they do **Figure 3-16** .

The <u>voluntary muscles</u>, which are under the control of a person's will, make possible all deliberate acts, including walking, chewing, swallowing, smiling, frowning, talking, and moving the eyeballs. Also called <u>skeletal muscles</u>, most voluntary muscles are attached by one or both ends to the skeleton by tendons. However, some muscles are attached to skin, cartilage, and special or-

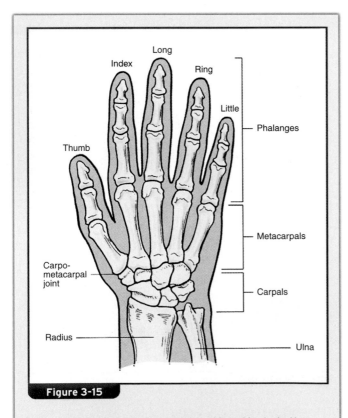

Figure 3-15

The principal bones in the wrist and hand include the carpals, the metacarpals, and the phalanges.

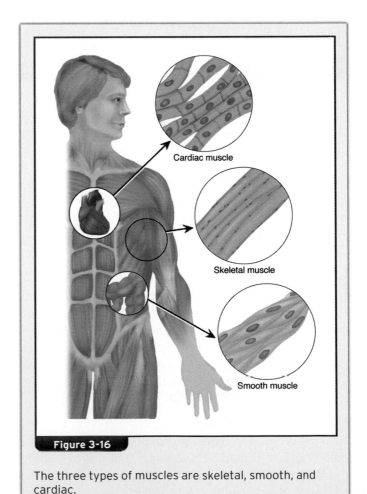

Figure 3-16

The three types of muscles are skeletal, smooth, and cardiac.

gans, such as the eyeball, or to other muscles, such as the tongue.

Muscles help to shape the body and to form its walls. Most skeletal muscles end in tough, whitish cords (tendons) that attach them to the bones they move. Tendons continue into the fascia, which covers the skeletal muscles. The fascia is much like the skin of a sausage in that it surrounds the muscle tissue. At either end of the muscle, the fascia extends beyond the muscle to attach to a bone. Tendons are covered with a synovial membrane, which secretes a lubricating substance, the synovial fluid. This makes it easier for the tendon to move when the muscle contracts or relaxes. Muscular contraction pulls the bone in the direction permitted by a joint.

When they are not working, muscles become comparatively slack. Normally, muscles never completely relax; some fibers are contracting all the time. They always have some tension (muscle tone). Loss of muscle tone can be a sign of nerve injury. Muscles can be injured in many ways. Overexerting a muscle can break fibers. Muscles can be bruised, crushed, cut, torn, or otherwise injured, with or without breaking the skin. Muscles injured in any of those ways are likely to become swollen, tender, painful, or weak.

A person has little or no control over the **smooth muscles** and usually is not conscious of them. Smooth muscles line the walls of tubelike structures such as the gastrointestinal tract, the urinary system, the blood vessels, and the bronchi of the lungs. Cardiac muscle is a specialized form of muscle found only in the heart. A continuous supply of oxygen and glucose is needed for cardiac muscle to work properly.

▶ The Skin

The skin covers the entire body, protecting the deep tissues from being injured, drying out, or being invaded by bacteria and other foreign bodies. The skin helps to regulate body temperature by aiding in the elimination of water and various salts. The skin senses heat, cold, touch, pressure, and pain and transmits that information to the brain and the spinal cord.

The skin **Figure 3-17** consists of two layers: the outer layer (**epidermis**) and the inner layer (**dermis**). The epidermis varies in thickness in different parts of the body (the palms and the soles of the feet are thickest), and its dead cells are constantly worn off. The dermis has a rich supply of blood vessels and nerve endings. Hair grows from the dermis through openings called hair follicles. Sweat glands and oil glands in the dermis empty onto the surface of the epidermis through pores in the skin. Beneath the dermis is the subcutaneous layer (under the skin), which is well supplied with fat cells and blood vessels.

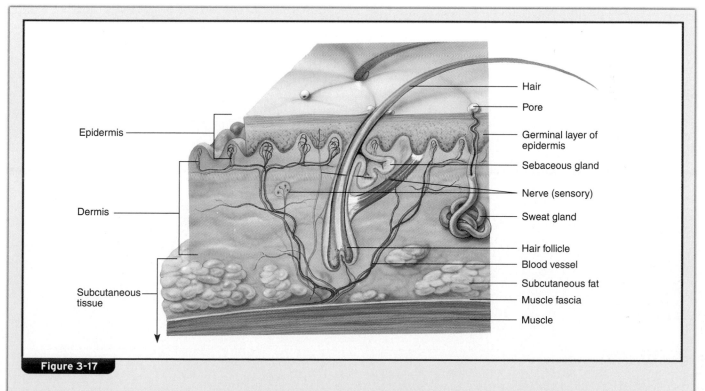

Epidermis
Dermis
Subcutaneous tissue

Hair
Pore
Germinal layer of epidermis
Sebaceous gland
Nerve (sensory)
Sweat gland
Hair follicle
Blood vessel
Subcutaneous fat
Muscle fascia
Muscle

Figure 3-17

The skin has two main layers: the epidermis and the dermis. Below the skin is a layer of subcutaneous tissue.

Sweat glands (perspiration) occur in nearly all parts of the skin. Sweat contains essentially the same minerals as blood plasma and urine, but it is more dilute. Normally, only traces of the waste products excreted in urine are in sweat. But when sweating is profuse or when the kidneys are diseased, the amounts of such wastes excreted in the sweat could be considerable. Several mineral salts are removed from the body in sweat. Chief among those in quantity is sodium chloride (the same mineral as common table salt).

▶ Ready for Review

- A first aider must be familiar with the basic structure and functions of the human body.
- The circulatory system is made up of the blood, heart, and the blood vessels.
- The nervous system is a complex collection of nerve cells that coordinate the work of all parts of the human body.
- The skeletal system is the bony framework that shapes the body.
- The muscle system lets the body move.
- Skin covers the entire body and protects the deep tissues.

▶ Vital Vocabulary

abdomen The body cavity that contains the major organs of digestion and excretion. It is located below the diaphragm and above the pelvis.

Adam's apple The projection on the anterior surface of the neck, formed by the thyroid cartilage over the larynx.

alveoli The air sacs of the lungs in which the exchange of oxygen and carbon dioxide takes place.

aorta The principal artery leaving the left side of the heart and carrying freshly oxygenated blood to the body.

arteries A blood vessel, consisting of three layers of tissue and smooth muscle, that carries blood away from the heart.

blood The fluid that circulates through the heart, arteries, capillaries, and veins carrying nutriment and oxygen to the body cells and removing waste products such as carbon dioxide and various metabolic products for excretion.

bones The hard form of connective tissue that constitutes most of the skeleton in humans.

brachial artery The artery of the arm that, in turn, branches at the elbow into the radial and ulnar arteries. Used to determine an infant's pulse.

brain The soft, large mass of nerve tissue that is contained in the cranium.

brain stem The area of the brain between the spinal cord and cerebrum, surrounded by the cerebellum; controls functions that are necessary for life, such as respirations.

capillary The small blood vessels through whose walls various substances pass into and out of the tissues and onto the cells.

carotid arteries The major arteries that supply blood to the head and brain.

central nervous system (CNS) The brain and spinal cord.

cerebellum One of the three major subdivisions of the brain; coordinates the various activities of the brain, particularly fine body movements.

cerebrospinal fluid (CSF) A clear, watery solution similar to blood plasma.

cerebrum The largest part of the three subdivisions of the brain, made up of several lobes that control movement, hearing, balance, speech, visual perception, emotions, and personality.

circulatory system The arrangement of connected tubes, including the arteries, arterioles, capillaries, venules, and veins, that moves blood, oxygen, nutrients, carbon dioxide, and cellular waste throughout the body.

clavicle The collarbone.

cranium The area of the head above the ears and eyes; the skull. The cranium contains the brain.

dermis The inner layer of the skin, containing hair follicles, sweat glands, nerve endings, and blood vessels.

diaphragm A muscular dome that forms the undersurface of the thorax, separating the chest from the abdominal cavity. Contraction of the diaphragm brings air into the lungs. Relaxation allows air to be expelled from the lungs.

dorsalis pedis artery The artery on the anterior (top) surface of the foot between the first and second metatarsals.

epidermis The outer layer of the skin, which is made up of cells that are sealed together to form a watertight protective covering for the body.

esophagus A collapsible tube that extends from the pharynx to the stomach; contractions of the muscle in the wall of the esophagus propel food and liquids through it to the stomach.

femoral artery The principal artery of the thigh. It supplies blood to the lower abdominal wall, external genitalia, and legs. It can be palpated in the groin area.

femur The thighbone; the longest and one of the strongest bones in the body.

floating ribs The 11th and 12th ribs, which do not attach to the sternum.

heart A hollow muscular organ that receives blood from the veins and propels it into the arteries.

humerus The supporting bone of the upper arm.

joint The place where two bones come into contact.

larynx The voice box.

ligament A band of the fibrous tissue that connects bones to bones. It supports and strengthens a joint.

nervous system The system that controls virtually all activities of the body, both voluntary and involuntary.

patella The kneecap; a specialized bone that lies within the tendon of the quadriceps muscle.

perfusion The circulation of oxygenated blood within an organ or tissue in adequate amounts to meet the cells' current needs.

plasma A sticky, yellow fluid that carries the blood cells and nutrients and transports cellular waste material to the organs of excretion.

platelets Tiny, disk-shaped elements that are much smaller than the cells; they are essential in the initial formation of a blood clot, the mechanism that stops bleeding.

posterior tibial artery The artery just posterior to the medial malleolus; supplies blood to the foot.

pulse The wave of pressure created as the heart contracts and forces blood out the left ventricle and into the major arteries.

radial artery The major artery in the forearm; it is palpable at the wrist on the thumb side.

radius The bone on the thumb side of the forearm.

red blood cells Cells that carry oxygen to the body's tissues; also called erythrocytes.

respiratory system All the structures of the body that contribute to the process of breathing, consisting of the upper and lower airways and their component parts.

skeletal muscle Muscle that is attached to bones and usually crosses at least one joint; striated, or voluntary, muscle.

skeleton The framework that gives us our recognizable form; also designed to allow motion of the body and protection of vital organs.

smooth muscle Nonstriated, involuntary muscle; it constitutes the bulk of the gastrointestinal tract and is present in nearly every organ to regulate automatic activity.

spinal cord An extension of the brain, composed of virtually all the nerves carrying messages between the brain and the rest of the body. It lies inside of and is protected by the spinal canal.

tibia The shinbone; the larger of the two bones of the lower leg.

trachea The windpipe; the main trunk for air passing to and from the lungs.

ulna The inner bone of the forearm, on the side opposite the thumb.

vein Any blood vessel that carries blood from the tissues to the heart.

voluntary muscle Muscle that is under direct voluntary control of the brain and can be contracted or relaxed at will; skeletal, or striated, muscle.

white blood cells Blood cells that play a role in the body's immune defense mechanisms against infection.

xiphoid process The lowest part of the sternum.

▶ Assessment in Action

Thanks to your friendly and engaging first aid and CPR instructor, you now have a firm grasp on how the human body works. Now you can watch those medical shows and decode some of their dialogue! As you settle into the couch next to your roommate to watch your favorite medical drama, you wonder if you'll ever have another opportunity to apply your new knowledge. During a commercial, such an opportunity arises when your roommate begins making coughing noises and slumps forward. *Directions:* Circle Yes if you agree with the statement, circle No if you disagree.

Yes   No   1. There is no cause to panic; the human body can survive for an hour without oxygen.

Yes   No   2. You should pinch your roommate's nose to see if he'll start breathing through his mouth.

Yes   No   3. Your roommate is probably dehydrated; you should coax some water down his throat.

Yes   No   4. Since your roommate's chest is not moving, he is not breathing.

Yes   No   5. If your roommate is not breathing, his body is not getting enough carbon dioxide into the lungs.

Answers: **1.** No; **2.** No; **3.** No; **4.** Yes; **5.** No

▶ Check Your Knowledge

Directions: Circle Yes if you agree with the statement, circle No if you disagree.

Yes   No   **1.** A first aider does not have to understand how the human body works in order to effectively provide care.

Yes   No   **2.** The human body can store oxygen for hours.

Yes   No   **3.** Blood is the delivery system for cells throughout the body.

Yes   No   **4.** The heart is a pear-shaped, muscular organ.

Yes   No   **5.** Once neurons have been destroyed, the body can replace them.

Yes   No   **6.** The automatic nervous system consists of a group of nerves that control heart rate, digestion, sweating, and other automatic body processes.

Yes   No   **7.** The adult skeleton has 208 bones.

Yes   No   **8.** A joint is where two or more bones meet or join.

Yes   No   **9.** There are three kinds of muscle: skeletal, smooth, and cardiac.

Yes   No   **10.** Skin transmits information to the brain and helps regulate body temperature.

Answers: **1.** No; **2.** No; **3.** Yes; **4.** Yes; **5.** No; **6.** Yes; **7.** No; **8.** Yes; **9.** Yes; **10.** Yes

4

Finding Out What's Wrong

▶ Checking the Victim

During emergency situations when panic exists, knowing what to do and what not to do is crucial. A victim assessment is a sequence of actions that helps determine what is wrong and thus ensures safe and appropriate first aid. Becoming familiar with the process of victim assessment will enable you to act quickly and decisively in hectic emergency situations. Victim assessment is an important first aid skill. It requires an understanding of each assessment step as well as decision-making skills.

Identifying what's wrong is the first step in providing first aid to an injured or ill victim. The goals of this identification are to:

- Detect life-threatening conditions rapidly and care for them as quickly as possible.
- Determine other problems needing care.
- Determine if the victim needs medical care, and if so, whether the victim should be transported by ambulance or private vehicle.

▶ Scene Size-Up

Every time you encounter a victim, first check out the scene. The <u>scene size-up</u> determines the safety of the scene, the <u>cause of injury</u> or <u>nature of illness</u>, and the number of victims. Without a scene size-up, a potentially hazardous situation could result in further injury to the victim or to you and others. If the scene appears hazardous, do not enter the area. You cannot help a victim if you become a victim yourself. Reduce exposure to potentially dangerous body substances that can carry disease. Disease transmission is very rare. Medical exam gloves should be worn when blood or other body fluid contact is possible.

The scene size-up is followed by the **initial check**. During the initial check, the first aider identifies and treats immediate life-threatening conditions involving problems with the victim's airway, breathing, and severe bleeding. Victims with immediate life-threatening conditions can die within minutes unless their problems are quickly recognized and treated. Determining whether the problem is an injury or an illness is also part of the initial check. If the scene size-up or initial check suggests serious illness or injury, call 9-1-1.

A **physical exam** and SAMPLE history follow the initial check. These procedures can reveal information that will help identify the injury or illness, its severity, and appropriate first aid. Detailed information is gained about the victim's injury (for example, painful ankle or bleeding nose) or chief complaint (for example, chest pain or itchy skin).

If two or more people are injured, attend to the quiet one first. A quiet victim might not be breathing or might not have a heartbeat. A victim who is talking, crying, or otherwise alert is obviously breathing.

▶ Initial Check

The initial check determines whether there are life-threatening problems requiring quick care. This step involves checking the victim's responsiveness, opening the airway, checking for breathing, and checking for severe bleeding. This step takes less than a minute to complete, unless first aid is required at any point. By the end of the initial check, the victim's problem will most likely be identified as an injury or an illness **Skill Drill 4-1**. During the initial check:

1. Determine if the victim is responsive: Call the victim in a tone of voice that is loud enough for the victim to hear. If the victim does not respond to the sound of your voice, gently tap or shake the victim's shoulder (**Step ❶**).
2. Ensure that the victim's airway is open: In the case of an unresponsive victim, open the airway by using the head tilt–chin lift technique (**Step ❷**).

3. Determine if the victim is breathing: Look, listen, and feel for signs of breathing (**Step ❸**).
4. Check for any obvious, severe bleeding (**Step ❹**).

General Impression of the Victim

As you approach the victim, form a **general impression** of the victim. This has also been referred to as a first impression, look test, and a gut reaction. Both the scene size-up and your general impression of the victim should help determine whether the victim is injured or if he or she is ill. If you are unable to determine whether the victim is ill or injured, treat as though he or she were injured. Impressions can come from the victim's position, the breathing sounds he or she is making, or from abnormal skin color.

Check Responsiveness

Victims can be *responsive* (they respond to the rescuer) or *unresponsive*. Not all responsive victims are fully alert and may respond to different levels of stimulation. The **AVPU scale** **Table 4-1** describes how responsive a victim is.

Table 4-1	The AVPU Scale	
A	Alert	The victim's eyes are open, and he or she can answer questions clearly. A victim who knows the day of the week, where she is (place), and her own name is said to be "alert and oriented."
V	Responsive to verbal stimulus	The victim might not know the day of the week, where he is, or his name, but does respond in some meaningful way when spoken to.
P	Responsive only to painful stimulus	The eyes do not open, and the victim does not respond to questions. The victim moves or cries out in response to a painful stimulus such as pinching the muscle above the clavicle, or firmly pinching the earlobe.
U	Unresponsive to any stimulus	The eyes do not open, and the victim does not respond to any stimulus.

skill drill

4-1   Initial Check

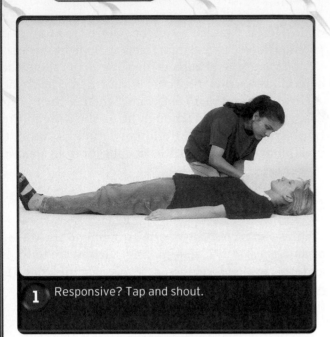

1 Responsive? Tap and shout.

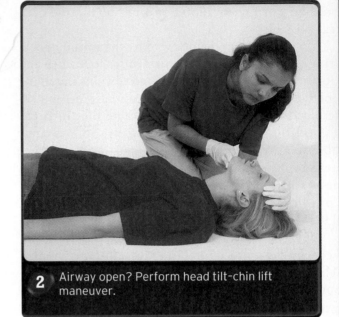

2 Airway open? Perform head tilt-chin lift maneuver.

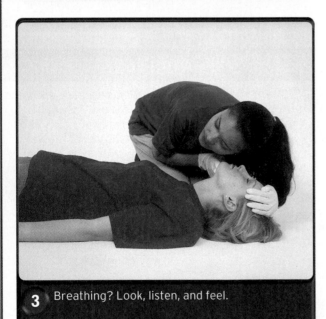

3 Breathing? Look, listen, and feel.

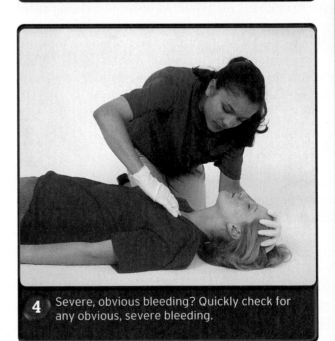

4 Severe, obvious bleeding? Quickly check for any obvious, severe bleeding.

For an alert victim, begin by introducing yourself. Tell the victim that you are trained in first aid, and ask permission to help. Ask the victim his or her name, if the victim knows where he or she is, the day of the week, and what happened. If the victim can talk, breathing and heartbeat are present. For a motionless victim, tap his or her shoulder and ask, "Are you okay?" If there is no response, evaluate the victim using the AVPU scale.

FYI

Verbal First Aid: What to Say to a Victim

Use these guidelines for gaining rapport and calming injured and ill victims:

1. Avoid negative statements that could add to a victim's distress and anxiety.
2. Your first words to a victim are very important.
3. Do not ask unnecessary questions unless it aids treatment or satisfies the victim's need to talk.
4. Tears and/or laughter can be normal—let the victim know this if such responses seem to make him or her feel embarrassed.
5. Stress the positive. For example, instead of "you will not have any pain," say, "the worst is over."
6. Do not deny the obvious. For example, instead of saying that "there is nothing wrong," say that "you've had quite a fall and probably don't feel too good, but we're going to look after you; you'll soon be feeling better."
7. Use the victim's name while providing first aid.

Open Airway

The airway must be open for breathing. If the victim is alert and able to answer questions without difficulty, the airway is open. If a responsive victim cannot talk, cry, or cough forcefully, the airway is probably obstructed and must be checked and cleared. In this case, abdominal thrusts (Heimlich maneuver) can be given to clear an obstructed airway in a responsive adult or child victim. Refer to chapter 5, where the Heimlich maneuver is described in detail.

In an unresponsive victim lying face up, open the airway using the head tilt–chin lift method (the latest guidelines do not recommend laypeople using the jaw-thrust technique when a neck injury is suspected—use the head tilt–chin lift method).

In an unresponsive victim lying face up, the most common airway obstruction is the tongue. Snoring is evidence of this. Because the tongue is attached to the lower jaw, any movement that brings the jaw forward will move the tongue away from the throat and therefore open the airway. Once the victim's airway is clear of obstruction, the initial check can continue.

It is difficult to assess and care for a victim who is not on her back (supine position). You will need to turn an unresponsive victim to the supine (on the back) position, but because of a possible neck or back injury this increases the chance of further damage. Moving the victim is best done by several people with the rule that the victim's navel and nose should be kept in a line and moved in unison. If you are the only help at the scene, turn the victim to the supine position if necessary to save the victim's life.

Check Breathing

See Table 4-2 for breathing sounds that might indicate a problem. Responsive victims with breathing difficulty, poor skin color, or decreased level on the AVPU scale need medical care.

Check for breathing in an unresponsive victim while opening the airway. Watch for the victim's chest to rise and fall as you place your ear next to the victim's mouth. Look, listen, and feel for 5 to 10 seconds to check for breathing. If the victim is not breathing, keep the airway open and breathe two breaths (each breath lasts 1 second) into the victim. Refer to chapter 5 for details. During this step, check for the presence of breathing or breathing difficulties.

Table 4-2   Breathing Sounds

Breathing Sounds	Possible Cause
Snoring	Airway partially blocked (usually by tongue)
Gurgling (breaths passing through liquid)	Fluids in throat
Crowing (birdlike sound)	Spasm of the larynx; foreign body
Wheezing	Spasm or partial obstruction in bronchi (asthma, emphysema)
Occasional, gasping breaths (known as agonal respirations)	Breathing after the heart has stopped

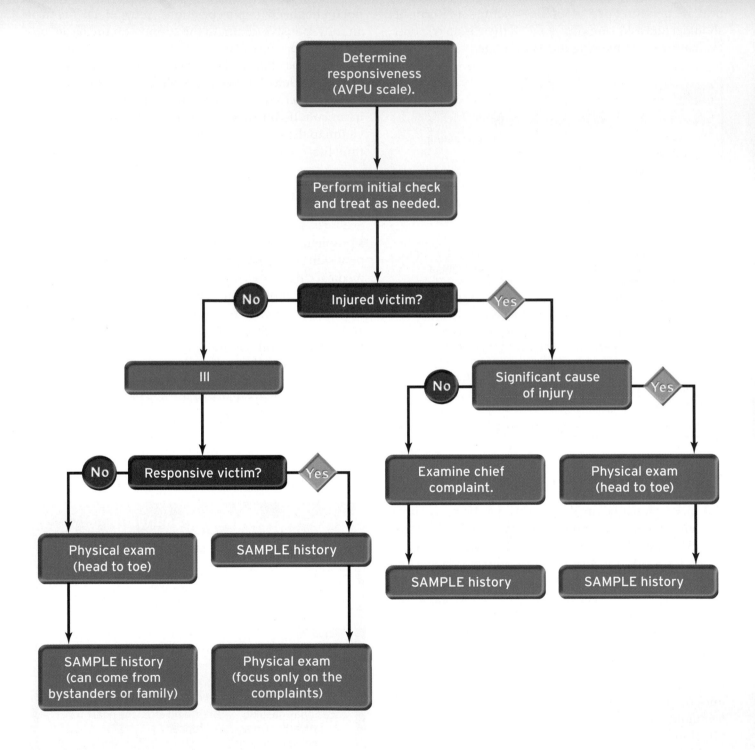

If the first breath does not go in, retilt the head and give another breath. If breath still will not go in, move to the chest and:

- give 30 chest compressions (same as CPR chest compressions—place your hands between the nipples and in the middle of the chest on the breastbone).
- look into the mouth for an object. If you see one, remove it. If you do not see one, give two breaths.

If the airway remains blocked, rotate through cycles of 30 chest compressions, looking into the mouth for an object, and two breaths until the object is removed or EMS personnel replace you.

Check for Severe Bleeding

Check for severe bleeding by quickly looking over the victim's entire body for blood (blood-soaked clothing or blood pooling on the floor or the ground). This is not a head-to-toe exam but a search for pools of blood around the victim or in the victim's clothing. In most cases, direct pressure with a hand and sterile dressing over the bleeding or a pressure bandage controls the bleeding. Life-threatening external bleeding is rare, but when found, it must be controlled immediately or the victim can bleed to death. Avoid contact with the victim's blood whenever possible by using medical exam gloves or extra layers of dressings or cloth.

Skin Condition

A quick check of the victim's skin can also provide information about the victim's condition Table 4-3. Check skin temperature, color, and condition. Skin color, especially in light-skinned people, reflects the circulation under the skin as well as oxygen status. For those with dark complexions, changes might not be readily apparent but can be assessed by the appearance of the nail beds, the inside of the mouth, and the inner eyelids.

You can get a rough idea of skin temperature by putting the back of your hand or wrist on the victim's forehead Table 4-4.

Some health care providers use the capillary refill. It can be performed by gently pressing a fingernail or toenail for a few seconds and then releasing the pressure. When released, the blanched skin should return to its normal color within two seconds (saying "capillary refill" takes two seconds). Anything more than two seconds indicates poor circulation, which needs medical attention. Some medical experts question the capillary refill test's reliability in adults because of various factors (for example, exposure to cold, heavy tobacco use).

Expose the Injury

Clothing might have to be removed to check for an injury and to give proper first aid. If you need to remove clothing, explain what you intend to do and why. Remove as much as necessary, try to maintain privacy, and prevent exposure to cold. Damage clothing only if necessary—cut along the seams Figure 4-1.

▶ Physical Exam

The goal of doing a hands-on physical exam is to identify immediately any potentially life-threatening illness or injury. It also helps provide an objective base on which to give first aid. A good physical exam is essential in discovering what is wrong.

Table 4-3

Skin Color	Possible Cause
Pink	Normal color in nonpigmented areas regardless of skin complexion—lining of the eyelids, inside mouth, fingernail beds
Red (flushed)	Dilated blood vessels; excess circulation to that part of the body
White (pale)	Constricted blood vessels from blood loss, shock, hypothermia, emotional distress
Blue (cyanosis)	Lack of oxygen in the blood from breathing or heart problems
Yellow (jaundice)	Liver disease or failure

Table 4-4

Skin Temperature/Moisture	Possible Cause
Warm and dry	Normal
Hot and dry or moist	Excessive body heat (heat stroke, high fever)
Cool and moist (clammy)	Poor circulation, heat exhaustion, shock, acute stress reaction
Cold and moist	Body is losing heat
Cold and dry	Exposed to cold and has lost considerable heat (hypothermia)

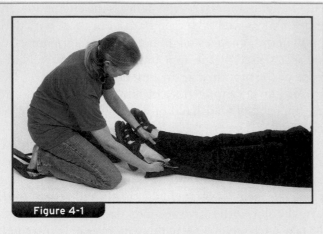

Figure 4-1

Expose the injury. Remove as much clothing as necessary, while trying to maintain privacy.

Table 4-5 Significant Causes of Injury
• Falls of more than 15 feet for adults, more than 10 feet for children, or more than three times the victim's height
• Vehicle collisions involving ejection, a rollover, high speed, a pedestrian, a motorcycle, or a bicycle
• Unresponsive or altered mental status
• Head trauma with altered mental status (V, P, or U on AVPU scale)
• Penetrations of the head, chest, or abdomen (for example, stab or gunshot wounds)
• Major burn injury
• Death of an occupant in the same vehicle

Most of the victims you are likely to see will *not* require a complete head-to-toe type of physical exam. Nevertheless, first aiders should know how to perform a complete physical exam. In most cases, only the victim's chief complaint requires attention. The chief complaint is the victim's major problem or chief concern. You can find it out in most cases by asking, "What's wrong?" or "What happened to you?"

Start by reconsidering the cause of injury that you identified during the scene size-up. This allows you to determine which procedures to use in checking an injured victim.

Determine if a significant cause of injury was involved Table 4-5 . In addition to the significant causes of injury, assume that a victim with a head injury also has a spinal injury until proven otherwise. About 15–20% of head injury victims also have a spinal injury.

For a responsive victim check for a spinal injury by asking:

- Can you feel me squeezing your fingers and toes?
- Can you wiggle your fingers and toes?
- Can you squeeze my hand, and can you push your foot against my hand?

For an unresponsive victim, check the spinal cord by stroking the bottom of the foot firmly toward the big toe with a key or similar sharp object. This is known as the Babinski reflex test. The normal response is an involuntary reflex that makes the big toe go down (except in in-fants, in whom it goes in the opposite direction). If the spinal cord or brain is injured, the toe will flex upward for both adults and children. If you suspect a spinal injury, do not move the victim's head or neck. Stabilize the victim against any movement, and tell him or her not to move.

A physical exam checks the victim's entire body from head to toe; you will note the victim's signs and symptoms:

- <u>Signs</u> = victim's conditions you can see, feel, hear, or smell.
- <u>Symptoms</u> = things the victim feels and is able to describe; known as the chief complaint.

To check a part of the body, look and feel for the following signs and symptoms of injury: deformities, open injuries, tenderness, and swelling. A physical exam might require removing some clothing, but could be impractical especially in a cold, windy environment. The mnemonic <u>DOTS</u> is helpful for remembering the signs of injury Figure 4-2 .

- D = Deformity—Abnormal shape of the body part (compare with uninjured part). Deformities occur when bones are broken or joints are dislocated.
- O = Open wounds—The skin is broken and there is bleeding.
- T = Tenderness—Sensitivity, discomfort, or pain when touched.
- S = Swelling—Area looks larger than usual. Caused by excess fluid in the tissue.

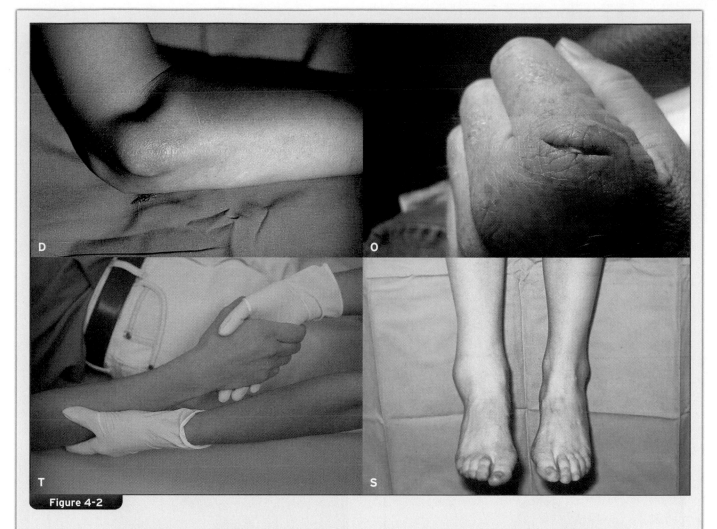

Figure 4-2

Examine an area by looking and feeling for: D = deformity; O = open wounds; T = tenderness; S = swelling.

Conducting a Physical Exam

To conduct a physical exam for an injury, follow the steps in `Skill Drill 4-2` :

1. Head: check for DOTS. Compare the pupils—they should be the same size and react to light. Check the ears and nose for clear or blood-tinged fluid. Check the mouth for objects that could block the airway, such as broken teeth (**Step ❶**).
2. Neck: check for DOTS. Look for a medical identification necklace (**Step ❷**).
3. Chest: check for DOTS. Gently squeeze inward (**Step ❸**).
4. Abdomen: check for DOTS. Gently push (**Step ❹**).

5. Pelvis: check for DOTS. Gently push downward and inward on the tops of the hips (**Steps ❺ₐ** and **❺ᵦ**).
6. Extremities: check both arms and legs for DOTS (**Step ❻**).
7. Back: if no spinal injury is suspected, turn the victim on his or her side and check for DOTS (**Step ❼**).

CAUTION

When Doing a Physical Exam
DO NOT aggravate injuries or contaminate wounds.
DO NOT move a victim with a possible spinal injury.

skill drill

4-2 **Physical Exam**

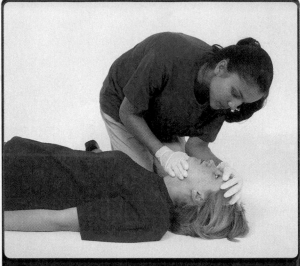

1 Head: check for DOTS. Compare the pupils; they should be the same size and react to light. Check the ears and nose for clear or blood-tinged fluid. Check the mouth for objects that could block the airway, such as broken teeth.

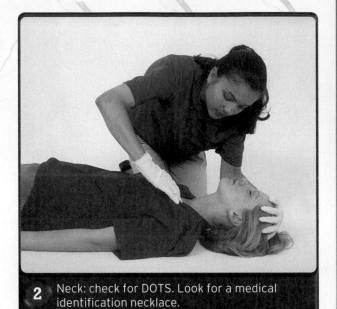

2 Neck: check for DOTS. Look for a medical identification necklace.

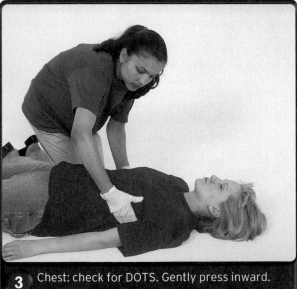

3 Chest: check for DOTS. Gently press inward.

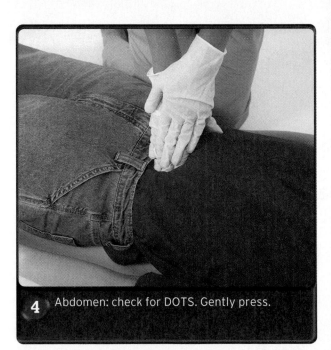

4 Abdomen: check for DOTS. Gently press.

skill drill

4-2   Physical Exam–Continued

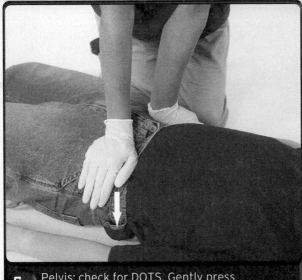

5a Pelvis: check for DOTS. Gently press downward and inward on the tops of the hips.

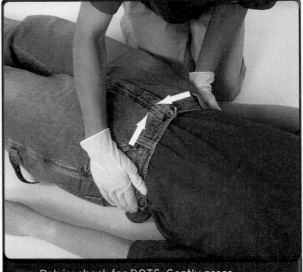

5b Pelvis: check for DOTS. Gently press downward and inward on the tops of the hips.

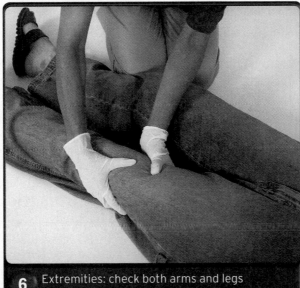

6 Extremities: check both arms and legs for DOTS.

7 Back: if no spinal injury is suspected, turn the victim on his or her side and check for DOTS.

Table 4-6 Sample History	
Description	**Sample Questions**
S = Symptoms	What's wrong? (known as the chief complaint)
A = Allergies	Are you allergic to anything?
M = Medications	Are you taking any medications? What are they for?
P = Past medical history	Have you had this problem before? Do you have other medical problems?
L = Last oral intake	When did you last eat or drink anything? What was it?
E = Events leading up to the illness or injury	Injury: How did you get hurt? Illness: What led to this problem?

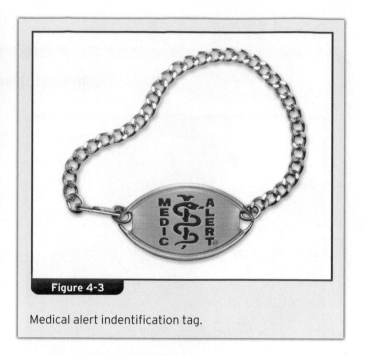

Figure 4-3

Medical alert indentification tag.

▶ SAMPLE History

The information in a SAMPLE history could help you to identify what is wrong with the victim and can indicate the needed first aid. It is called a **SAMPLE history** because the letters in the word SAMPLE stand for the elements of the history (Table 4-6). If the victim is unresponsive or is a child, you might be able to obtain the SAMPLE history information from family, friends, or bystanders.

▶ Medical Identification Tags

Look for a medical identification tag or for a medical information card in the victim's wallet or purse (this might be illegal in some states). It can be beneficial in identifying allergies, medications, or medical history (Figure 4-3). A medical identification tag, worn as a necklace or as a bracelet, contains the wearer's medical problem(s) and a 24-hour telephone number that offers, in case of an emergency, access to the victim's medical history plus names of doctors and close relatives. Necklaces and bracelets are durable, instantly recognizable, and less likely than cards to be separated from the victim in an emergency. Always look for victim identification in the presence of another person at the scene.

▶ Putting It All Together

The victim assessment will be influenced by whether the victim is suffering from an illness or an injury, whether the victim is responsive or unresponsive, and whether life-threatening conditions are present. Remember to first conduct an initial check and correct any problems you uncover before gong on with the assessment.

Different problems and conditions require different approaches for determining what is wrong. Not all parts of the assessment will apply to every victim, and the sequencing can vary depending on the victim's problem. Most victims do not require a complete assessment. For example, a victim who cuts a finger while whittling a stick will not require a complete assessment, but a victim with a cut finger from slipping and falling 20 feet down a mountainside will, because other injuries might be present. Table 4-7 gives the sequence for various types of victims.

A victim assessment can provide important information about a problem and help you determine how you treat it and whether medical care is needed. If the victim requires medical care, pass what you found during the assessment to the EMS or health care providers. Provide the following information:

1. Victim's chief complaint
2. Responsiveness (AVPU scale)
3. Initial check (breathing and severe bleeding status)
4. Physical exam findings
5. SAMPLE history
6. Any first aid that has been provided

Table 4-7   Sequence of Victim Assessment

Injured Victim			Ill Victim	
Unresponsive	Responsive		Unresponsive	Responsive
	With Significant COI*	Without Significant COI*		
• Initial check • Physical exam using DOS of DOTS • SAMPLE history from others	• Initial check • Physical exam using DOTS • SAMPLE history	• Initial check • Examine chief complaint • SAMPLE history	• Initial check • Physical exam using DOS of DOTS • SAMPLE history from others	• Initial check • SAMPLE history • Examine chief complaint

*COI–Cause of injury

▶ What to Do Until Medical Help Is Available

The initial check, physical exam, and SAMPLE history are done quickly so that injuries and illnesses can be identified and given first aid and, if necessary, transportation can be arranged. After the most serious problems have been cared for, regularly recheck an alert victim who has a serious injury or illness every 15 minutes, and at least every five minutes for an unresponsive victim or one having breathing difficulties, major blood loss, or a significant cause of injury. When in doubt, keep checking the victim every five minutes or as frequently as possible.

▶ Triage: What to Do with Multiple Victims

You might encounter emergency situations in which there are two or more victims. This is often the case in multiple-car collisions or disasters. After making a quick scene size-up, decide who must be cared for and transported first. This process of prioritizing victims is called **triage**.

Various systems have been used to establish priorities. To find those needing immediate care for life-threatening conditions, tell all victims who can get up and walk to move to a specific area. Victims who can get up and walk rarely have life-threatening injuries. These victims (the walking wounded) are classified as delayed priority (see below). Do not force a victim to move if he or she complains of pain.

Find the life-threatened victims by performing only the initial survey on all remaining victims. Go to mo-

tionless victims first. You must move rapidly (spend less than 60 seconds with each victim) from one victim to the next until all have been checked. Classify victims according to the following care and transportation priorities:

1. *Immediate care.* Victims who have life-threatening injuries but can be saved:
   ◦ Breathing difficulties (abnormal breath sounds or not breathing)
   ◦ Severe chest pain
   ◦ Uncontrolled or massive bleeding
   ◦ Unresponsive
2. *Urgent care.* Victims who do not fit into the immediate or delayed categories. Care and transportation can be delayed up to 1 hour.
3. *Delayed care.* Victims with minor injuries. Care and transportation can be delayed up to 3 hours.
4. *Dead.* Victims who are obviously dead, or unlikely to survive.

Recheck victims regularly for changes in their condition. Only after those with immediate life-threatening conditions receive care should those with less serious conditions be given care. You will usually be relieved from triage responsibility when more highly trained emergency personnel arrive on the scene. You might then be asked to provide first aid, to help move victims, or to help with ambulance or helicopter transportation.

Advantages of the Left-Side Position

Left-side positioning **Figure 4-4** is referred to by several terms: recovery position, left lateral recumbent position, left lateral decubitus position, and stable-side position.

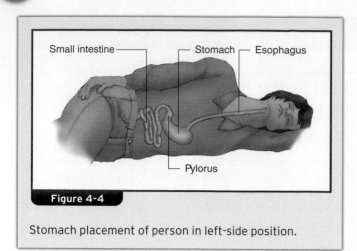

Figure 4-4

Stomach placement of person in left-side position.

Positioning a person on his or her left side has several advantages:

- It keeps the airway open in an unresponsive, breathing victim without a spinal injury.
- It delays vomiting by placing the esophagus above the stomach.
- It delays a poison's effects by retaining the poison in the stomach. A poison can be better dealt with in the stomach than in the small intestines.
- It relieves pressure on a pregnant woman's vena cava (the body's largest vein). Many pregnant women will pass out or at least feel dizzy if they lie supine (on their backs) because of the reduced blood flow.

▶ Ready for Review

- Victim assessment is a sequence of actions that helps determine what is wrong and thus ensures safe and appropriate first aid.
- Every time you encounter a victim, first check out the scene.
- The initial check determines whether there are life-threatening problems requiring quick care.
- The goal of a hands-on physical exam is to identify immediately any potentially life-threatening illness or injury.
- The information in a SAMPLE history can help you to identify what is wrong with the victim and can indicate the needed first aid.
- Look for medical identification tags on the victim.
- Victim assessment will be influenced by whether the victim is suffering from an illness or injury, whether the victim is responsive or unresponsive, and whether life-threatening conditions are present.
- Triage is the process of prioritizing victims.

▶ Vital Vocabulary

AVPU scale A method of assessing a victim's level of responsiveness; used mainly during the initial check.

cause of injury The force that causes an injury.

DOTS A mnemonic for assessment in which each area of the body is evaluated for deformities, open wounds, tenderness, and swelling.

general impression The part of the victim assessment that helps identify any immediately or potentially life-threatening conditions.

initial check A step of the victim assessment in which a first aider checks for life-threatening injuries and gives care for any that are found.

nature of illness The general type of illness a victim is experiencing.

physical exam Part of the victim assessment process in which a detailed, area-by-area exam is performed on victims whose problems cannot be readily identified or when more specific information is needed about a problem.

SAMPLE history A brief history of a victim's condition to determine symptoms, allergies, medications, pertinent past history, last oral intake, and event leading to the illness/injury.

scene size-up A quick assessment of the scene and the surroundings for its safety, the cause of injury or nature of illness, and number of victims before starting first aid.

sign Evidence of an injury or disease which can be seen, heard, or felt.

symptom What a victim tells a first aider about what he feels.

triage A system of placing priorities for first aid and/or transportation in cases when two or more people are injured or suddenly ill.

▶ Assessment in Action

The light in the upstairs hall has gone out and your roommate doesn't want to wait for the landlord to change the light bulb. He gets a ladder out of the basement and attempts to change the light bulb himself. Unfortunately he slips and falls off of the ladder while climbing down. You hear a loud thud and run out into the hallway to find your roommate lying on the floor motionless. You notice his medical identification bracelet.

Directions: Circle Yes if you agree with the statement, circle No if you disagree.

Yes No 1. After confirming that the scene is safe, you next check the medical identification bracelet as a clue for finding out what's wrong.

Yes No 2. If he was unresponsive, you would first look at and feel his legs for a broken bone.

Yes No 3. If he was responsive, you would first ask about his health history.

Yes No 4. The physical exam should be started at the victim's head.

Yes No 5. A medical identification tag lists the victim's medical problems.

Answers: **1.** No; **2.** No; **3.** No; **4.** Yes; **5.** Yes

prep kit

▶ Check Your Knowledge

Directions: Circle Yes if you agree with the statement, circle No if you disagree.

Yes No **1.** The purpose of an initial check is to find life-threatening conditions.

Yes No **2.** A quiet, motionless victim could indicate a breathing problem.

Yes No **3.** Most injured victims require a complete physical exam.

Yes No **4.** For a physical exam, you usually begin at the head and work down the body.

Yes No **5.** If the victim is not breathing, give two breaths before giving chest compression.

Yes No **6.** The mnemonic DOTS helps in remembering what information to obtain about the victim's history that could be useful.

Yes No **7.** For all injured and suddenly ill persons, look for a medical identification tag during a physical exam.

Yes No **8.** The mnemonic SAMPLE can remind you how to examine an area for signs of an injury.

Yes No **9.** If there is more than one victim, go to the quiet, motionless victim first.

Yes No **10.** A gurgling sound heard while checking for breathing indicates possible fluid in the throat.

Answers: **1.** Yes; **2.** Yes; **3.** No; **4.** Yes; **5.** Yes; **6.** No; **7.** Yes; **8.** No; **9.** Yes; **10.** Yes

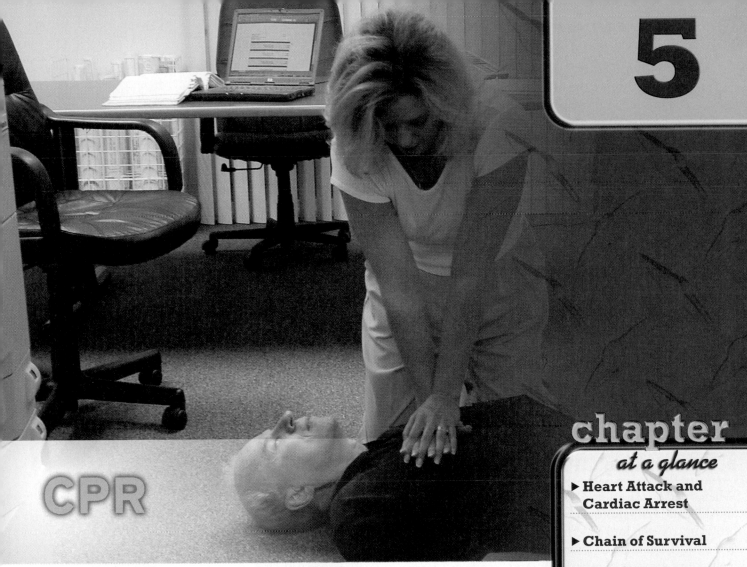

CPR

▶ Heart Attack and Cardiac Arrest

A <u>heart attack</u> occurs when heart muscle tissue dies because its blood supply is severely reduced or stopped. This often occurs because of a clot in one or more coronary arteries. The signs of a heart attack and the steps for caring for a heart attack are discussed in detail in Chapter 17. If damage to the heart muscle is too severe, the victim's heart can stop beating—a condition known as <u>cardiac arrest</u>. Sudden cardiac arrest is a leading cause of death in the United States, affecting about 250,000 people yearly in out-of-hospital locations.

▶ Chain of Survival

Few victims experiencing sudden cardiac arrest outside of a hospital survive unless a rapid sequence of events takes place. The <u>chain of survival</u> is a way of describing the ideal sequence of care that should take place when a cardiac arrest occurs.

The four links in the chain of survival are as follows:

1. *Early access:* Recognizing the emergency and immediately calling 9-1-1 to activate emergency medical services (EMS).
2. *Early CPR:* Cardiopulmonary resuscitation (<u>CPR</u>) supplies a minimal amount of blood to the heart and brain. It buys time until a defibrillator and EMS personnel are available. It can double or triple the victim's chances of survival.

3. *Early defibrillation:* Administering a shock to the heart can restore the heartbeat in some victims. It can produce survival rates as high as 50–75%.

4. *Early advanced care:* Health care providers give advanced cardiac life support to victims of sudden cardiac arrest. This includes providing IV fluids, medications, and advanced airway devices.

If any one of these links in the chain is broken (absent), the chance that the victim will survive is greatly decreased. If all links in the chain are strong, the victim has the best possible chance of survival.

FYI

Defibrillation

Most adults in cardiac arrest need defibrillation. Early defibrillation is the single most important factor in surviving cardiac arrest. Chapter 6 provides information on automated external defibrillators (AEDs).

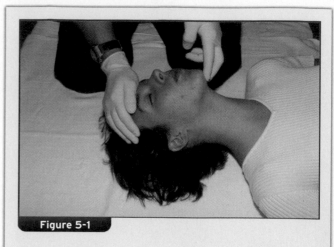

Figure 5-1

The head tilt-chin lift maneuver is a simple method for opening the airway.

▶ Performing CPR

When a person's heart stops beating, he or she needs CPR, an AED, and EMS professionals quickly. CPR consists of breathing oxygen into a victim's lungs and moving blood to the heart and brain by giving **chest compressions**. CPR techniques are very similar for infants (birth to 1 year), children (ages 1–8), and adults (age 8 and older), with just a few slight variations.

Check for Responsiveness

When the scene is safe, check for responsiveness by tapping the victim's shoulder and asking if he or she is okay. If the victim does not respond, ask a bystander to call 9-1-1. If you are alone with an adult and a phone is nearby, call 9-1-1. If you are alone with an unresponsive child or infant, give CPR for 2 minutes (five cycles), and then call 9-1-1.

Open the Airway and Check for Breathing

Before starting CPR, open the victim's airway and check to see if the victim is breathing. Open the airway by tilting the head back and lifting the chin **Figure 5-1**. This moves the tongue away from the back of the throat, allowing air to enter and escape the lungs. The procedure can be done for injured or uninjured victims.

While performing the head tilt–chin lift maneuver, check for breathing by placing your ear next to the victim's mouth. Look at the victim's chest to rise and fall and

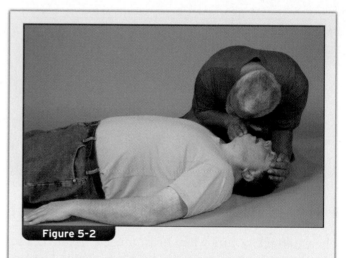

Figure 5-2

Look, listen, and feel for signs of normal breathing.

listen and feel for breathing. Look, listen and feel for signs of normal breathing for 5 to 10 seconds **Figure 5-2**.

Rescue Breaths

If the victim is not breathing, you must provide **rescue breaths**. With the airway open, pinch the victim's nose and make a tight seal over the victim's mouth with your mouth. Give one breath lasting 1 second, take a normal breath for yourself (not a deep breath), and then give another breath like the first one. Each rescue breath should make the victim's chest rise. Other methods of rescue breathing are as follows:

- Mouth-to-barrier device
- Mouth-to-nose method
- Mouth-to-stoma method

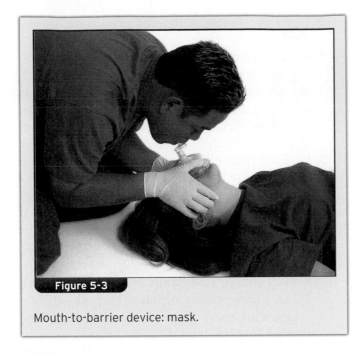

Figure 5-3

Mouth-to-barrier device: mask.

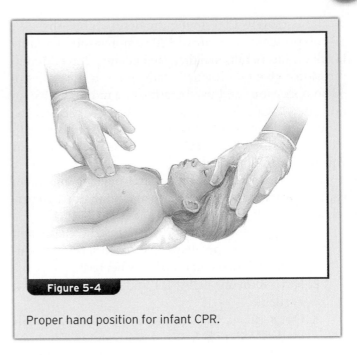

Figure 5-4

Proper hand position for infant CPR.

Mouth-to-Barrier Device

A barrier device is placed in the victim's mouth or over the victim's mouth and nose as a precaution against infection. There are several different types of barrier devices (for example, face shields and face masks), and all are easy to use with little modification to the mouth-to-mouth method 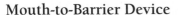.

Mouth-to-Nose Method

If you cannot open the victim's mouth, the teeth are clenched shut, the mouth is severely injured, or you cannot make a good seal with the victim's mouth (for example, because there are no teeth), use the mouth-to-nose method. With the head tilted back, push up on the victim's chin to close the mouth. Make a seal with your mouth over the victim's nose and provide rescue breaths.

Mouth-to-Stoma Method

Some diseases of the vocal cords result in surgical removal of the larynx. People who have this surgery breathe through a small, permanent opening in the neck called a stoma. To perform mouth-to-stoma breathing, close the victim's mouth and nose and breathe through the opening in the neck.

Chest Compressions

Chest compressions move a small but critical amount of blood to the heart and brain. Perform chest compressions with two hands for an adult, one or two hands for a child, and two fingers for an infant. Effective compressions require rescuers to push hard and fast. The chest of an adult should be compressed 1.5 to 2 inches, and the chest of a child or infant should be compressed one third to one half the depth of the chest. The chest should be allowed to return to its normal depth after each compression. The desired position for adult and child chest compressions is in the center of the chest between the nipples; for infants, it is just below the nipple line **Figure 5-4**. The victim should be on a hard, flat surface (for example, the floor) and on his or her back.

FYI

Avoiding Stomach Distention
Rescue breaths can cause stomach distention. Minimize this problem by limiting the breaths to the amount needed to make the chest rise. Avoid overinflating the victim's lungs by just taking a normal breath yourself before breathing into the victim. Gastric distention can cause regurgitation of stomach contents and complicate care.

CAUTION

First aiders DO NOT:
Check for a pulse or other signs of circulation (for example, movement).
Give rescue breaths without chest compressions.
Use a jaw thrust to open the airway—only health care providers use this maneuver.

Immediately after giving the first two breaths, give 30 compressions at a rate of 100 compressions a minute for all victims (adults, children, and infants). After 30 compressions, give two rescue breaths. Repeat the cycles of 30 compressions and two breaths for 2 minutes (five total cycles). Check for breathing after every 5 cycles. Continue the cycles of CPR until an AED becomes available, the victim shows signs of life, EMS takes over, or you are too tired to continue.

Over the years, CPR procedures have changed, becoming easier for people to learn and remember. To perform adult CPR, follow the steps in **Skill Drill 5-1** :

1. Check responsiveness by tapping the victim and asking, "Are you okay?" If the victim is unresponsive, roll him or her onto his or her back.
2. Have someone call 9-1-1 and retrieve an AED if available.
3. Open the airway using the head tilt–chin lift method (**Step ❶**).
4. Check for breathing for 5 to 10 seconds by looking for chest rise and fall and listening and feeling for breathing (**Step ❷**). If the victim is breathing, place him or her in the recovery position. If the victim is not breathing, go to the next step.
5. Give two rescue breaths (1 second each), making the chest rise (**Step ❸**). If the first breath does not cause the chest to rise, retilt the head and try the breath again and then proceed to the next step. If both breaths cause the chest to rise, go to the next step.
6. Perform CPR.
   - Place the heel of one hand on the center of the chest between the nipples. Place the other hand on top of the first hand (**Step ❹**).
   - Depress the chest 1.5 to 2 inches.
   - Give 30 chest compressions at a rate of about 100 per minute.
   - Open the airway, and give two breaths (1 second each). For airway obstruction, look for object in mouth before giving two rescue breaths.
7. Continue cycles of 30 chest compressions and two breaths for 2 minutes (about four more cycles), or until an AED is available, the victim is breathing, EMS takes over, or you are too tired to continue (**Step ❺**).

To perform CPR on a child, follow the steps in **Skill Drill 5-2** :

1. Check responsiveness by tapping the victim and shouting, "Are you okay?" If the victim is unresponsive, roll her onto her back.
2. Have someone call 9-1-1 and retrieve an AED if available.
3. Open the airway using the head tilt–chin lift method (**Step ❶**).
4. Check for breathing for 5 to 10 seconds by looking for chest rise and fall and listening and feeling for breathing (**Step ❷**). If the victim is breathing, place him or her in the recovery position. If the victim is not breathing, go to the next step.
5. Give two rescue breaths (1 second each), making the chest rise (**Step ❸**). If the first breath does not cause the chest to rise, retilt the head and try the breath again, then proceed to the next step. If both breaths cause the chest to rise, go to the next step.
6. Perform CPR.
   - Place one or two hands on the center of the chest between the nipples (**Step ❹**). If two hands are used, place one hand on top of the other as in adult CPR.
   - Depress chest one third to one half the depth of the chest.
   - Give 30 chest compressions at a rate of about 100 per minute.
   - Open the airway and give two breaths (1 second each). For airway obstruction, look for object in mouth before giving two breaths.
7. Continue cycles of 30 chest compressions and two breaths for 2 minutes (about four more cycles), or until an AED is available, the victim is breathing, EMS takes over, or you are too tired to continue (**Step ❺**).

To perform CPR on an infant, follow the steps in **Skill Drill 5-3** :

1. Check responsiveness by tapping the victim and shouting, "Are you okay?" If the victim is unresponsive, roll him onto his back.
2. Have someone call 9-1-1.
3. Open the airway by tilting the head back slightly and lifting the chin (**Step ❶**).
4. Check breathing for 5 to 10 seconds by looking for chest rise and fall and listening and feeling for breathing (**Step ❷**). If the victim is breathing, place him or her in the recovery position. If the victim is not breathing, go on to the next step.
5. Give two rescue breaths (1 second each), making the chest rise (**Step ❸**). If the first breath does not cause the chest to rise, retilt the head and try the breath again and then proceed to the next step. If both breaths cause the chest to rise, go to the next step.

skill drill

5-1 Adult CPR

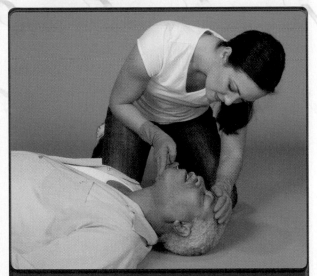

1 Check responsiveness. If the victim is unresponsive, roll him onto his back. Have someone call 9-1-1 and retrieve an AED if available.
Open the airway using the head tilt-chin lift method.

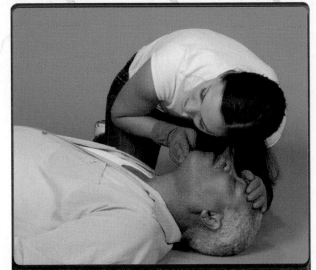

2 Check for breathing for 5 to 10 seconds. If the victim is breathing, place him or her in the recovery position. If the victim is not breathing, go to the next step.

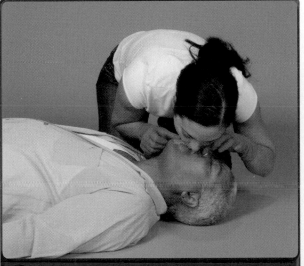

3 Give two rescue breaths (1 second each). If the first breath does not cause the chest to rise, retilt the head and try the breath again and then proceed to the next step. If both breaths cause the chest to rise, go to the next step.

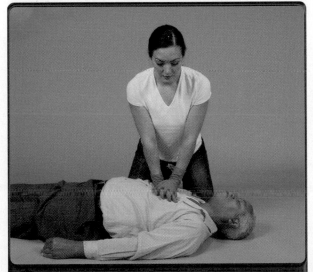

4 Perform CPR.

5 Continue cycles of chest compressions and breaths for 2 minutes (about four more cycles), or until an AED is available, the victim is breathing, EMS takes over, or you are too tired to continue.

5-2 Child CPR

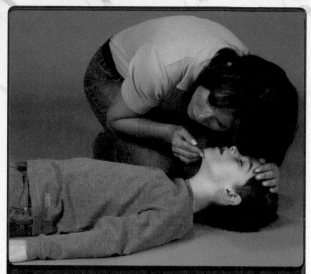

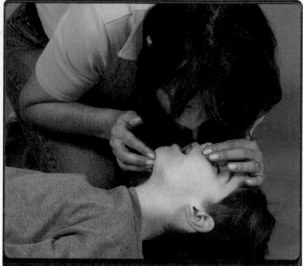

1 Check responsiveness. If the victim is unresponsive, roll her onto her back.

Have someone call 9-1-1 and retrieve an AED if available.

Open the airway using the head tilt-chin lift method.

2 Check for breathing for 5 to 10 seconds. If the victim is breathing, place him or her in the recovery position. If the victim is not breathing, go to the next step.

3 Give two rescue breaths (1 second each), making the chest rise. If the first breath does not cause the chest to rise, retilt the head and try the breath again and then proceed to the next step. If both breaths cause the chest to rise, go to the next step.

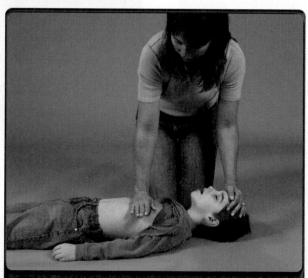

4 Perform CPR.

5 Continue cycles of chest compressions and breaths for 2 minutes (about four more cycles), or until an AED is available, the victim is breathing, EMS takes over, or you are too tired to continue. Use 1 or 2 hands for compressions.

skill drill

5-3 Infant CPR

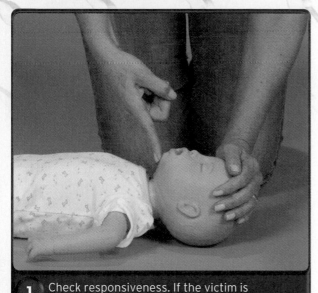

1 Check responsiveness. If the victim is unresponsive, roll him onto his back.

Have someone call 9-1-1.

Open the airway by tilting the head back slightly and lifting the chin.

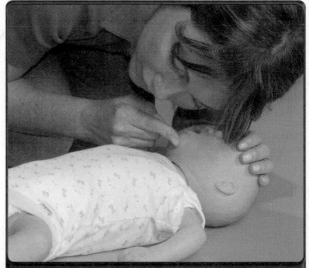

2 Check breathing for 5 to 10 seconds. If the victim is breathing, place him in the recovery position. If the victim is not breathing, go on to the next step.

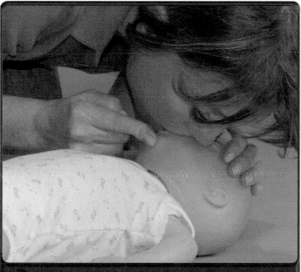

3 Give two rescue breaths (1 second each). If the first breath does not cause the chest to rise, retilt the head and try the breath again and then proceed to the next step. If both breaths cause the chest to rise, go to the next step.

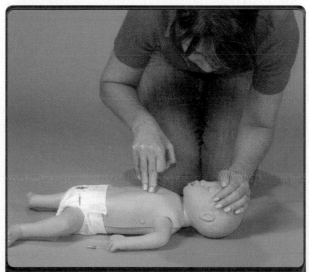

4 Perform CPR.

5 Continue cycles of chest compressions and breaths for 2 minutes (about four more cycles) until the infant starts breathing, EMS arrives, or you are too tired to continue.

6. Perform CPR.
   - Place two fingers on the breastbone just below the nipple line (one finger even with the line) (Step ❹).
   - Depress chest one third to one half the depth of the chest.
   - Give 30 chest compressions at a rate of about 100 per minute.
   - Open the airway and give two breaths (1 second each).
7. Continue cycles of 30 chest compressions and two breaths for 2 minutes (about four more cycles) until the infant starts breathing, EMS arrives, or you are too tired to continue (Step ❺).

FYI

Compression-Only CPR

Mouth-to-mouth rescue breathing has a long safety record for victims and rescuers. But fear of infectious diseases causes some to be reluctant to give mouth-to-mouth rescue breaths to strangers. To avoid the chance that the victim will not receive any care, compression-only CPR can be considered in these circumstances:

- Rescuer is unwilling or unable to perform mouth-to-mouth rescue breathing.
- Untrained bystander is following dispatcher-assisted CPR instructions.

▶ Airway Obstruction

People can choke on all kinds of objects. Foods such as candy, peanuts, and grapes are major offenders because of their shapes and consistencies. Nonfood choking deaths are often caused by balloons, balls and marbles, toys, and coins inhaled by children and infants.

Recognizing Airway Obstruction

An object lodged in the airway can cause a mild or severe airway obstruction. In a mild airway obstruction, good air exchange is present. The victim is able to make forceful coughing efforts in an attempt to relieve the obstruction. The victim should be encouraged to cough. A victim with a severe airway obstruction will have poor air exchange. The signs of a severe airway obstruction include the following:

- Breathing becoming more difficult
- Weak and ineffective cough

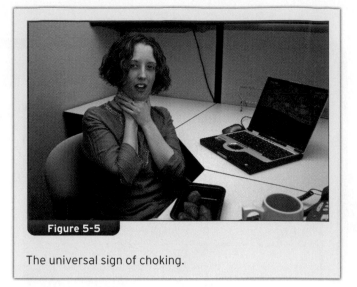

Figure 5-5

The universal sign of choking.

- Inability to speak or breathe
- Skin, fingernail beds, and the inside of the mouth appear bluish gray (indicating cyanosis)

Choking victims sometimes clutch their necks to communicate that they are choking. This motion is known as the universal distress signal for choking. The victim becomes panicked and desperate **Figure 5-5**.

Caring for a Person with an Airway Obstruction

For a responsive adult or child with a severe airway obstruction, ask the victim "Are you choking?" If the victim is unable to respond verbally, but nods yes, provide care for the victim. Move behind the victim and reach around the victim's waist with both arms. Place a fist with the thumb side against the victim's abdomen, just above the navel. Grasp the fist with your other hand and press into the abdomen with quick inward and upward thrusts (this is the Heimlich maneuver). Continue thrusts until the object is removed or the victim becomes unresponsive.

For a responsive infant with a severe airway obstruction, give back blows and chest thrusts instead of abdominal thrusts to relieve the obstruction. Support the infant's head and neck and lay the infant face down on your forearm, then lower your arm to your leg. Give up to five back blows between the infant's shoulder blades with the heel of your hand **Figure 5-6**. While supporting the back of the infant's head, roll the infant face up and give up to five chest thrusts with two fingers on the infant's sternum in the same location used for CPR **Figure 5-7**. Repeat these steps until the object is removed or the infant becomes unresponsive.

Adult CPR

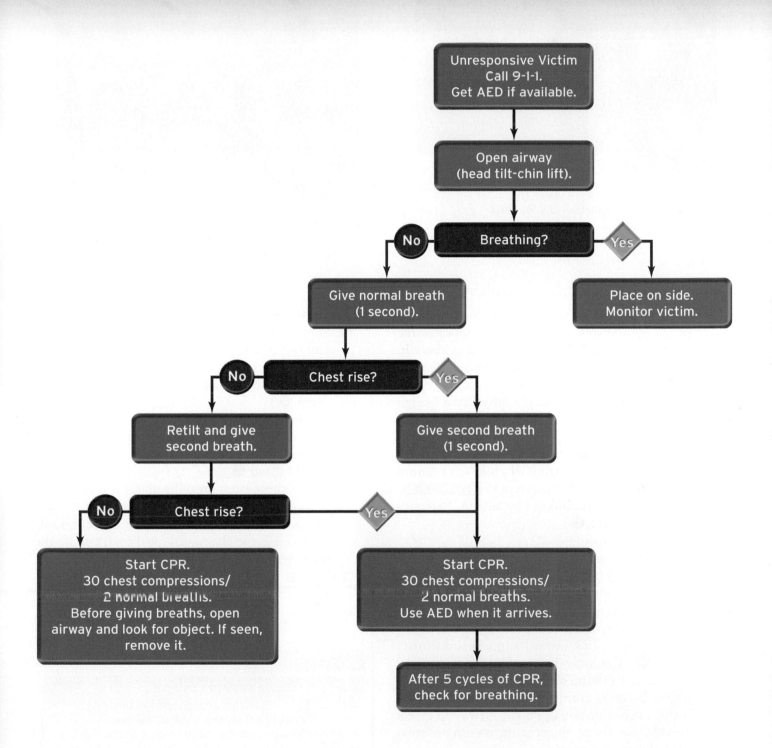

Unresponsive Victim
Call 9-1-1.
Get AED if available.

↓

Open airway
(head tilt-chin lift).

↓

No — Breathing? — **Yes**

Give normal breath
(1 second).

Place on side.
Monitor victim.

No — Chest rise? — **Yes**

Retilt and give
second breath.

Give second breath
(1 second).

No — Chest rise? — **Yes**

Start CPR.
30 chest compressions/
2 normal breaths.
Before giving breaths, open
airway and look for object. If seen,
remove it.

Start CPR.
30 chest compressions/
2 normal breaths.
Use AED when it arrives.

↓

After 5 cycles of CPR,
check for breathing.

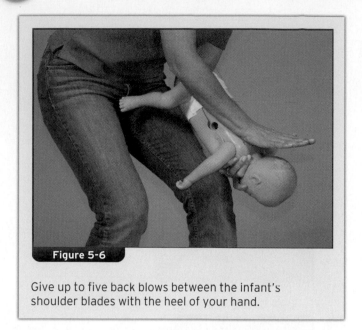

Figure 5-6

Give up to five back blows between the infant's shoulder blades with the heel of your hand.

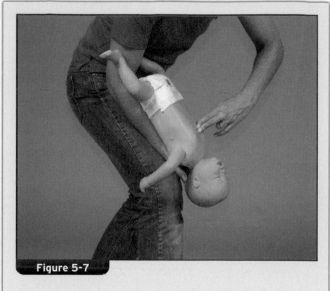

Figure 5-7

Give up to five chest thrusts with two fingers on the infant's sternum in the same location used for CPR.

If you are caring for an unresponsive, nonbreathing victim of any age and your first breath does not cause the chest to rise, retilt the head and try a second breath. Whether the second breath is successful or not, perform CPR—30 compressions and two breaths for five cycles (2 minutes). Since the victim might have had a foreign body airway obstruction, look for an object in the victim's mouth and, if you see it, remove it before giving the two breaths during the cycles of CPR. To relieve airway obstruction in a responsive adult or child who cannot speak, breathe, or cough, follow the steps in **Skill Drill 5-4**:

1. Check victim for choking by asking, "Are you choking?" (**Step ❶**).
2. Have someone call 9-1-1.
3. Position yourself behind the victim and locate the victim's navel (**Step ❷**).
4. Place a fist with thumb side against the victim's abdomen just above the navel (**Step ❸**), grasp it with the other hand, and press into victim's abdomen with quick inward and upward thrusts (**Step ❹**). Continue thrusts until the object is removed or the victim becomes unresponsive. If the victim becomes unresponsive, call 9-1-1 and give CPR. Each time you open the airway to give a breath, look for an object in the mouth or throat and, if seen, remove it.

To relieve airway obstruction in a responsive infant who cannot cry, breathe, or cough, follow the steps in **Skill Drill 5-5**:

1. Have someone call 9-1-1 (**Step ❶**).
2. Support the infant's head and neck and lay the infant face down on your forearm, then lower your arm to your leg. Give five back blows between the infant's shoulder blades with the heel of your hand (**Step ❷**).
3. While supporting the back of the infant's head, roll the infant face up and give five chest thrusts on the infant's sternum in the same location used in CPR (**Step ❸**).
4. Repeat these steps until the object is removed. If the infant becomes unresponsive, begin CPR. Each time you open the airway to give a breath, look for an object in the mouth or throat, and if you see it, remove it (**Step ❹**).

Table 5-1 provides a review of CPR and the steps to take in the event of an airway obstruction for victims of all ages.

FYI

The Tongue and Airway Obstruction

Airway obstruction in an unresponsive victim lying on his or her back is usually the result of the tongue relaxing in the back of the mouth, restricting air movement. Opening the airway with the head tilt-chin lift method could be all that is needed to correct this problem.

skill drill

5-4 | Airway Obstruction in a Responsive Adult or Child

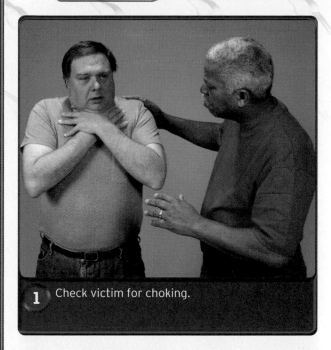

1 Check victim for choking.

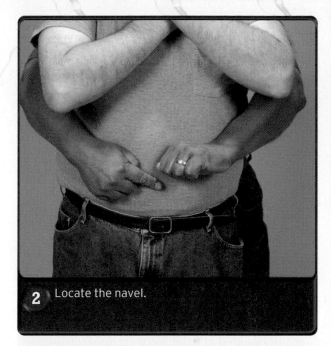

2 Locate the navel.

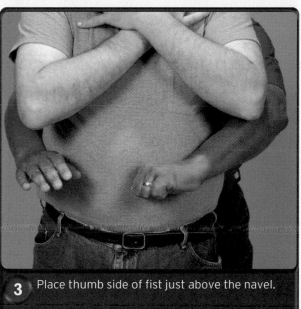

3 Place thumb side of fist just above the navel.

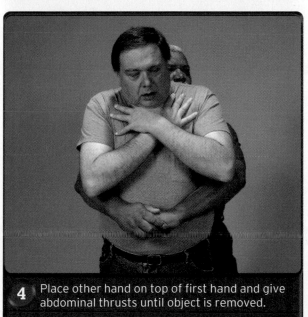

4 Place other hand on top of first hand and give abdominal thrusts until object is removed.

skill drill

5-5   Airway Obstruction in a Responsive Infant

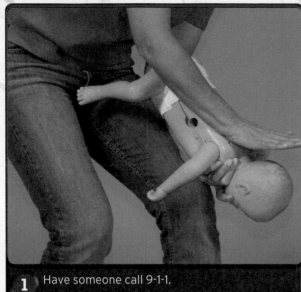

1 Have someone call 9-1-1.

2 Give five back blows between the infant's shoulder blades with the heel of your hand.

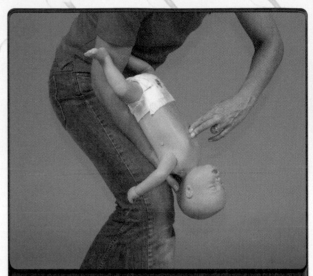

3 Give five chest thrusts on the infant's sternum in the same location used in CPR.

4 Repeat these steps until the object is removed. If the infant becomes unresponsive, begin CPR. Each time you open the airway to give a breath, look for an object in the mouth or throat, and if you see it, remove it.

Table 5-1   CPR and Airway Obstruction Review

These eight steps are the same for *all* motionless victims regardless of age:

1. *Check responsiveness:* Tap a shoulder and ask if the victim is okay. If the victim is unresponsive, have someone call 9-1-1.
2. *Open airway:* Head tilt–chin lift maneuver.
3. *Check breathing:* Look at the chest to see it rise and fall, and listen and feel for breathing for 5-10 seconds.
4. *Place victim in recovery position:* If victim is breathing but unresponsive, place him or her in recovery position.
5. *Give breaths:* If victim is not breathing, give two breaths (1 second per breath).
6. *Perform CPR:* If breaths cause the chest to rise, begin CPR—cycles of 30 chest compressions and two breaths for five cycles (2 minutes). Rate should be 100 compressions per minute. Recheck breathing after every five cycles.
7. *Retilt and retry:* If first breath does not cause the chest to rise, retilt victim's head and try a second breath.
8. *Perform CPR:* Whether the second breath is successful or not, perform CPR—30 compressions and 2 breaths for five cycles (2 minutes). In the case of an unresponsive victim with an airway obstruction, look for an object in the victim's mouth before giving the two breaths, and remove it if you see it.

Action	Adult (≥ 8 years)	Child (1-8 years)	Infant (< 1 year)
1. Breathing methods	Mouth-to-barrier device Mouth-to-mouth Mouth-to-nose Mouth-to-stoma	Mouth-to-barrier device Mouth-to-mouth Mouth-to-nose Mouth-to-stoma	Mouth-to-mouth and nose Mouth-to-barrier device Mouth-to-nose
2. Chest compressions			
Locations	On the breastbone, between nipples	On the breastbone, between nipples	On the breastbone, just below nipple line
Method	Two hands: Heel of one hand on breastbone between nipples; other hand on top	One or two hands	Two fingers
Depth	1.5 to 2 inches	One third to one half the depth of the chest	One third to one half the depth of the chest
Rate	100 per minute	100 per minute	100 per minute
Ratio of chest compressions to breaths	30:2	30:2	30:2
3. When to activate EMS when alone	Immediately after determining unresponsiveness	After 5 cycles of CPR	After 5 cycles of CPR
4. Use of AED	Yes; deliver one shock as soon as possible, followed by 5 cycles of CPR	Yes; use special electrode pads if available	No
5. Responsive victim and airway obstruction	Heimlich maneuver	Heimlich maneuver	Back blows and chest thrusts

prep kit

▶ Ready for Review

- A heart attack occurs when heart muscle tissue dies because the blood supply is severely reduced or stopped.
- The four links in the chain of survival are early access, early CPR, early defibrillation, and early advanced care.
- CPR consists of breathing oxygen into a victim's lungs and moving blood to the heart and brain by giving chest compressions.
- The signs of a severe airway obstruction include difficult breathing, weak and ineffective cough, inability to speak or breathe, and signs of cyanosis.

▶ Vital Vocabulary

airway obstruction A blockage, often the result of a foreign body, in which air flow to the lungs is reduced or completely blocked.

cardiac arrest Stoppage of the heartbeat.

chain of survival A four-step concept to help improve survival from cardiac arrest: early access, early CPR, early defibrillation, and early advanced care.

chest compressions Depressing the chest and allowing it to return to its normal position as part of CPR.

CPR Cardiopulmonary resuscitation; the act of providing rescue breaths and chest compressions for a victim in cardiac arrest.

heart attack Death of a part of the heart muscle.

rescue breaths Breathing for a person who is not breathing.

▶ Assessment in Action

You are at a local health club when you overhear someone in the weight room nearby shouting for help. You enter the room and see a person lying motionless on the floor. You quickly confirm that he is unresponsive.

Directions: Circle Yes if you agree with the statement, circle No if you disagree.

Yes	No	1. The next thing to do is to start chest compressions.
Yes	No	2. The ratio of chest compressions to rescue breaths is 15 to 2.
Yes	No	3. Compression depth for an adult is one third the depth of the chest.
Yes	No	4. Open the airway using the head tilt–chin lift method.
Yes	No	5. Continue CPR until an AED becomes available or EMS personnel arrive.

Answers: 1. No; 2. No; 3. No; 4. Yes; 5. Yes

▶ Check Your Knowledge

Directions: Circle Yes if you agree with the statement, circle No if you disagree.

Yes	No	1. Take 5 to 10 seconds when checking for breathing.
Yes	No	2. After you determine that an adult victim is unresponsive, the next step is to call 9-1-1.
Yes	No	3. Tilting the head back and lifting the chin helps move the tongue and open the airway.
Yes	No	4. If you determine that a victim is not breathing, begin chest compressions.
Yes	No	5. Do not start chest compressions until you have checked for a pulse.
Yes	No	6. For all victims (adult, child, infant) needing CPR, give 30 compressions followed by two breaths.
Yes	No	7. Use two fingers when performing CPR on an infant.
Yes	No	8. A sign of choking is that the victim is unable to speak or cough.
Yes	No	9. To give abdominal thrusts to a responsive choking victim, place your fist below the victim's navel.
Yes	No	10. When giving abdominal thrusts to a responsive choking victim, repeat the thrusts until the object is removed or the victim becomes unresponsive.

Answers: 1. Yes; 2. Yes; 3. Yes; 4. No; 5. No; 6. Yes; 7. Yes; 8. Yes; 9. No; 10. Yes

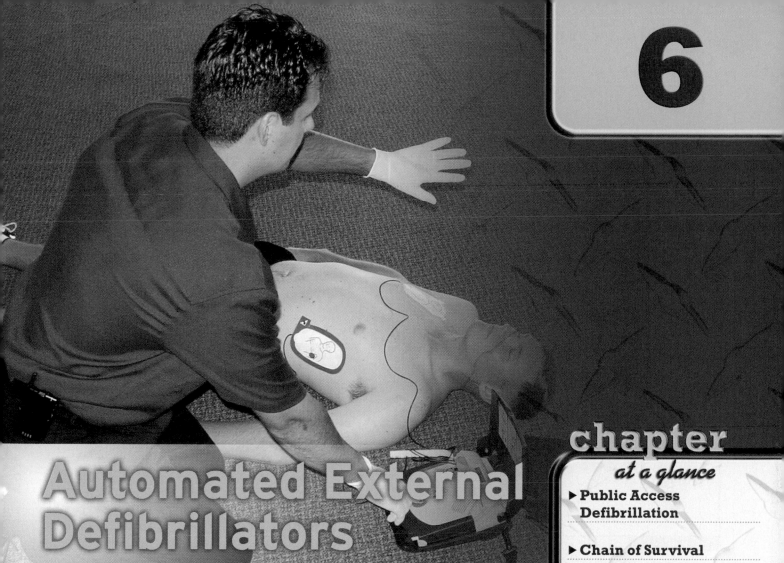

Automated External Defibrillators

▶ Public Access Defibrillation

Sudden cardiac death remains an unresolved public health crisis. A victim's chances for survival are dramatically improved through early cardiopulmonary resuscitation (CPR) and early <u>defibrillation</u> with the use of an <u>automated external defibrillator (AED)</u>. To be effective, defibrillation must be used in the first few minutes following cardiac arrest. The implementation of state public access defibrillation (PAD) laws and the Food and Drug Administration's (FDA) approval of home use AEDs have made this important care step available to many rescuers in many places, including the following **Figure 6-1** :

- Airports and airplanes
- Stadiums
- Health clubs
- Golf courses
- Schools
- Government buildings
- Offices
- Homes

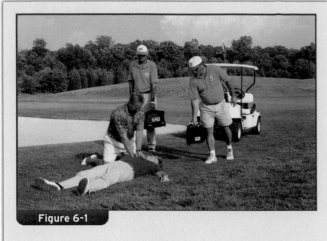

Figure 6-1

AEDs are available in many places for use by trained rescuers.

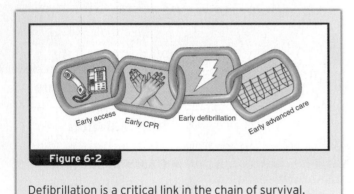

Figure 6-2

Defibrillation is a critical link in the chain of survival.

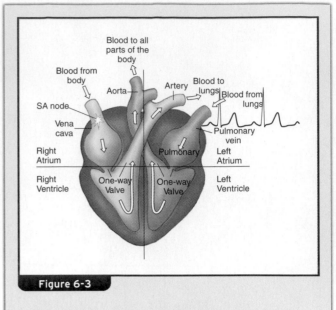

Figure 6-3

The sinoatrial (SA) node is the primary heart pacemaker, which sends electrical impulses to contract the heart's chambers in a coordinated manner.

▶ Chain of Survival

The chain of survival is a concept that recognizes the importance of four critical components in saving the life of a victim of cardiac arrest. Early defibrillation is the third link in this chain **Figure 6-2** :

1. Early access
2. Early CPR
3. Early defibrillation
4. Early advanced care

▶ How the Heart Works

The heart is an organ with four hollow chambers. The two chambers on the right side receive blood from the body and send it to the lungs for oxygen. The two chambers on the left side of the heart receive freshly oxygenated blood from the lungs and send it back out to the body.

The heart has a unique electrical system that controls the rate at which the heart beats, as well as the amount of work the heart performs. In the right upper chamber of the heart, there is a collection of special pacemaker cells. About 60 to 100 times a minute, these cells emit electrical impulses that cause the other heart muscle cells to contract in a coordinated manner **Figure 6-3** .

Because the heart contracts approximately every second, it needs an abundant supply of oxygen, which it gets through the coronary arteries. These arteries run along the outside of the heart muscle and branch into smaller vessels. These arteries sometimes become diseased (with atherosclerosis), resulting in a lack of oxygen to the pacemaker cells, which can cause abnormal electrical activity in the heart.

When Normal Electrical Activity Is Interrupted

Ventricular fibrillation (also known as *V-fib*) is the most common abnormal heart rhythm in cases of sudden cardiac arrest in adults **Figure 6-4** . The organized wave of electrical impulses that cause the heart muscle to contract and relax in a regular fashion is lost when the heart is in ventricular fibrillation. As a result, the lower chambers of the heart quiver and cannot pump blood, so circulation is lost (there is no pulse). A second, potentially life-threatening, electrical problem is ventricular tachycardia (*V-tach*), in which the heart beats too fast to pump blood effectively **Figure 6-5** .

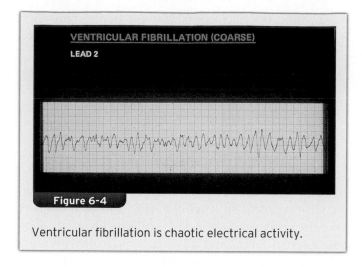

Ventricular fibrillation is chaotic electrical activity.

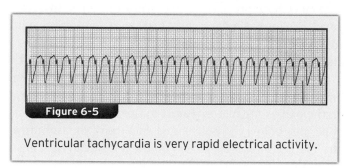

Ventricular tachycardia is very rapid electrical activity.

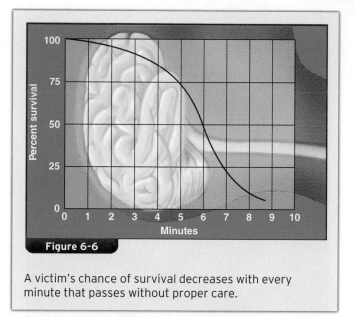

A victim's chance of survival decreases with every minute that passes without proper care.

▶ Care for Cardiac Arrest

When the heart stops beating, the blood stops circulating, cutting off all oxygen and nourishment to the entire body. In this situation, time is a crucial factor. For every minute that defibrillation is delayed, the victim's chance of survival decreases by 7–10% **Figure 6-6** . CPR is the initial care for cardiac arrest until a defibrillator is available. Perform cycles of chest compressions and breaths until an AED is ready to be connected to the victim.

▶ About AEDs

An AED is an electronic device that analyzes the heart rhythm and, if necessary, delivers an electrical shock, known as defibrillation, to the heart of a person in cardiac arrest. The purpose of this shock is to correct one of the abnormal electrical disturbances previously discussed and to reestablish a heart rhythm that will result in normal electrical and pumping function.

All AEDs are attached to the victim by a cable connected to two adhesive pads (electrodes) placed on the victim's chest. The pad and cable system sends the electrical signal from the heart into the device for analysis

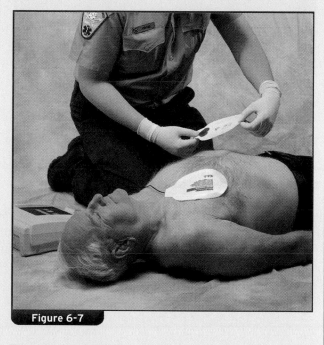

Two adhesive pads are placed on the victim's chest and connected by a cable to the AED.

and delivers the electric shock to the victim when needed **Figure 6-7** .

AEDs have built-in rhythm analysis systems that determine whether the victim needs a shock. This system enables first aiders and other rescuers to deliver early defibrillation with only minimal training. AEDs also record the victim's heart rhythm (known as an electrocardiogram, or ECG), shock data, and other information about the device's performance (for example, the date, time, and number of shocks supplied) **Figure 6-8** .

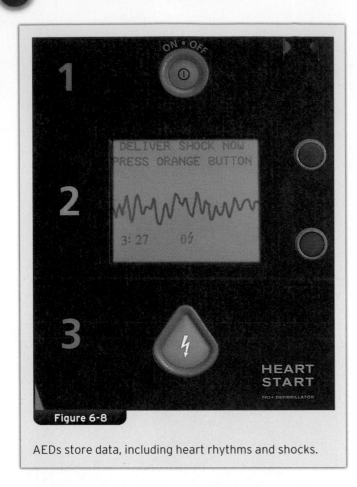

Figure 6-8

AEDs store data, including heart rhythms and shocks.

Common Elements of AEDs

Many different AED models exist. The principles for use are the same for each, but the displays, controls, and options vary slightly. You will need to know how to use your specific AED. All AEDs have the following elements in common:

- Power on/off mechanism
- Cable and pads (electrodes)
- Analysis capability
- Defibrillation capability
- Prompts to guide you
- Battery operation for portability

▶ Using an AED

Once you have determined the need for the AED (victim unresponsive and not breathing), the basic operation of all AED models for anyone over 1 year of age follows this sequence **Skill Drill 6-1**:

1. Perform CPR until an AED is available (Step ❶).
2. Once the AED is available, turn the equipment on (Step ❷).

3. Apply the electrode pads to the victim's bare chest and the cable to the AED (Step ❸). If available, use child pads for a child.
4. Stand clear and analyze the heart rhythm (Step ❹).
5. Deliver a shock if indicated (Step ❺).
6. Perform CPR for 2 minutes (five cycles) (Step ❻).
7. Check the victim and repeat the analysis, shock, and CPR steps as needed (Step ❼).

Some AEDs are powered on by pressing an on/off button. Others power on when the AED case lid is opened. Once the power is on, the AED will quickly go through some internal checks and will then begin to provide voice and screen prompts. Expose the victim's chest. The skin must be fairly dry so that the pads will adhere and conduct electricity properly. If necessary, dry the skin with a towel. Because excessive chest hair can also interfere with adhesion and electrical conduction, you might need to quickly shave the area where the pads are to be placed.

Remove the backing from the pads and apply them firmly to the victim's bare chest according to the diagram on the pads. One pad is placed to the right of the breastbone, just below the collarbone and above the right nipple. The second pad is placed on the left side of the chest, left of the nipple and above the lower rib margin.

Make sure the cable is attached to the AED, and stand clear for analysis of the heart's electrical activity. No one should be in contact with the victim at this time, or later if a shock is indicated.

The AED will advise if a shock is needed. Deliver the shock after verifying that no one is in contact with the victim. Begin CPR immediately following the shock for 2 minutes (five cycles). Following CPR, recheck to see if the victim is breathing and reanalyze the rhythm. If the shock worked, the victim will begin to regain signs of life. Continue providing care until EMS personnel arrive and take over.

▶ Special Considerations

There are several special situations that you should be aware of when using an AED. These include the following:

- Water
- Children
- Medication patches
- Implanted devices

Water

Because water conducts electricity, it can provide an energy pathway between the AED and the rescuer or bystanders. Remove the victim from freestanding water.

skill drill

6-1 | **Using an AED**

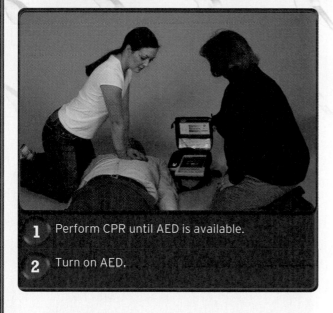

1 Perform CPR until AED is available.

2 Turn on AED.

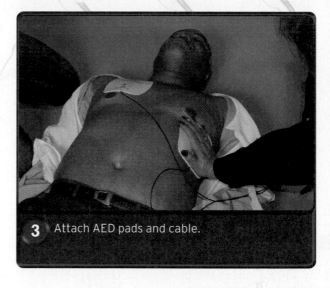

3 Attach AED pads and cable.

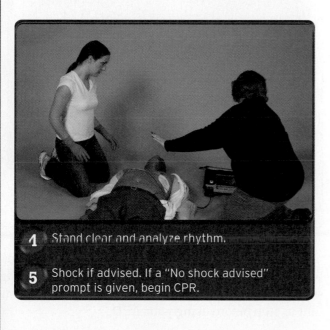

4 Stand clear and analyze rhythm.

5 Shock if advised. If a "No shock advised" prompt is given, begin CPR.

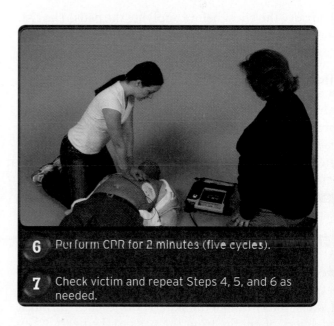

6 Perform CPR for 2 minutes (five cycles).

7 Check victim and repeat Steps 4, 5, and 6 as needed.

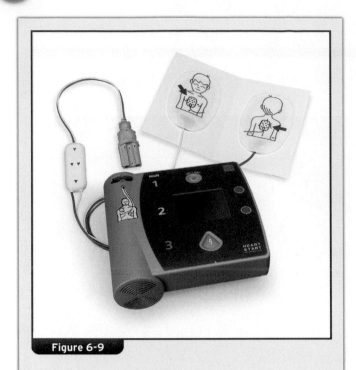

Figure 6-9

If your AED has child pads, use them according to the manufacturer's instructions.

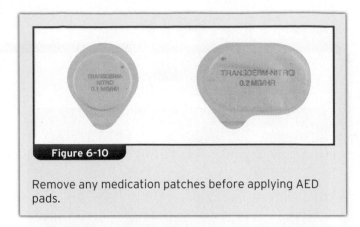

Figure 6-10

Remove any medication patches before applying AED pads.

Quickly dry the chest before applying the pads. The risk to the rescuers and bystanders is very low if the chest is dry and the pads are secured to the chest.

Children

Cardiac arrest in children is usually caused by an airway or breathing problem, rather than a primary heart problem as in adults. AEDs can deliver energy levels appropriate for children aged 1 year or older. If your AED has special pediatric pads and cable, use these for the child **Figure 6-9**. If the pediatric equipment is not available, use an adult AED and pads.

Medication Patches

Some people wear an adhesive patch containing medication (such as nitroglycerin, nicotine, or pain medication) that is absorbed through the skin. These patches can block the delivery of energy from the pads to the heart. They need to be removed if they are located where the AED pads go; wipe the skin dry before attaching the AED pads. **Figure 6-10**.

Implanted Devices

Implanted pacemakers and defibrillators are small devices placed underneath the skin of people with certain types of heart disease **Figure 6-11**. These devices can often be seen or felt when the chest is exposed. Avoid plac-

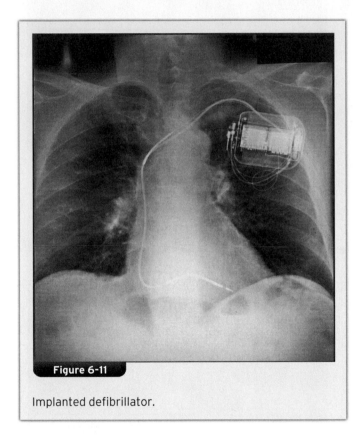

Figure 6-11

Implanted defibrillator.

ing the pads directly over these devices whenever possible. If an implanted defibrillator is discharging, you might see the victim twitching periodically. Allow the implanted unit to stop before using your AED.

▶ AED Maintenance

Daily inspection of your AED can ensure that the device has the necessary supplies and is in proper working condition **Figure 6-12**. AEDs conduct automatic internal checks and provide visual indications that the unit is ready and functioning properly. You do not need to turn the device on daily to check it as part of any inspection. Doing so will only wear down the battery.

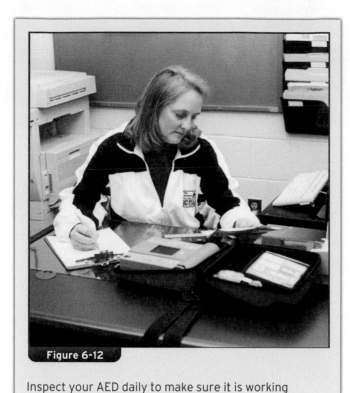

Figure 6-12

Inspect your AED daily to make sure it is working properly and has the necessary supplies.

AED supplies should include items such as the following:

- Two sets of electrode pads with expiration dates that are not expired
- Extra battery
- Razor
- Hand towel

Other items that should be considered are a breathing device (for example, a mask or shield) and medical exam gloves.

▶ Cardiac Arrest

What to Look For	What to Do
Unresponsiveness Not breathing	1. Perform CPR until an AED is available. 2. Turn on the AED. 3. Apply the pads. 4. Analyze the heart rhythm. 5. Administer a shock if needed. 6. Perform CPR for 2 minutes (five cycles). 7. Recheck.

AED Skill Checklist

Student's Name _____ Date _____

Skills	Satisfactory	Unsatisfactory
Check for Scene Safety	◯	◯

Initial check and care:
If two rescuers are involved, one assesses and performs CPR while the other applies the AED.

	Satisfactory	Unsatisfactory
• Establish unresponsiveness.	◯	◯
• Have someone call 9-1-1 and get AED.	◯	◯
• Open airway.	◯	◯
• Check for breathing (5–10 seconds).	◯	◯
• Give two breaths (1 second each).	◯	◯
• Begin CPR until an AED is available.	◯	◯

Defibrillation:

	Satisfactory	Unsatisfactory
• Turn AED power on.	◯	◯
• Ensure skin surface is dry.	◯	◯
• Apply electrode pads correctly.	◯	◯
• Ensure electrode cable is plugged in.	◯	◯
• Stand clear while analyzing.	◯	◯
• If shock is indicated:	◯	◯
a. Remain clear.	◯	◯
b. Deliver shock.	◯	◯
c. Perform 2 minutes of CPR.	◯	◯
d. Reanalyze.	◯	◯
• If shock is indicated, repeat steps a through d.	◯	◯
• If no shock is indicated:	◯	◯
a. Check victim for breathing.	◯	◯
b. If victim is not breathing, perform 2 minutes of CPR and reanalyze.	◯	◯

Pass _____   Fail _____

▶ Ready for Review

- Sudden cardiac death remains an unresolved public health crisis.
- A victim's chances for survival are dramatically improved through early CPR and early defibrillation.
- The links in the chain of survival are early access, early CPR, early defibrillation, and early advanced care.
- Because the heart contracts approximately every second, it needs an abundant supply of oxygen.
- CPR is the initial care for cardiac arrest until a defibrillator is available.
- An AED is an electronic device that analyzes the heart rhythm and delivers an electrical shock to the heart of a person in cardiac arrest.
- There are several special situations to be aware of when using an AED, including: water, children, medication patches, and implanted devices.
- Periodic inspection of the AED can ensure that the device has the necessary supplies and is in proper working condition.

▶ Vital Vocabulary

<u>automated external defibrillator (AED)</u> Device capable of analyzing the heart rhythm and providing a shock.
<u>defibrillation</u> The electrical shock administered by an AED to reestablish a normal heart rhythm.

▶ Assessment in Action

A 45-year-old professor suddenly collapses during lunch in the cafeteria. You and several other students witness this event. You check the victim and determine that he is not breathing. Your school has recently implemented an AED program, and you and other students have been trained. This person needs your help to save his life.
Directions: Circle Yes if you agree with the statement, circle No if you disagree.

Yes   No   1. As soon as you determine that the victim is unresponsive, you should send someone to call 9-1-1 and another to retrieve the AED.

Yes   No   2. CPR should be performed for at least 2 minutes even if the AED is readily available.

Yes   No   3. The AED pads can be applied over the top of the victim's shirt.

Yes   No   4. AED can indicate improper placement or poor connection of pads.

Yes   No   5. This victim is not old enough to require the use of an AED.

Answers: 1. Yes; 2. No; 3. No; 4. Yes; 5. No

▶ Check Your Knowledge

Directions: Circle Yes if you agree with the statement, circle No if you disagree.

Yes   No   1. The earlier defibrillation occurs, the better the victim's chance of survival.

Yes   No   2. An AED is only to be applied to a victim who is unresponsive and not breathing.

Yes   No   3. CPR is not needed if you are sure an AED will be available in 3 to 4 minutes.

Yes   No   4. AEDs require the operator to know how to interpret heart rhythms.

Yes   No   5. Because all AEDs are different, the basic steps of operation are also different.

Yes   No   6. The AED pads (electrodes) need to be attached to a dry chest.

Yes   No   7. Two electrode pads are placed on the left side of the victim's chest.

Yes   No   8. Batteries and pads have expiration dates of which you should be aware.

Yes   No   9. An AED can still be used if an implanted pacemaker is present.

Yes   No   10. You need to turn the AED on daily as part of a routine inspection.

Answers: 1. Yes; 2. Yes; 3. No; 4. No; 5. No; 6. Yes; 7. No; 8. Yes; 9. Yes; 10. No

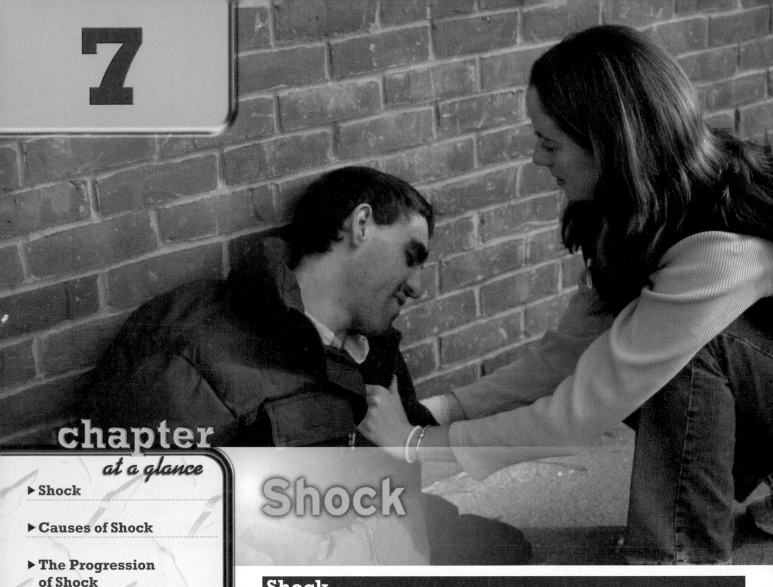

7

chapter
at a glance

Shock

Shock

Perfusion is when adequate blood and oxygen are provided to all cells in different tissues and organs in the body. Shock occurs when the body's tissues do not receive enough oxygenated blood. Do not confuse this with electric shock or being shocked, as in being scared or surprised. <u>Shock</u> (hypoperfusion) describes a state of collapse and failure of the cardiovascular system in which blood circulation decreases and eventually ceases. Shock can be associated with a wide variety of conditions—from a heart attack to an allergic reaction.

▶ Causes of Shock

Understanding the basic physiologic causes of shock will better prepare you to treat it. The damage caused by shock depends on which body part is deprived of oxygen and for how long. For example, without oxygen, the brain will be irreparably damaged in 4 to 6 minutes, the abdominal organs in 45 to 90 minutes, and the skin and muscle cells in 3 to 6 hours.

To understand shock, think of the circulatory system as having three components: a working pump (the heart), a network of pipes (the blood vessels), and an adequate amount of fluid (the blood) pumped through the pipes. Damage to any of these components can deprive tissues of blood and produce the condition known as shock. These three parts can be referred to as the perfusion triangle **Figure 7-1**. When a victim is in shock, one or more of the three sides is not working properly.

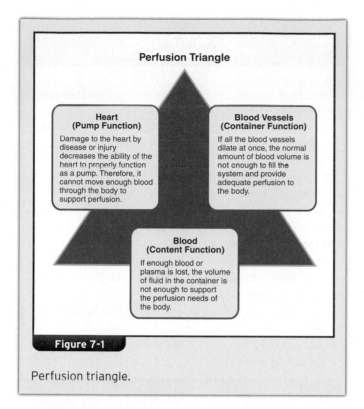

Figure 7-1

Perfusion triangle.

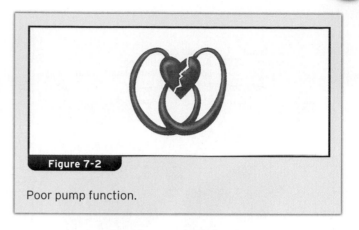

Figure 7-2

Poor pump function.

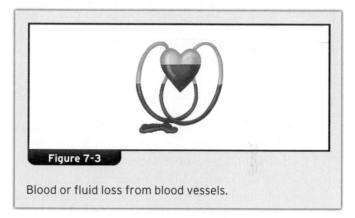

Figure 7-3

Blood or fluid loss from blood vessels.

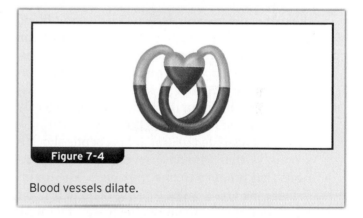

Figure 7-4

Blood vessels dilate.

Causes of shock can be both cardiovascular and non-cardiovascular. The noncardiovascular causes of shock are respiratory insufficiency, psychogenic shock, and **anaphylaxis**, an extreme allergic reaction to a foreign substance. There are three major cardiovascular causes of shock:

- *Poor pump function.* If damaged by disease or injury, the heart might not generate sufficient energy to move blood through the system (for example, cardiogenic shock) **Figure 7-2** .
- *Blood or fluid loss from blood vessels.* If enough blood or plasma is lost, the volume of fluid left in the vascular system is inadequate to perfuse all tissues and organs (for example, hemorrhagic shock) **Figure 7-3** .
- *Poor vessel function.* With widespread vessel dilation, the normal volume of blood will be insufficient to fill the system and provide efficient perfusion (for example, neurogenic shock) **Figure 7-4** .

Cardiovascular Causes of Shock

- *Pump failure.* Cardiogenic shock is caused by inadequate function of the heart, or pump failure. Circulation requires the constant pumping action of a normal heart muscle. Many diseases can cause destruction or inflammation of this muscle. The

heart can adapt somewhat to these problems, but if too much muscle damage occurs, as sometimes happens in a heart attack, the heart no longer functions well. The major effect is the backup of blood into the lungs. The resulting buildup of fluid in the lungs is called pulmonary edema.

- *Content failure.* In injuries, shock is most often the result of fluid or blood loss. This type of shock is called hypovolemic (low-volume) shock or hemorrhagic shock. The loss can be due to internal or external bleeding. Hypovolemic shock also occurs with severe thermal burns. Plasma, the fluid

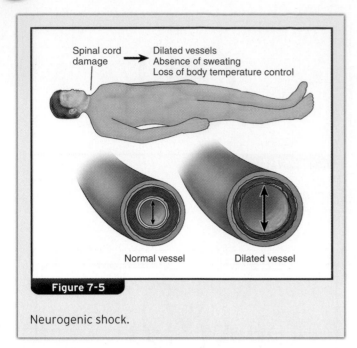

Spinal cord damage → Dilated vessels
Absence of sweating
Loss of body temperature control

Normal vessel   Dilated vessel

Figure 7-5

Neurogenic shock.

Table 7-1	**Signs and Symptoms of Anaphylactic Shock**

Skin
- Flushing, itching, or burning, especially over the face and upper chest
- Hives, which can spread over large areas of the body
- Swelling, especially of the face, tongue, and lips
- Bluish lips (cyanosis)

Circulatory system
- Weak pulse (you might be barely able to feel it)
- Dizziness
- Fainting and unresponsiveness

Respiratory system
- Sneezing or itching in the nostrils
- Tightness in the chest, with a persistent, dry cough
- Breathing difficulty
- Secretions of fluid and mucus into the throat and lungs
- Wheezing (forced expirations during breathing)
- Breathing stops

portion of the blood, leaks from the circulatory system into burned tissues adjacent to the injury. Dehydration aggravates shock. In all these circumstances, the common factor is an insufficient volume of blood within the vascular system to provide adequate perfusion to the tissues.

- *Poor vessel function.* Spinal cord damage can injure the part of the nervous system that controls blood vessel size and muscle tone. Neurogenic shock can result. Cut off from their impulses to contract, muscles in the blood vessels dilate (relax) widely, increasing the size and capacity of the vascular system. The blood in the body can no longer fill the enlarged vessels **Figure 7-5** .
- *Combined vessel and content failure.* Septic shock is seen in victims who have severe bacterial infections that produce toxins (poisons). The toxins damage the vessel walls, causing them to become leaky and making them unable to contract well. Widespread vessel dilation, combined with the loss of plasma through injured vessel walls, results in shock. Septic shock is almost always a complication of a serious illness, injury, or surgery. Septic shock also occurs with anaphylaxis.

Noncardiovascular Cause of Shock

- *Respiratory insufficiency.* A severe chest injury or an airway obstruction can make a victim unable to breathe adequately. Insufficient oxygen in the blood can produce shock as rapidly as vascular causes, even when cardiovascular function is normal. This is why the first two steps in resuscitation are always opening an airway and rescue breaths.

Circulation of nonoxygenated blood will not benefit the victim.
- *Anaphylactic shock.* Anaphylaxis, or anaphylactic shock, occurs when the immune system reacts violently to a substance to which it has already been sensitized. Severe allergic reactions commonly follow exposure by one of these:
  - medications (penicillin and related drugs, aspirin, sulfa drugs)
  - food (shellfish, nuts—especially peanuts, eggs)
  - insect stings (honeybee, wasp, yellow jacket, hornet, fire ant)
  - plant pollen

Anaphylactic reactions can develop in minutes or even seconds after contact with the substance to which a victim is sensitized. The signs of such allergic reactions are distinct from those of other forms of shock. **Table 7-1** shows the signs and symptoms of anaphylactic shock.

In anaphylactic shock, although there is no loss of blood, no vascular damage, and only a slight possibility of cardiac muscular injury, the widespread vascular dilation causes poor oxygenation and poor perfusion of tissues, which can easily cause death.

- *Psychogenic shock.* Psychogenic shock is a sudden nervous system reaction that produces a temporary vascular dilation, resulting in fainting, or syncope. Blood pools in the dilated vessels, reducing the blood supply to the brain, and the victim becomes unresponsive. Causes of fainting (psy-

Table 7-2 Progression of Shock

Compensated Shock	Decompensated Shock
• Agitation	• Difficulty breathing
• Anxiety	• Ashen, mottled, or cyanotic skin
• Restlessness	• Dull eyes, dilated pupils
• Feeling of impending doom	
• Altered mental status	
• Weak, rapid, or absent pulse	
• Clammy (pale, cool, moist) skin	
• Paleness, with cyanosis about the lips	
• Shallow, rapid breathing	
• Shortness of breath	
• Nausea or vomiting	
• Capillary refill longer than 2 seconds in infants and children	
• Thirst	

chogenic shock) range from fear, bad news, or unpleasant sights (often the sight of blood).

▶ The Progression of Shock

Although shock itself cannot be seen, you can see its signs and symptoms progress Table 7-2 . The early stage of shock, when the body can still compensate for blood loss, is called compensated shock. The late stage, when blood pressure is falling, is decompensated shock. The final stage, when shock is terminal, is called irreversible shock. Even transfusion will not save the victim's life at this point.

FYI

Red Flags for Shock

Shock is seen in both injured and suddenly ill victims. Anticipate and expect shock if a victim has any of these conditions:

• Massive external or internal bleeding
• Multiple severe fractures
• Abdominal or chest injury
• A severe infection
• Sign of a heart attack
• Anaphylaxis

▶ Care for Shock

Because every injury affects the circulatory system to some degree, first aiders should automatically treat injured vic-

tims for shock. Shock is one of the most common causes of death in an injured victim. Even if an injured victim does not have signs or symptoms of shock, first aiders should care for shock. You can prevent shock from getting worse; first aiders cannot reverse it.

General Care for Shock

1. Protect yourself against disease by wearing medical exam gloves.
2. Monitor breathing and provide care if needed.
3. Control all obvious external bleeding.
4. Place the victim on his or her back (supine position). Those having a heart attack or those with lung disease breathe easier in a half-sitting position).
5. Raise the victim's legs 6 to 12 inches. This helps stop bleeding in the lower extremities and allows the blood to drain from the legs back to the heart Figure 7-6 . Do not move the victim if there are suspected fractures or head, spine, or torso injuries.
6. Splint any bone or joint injuries to minimize pain and bleeding. This also prevents further damage to tissues.
7. Keep the victim warm. Place blankets under and over the victim. Do not use external heat sources (for example, hot water bottles or heating pads).
8. Handle the victim gently.
9. Seek medical care. Depending upon the problem, it might require calling 9-1-1 or transporting a victim using a private vehicle if EMS is not available.

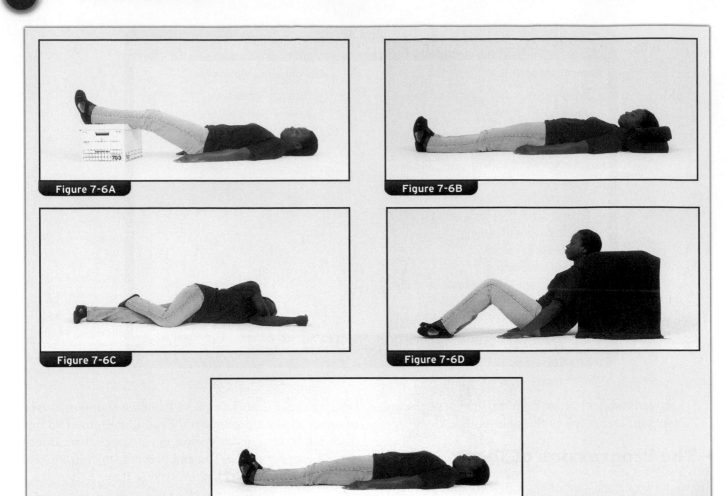

Figure 7-6A

Figure 7-6B

Figure 7-6C

Figure 7-6D

Figure 7-6E

Shock positions. **A.** Usual shock position. **B.** For a victim with head injury, elevate the head (if spinal injury is not suspected). **C.** Position an unresponsive or stroke victim in the recovery position. **D.** Use a half-sitting position for victims with breathing difficulties, chest injuries, or a heart attack. **E.** Keep the victim flat if a spinal injury or leg fracture is suspected.

CAUTION

DO NOT place victims with breathing difficulties, chest injuries, penetrating eye injuries, or heart attacks on their backs. Place them in a half-sitting position to help breathing.

DO NOT give the victim anything to eat or drink. It could cause nausea and vomiting. It could also cause complications if surgery is needed.

DO NOT raise the legs more than 12 inches because that will affect the victim's breathing by pushing the abdominal organs up against the diaphragm.

DO NOT lift the foot of a bed or stretcher—breathing will be affected, and the blood flow from the brain could be retarded and lead to brain swelling.

DO NOT raise the legs of a victim with head injuries, stroke, chest injuries, breathing difficulty, or those of a victim in whom a heart attack is suspected.

DO NOT use external heat sources (such as hot water bottles or heating pads).

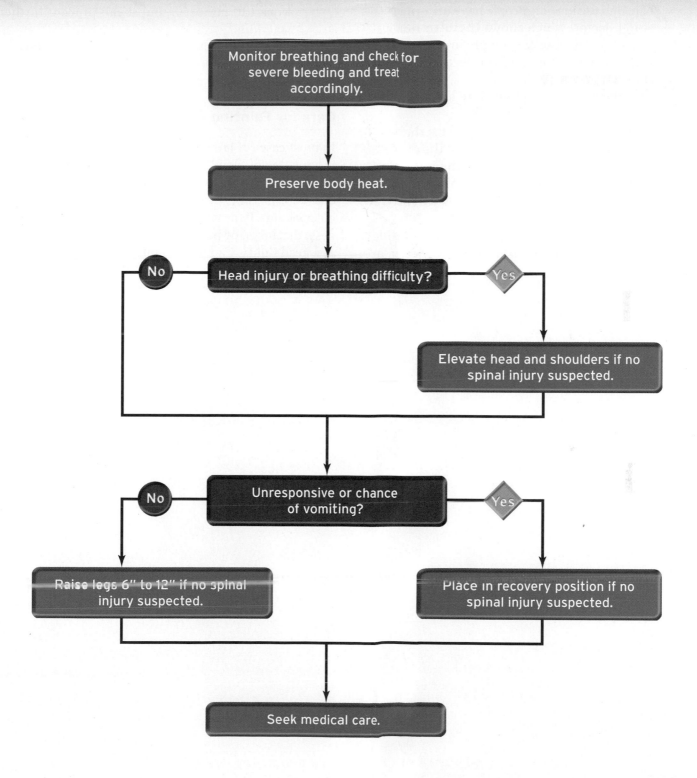

Monitor breathing and check for severe bleeding and treat accordingly.

Preserve body heat.

Head injury or breathing difficulty?

No

Yes — Elevate head and shoulders if no spinal injury suspected.

Unresponsive or chance of vomiting?

No — Raise legs 6" to 12" if no spinal injury suspected.

Yes — Place in recovery position if no spinal injury suspected.

Seek medical care.

Care for Anaphylaxis

1. Monitor breathing and if necessary, give CPR.
2. Call 9-1-1 immediately.
3. If the victim has his own prescribed epinephrine, help him use it. Some people have an **epinephrine auto-injector**, which allows them to administer an emergency dose of epinephrine. If you are assisting with or using an auto-injector, follow these steps Skill Drill 7-1 :

   a. Remove the safety cap. The auto-injector is now ready for use (**Step ❶**).
   b. Support the victim's thigh and place the black tip of the auto-injector lightly against the outer thigh.
   c. Using a quick motion, push the auto-injector firmly against the thigh and hold it in place for several seconds (**Step ❷**). This will inject the medication.
   d. Remove the auto-injector from the thigh. Carefully reinsert the used auto-injector, needle first, into the carrying tube (**Step ❸**). A small amount of medication will remain in the device, but the device cannot be reused.

4. Give an antihistamine (such as Benadryl)—it is not life saving because it takes too long to work (20 minutes), but it can prevent further reactions.
5. Keep a responsive victim sitting up to help breathing. Place an unresponsive victim on his or her side (recovery position).

Care for Fainting (Psychogenic Shock)

In most cases of fainting, once the victim collapses and is lying down, blood circulation to the brain is restored and responsiveness usually returns. If the victim fell, check for possible head and spine injuries, especially in older victims. If the victim is unable to walk without weakness, dizziness, or pain, suspect another problem, such as a head injury. Call 9-1-1 immediately.

skill drill

7-1   Using an Epinephrine Auto-Injector

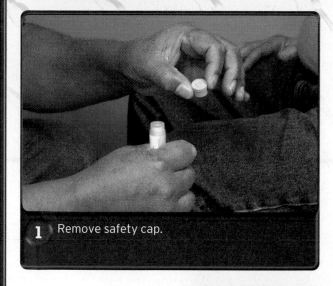

1 Remove safety cap.

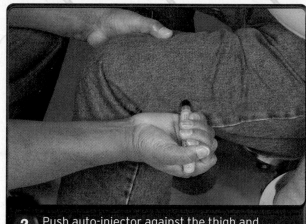

2 Push auto-injector against the thigh and hold in place for several seconds.

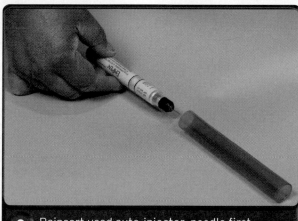

3 Reinsert used auto-injector, needle first, into the carrying tube.

▶ Shock

What to Look For

- Agitation
- Anxiety
- Restlessness
- Feeling of impending doom
- Altered mental status
- Weak, rapid, or absent pulse
- Clammy (pale, cool, moist) skin
- Paleness, with cyanosis about the lips
- Shallow, rapid breathing
- Shortness of breath
- Nausea or vomiting

What to Do

1. Wear medical exam gloves.
2. Monitor breathing and provide care if needed.
3. Control all obvious bleeding.
4. Place the victim on his or her back. (Those having a heart attack or those with lung disease breathe easier in a half-sitting position).
5. Raise the victim's legs 6 to 12 inches. Do not move the victim if there are suspected fractures or head, spine, or torso injuries.
6. Splint any bone or joint injuries.
7. Place blankets under and over the victim.
8. Handle the victim gently.
9. Seek medical care by calling 9-1-1 if signs of shock are present.

▶ Anaphylaxis

What to Look For

Skin
- Flushing, itching, or burning, especially over the face and upper chest
- Hives, which can spread over large areas of the body
- Swelling, especially of the face, tongue, and lips
- Bluish lips (cyanosis)

Circulatory system
- Weak pulse (you might be barely able to feel it)
- Dizziness
- Fainting and unresponsiveness

Respiratory system
- Sneezing or itching in the nostrils
- Tightness in the chest, with a persistent dry cough
- Breathing difficulty
- Secretions of fluid and mucus into the throat and lungs
- Wheezing (forced expirations during breathing)
- Breathing stops

What to Do

1. Monitor breathing, and if necessary, give CPR.
2. Call 9-1-1 immediately.
3. If the victim has his or her own prescribed epinephrine, help the victim use it. If you are assisting with or using an auto-injector, follow the container's instructions.
4. Give an antihistamine (such as Benadryl)—it is not life saving because it takes too long to work (20 minutes), but can prevent further reactions.
5. Keep a responsive victim sitting up to help breathing. Place an unresponsive victim on his or her side (recovery position).

▶ Ready for Review

- Shock is a state of collapse and failure of the cardiovascular system in which blood circulation decreases and eventually ceases.
- The damage caused by shock depends on which body part is deprived of oxygen and for how long.
- Causes of shock can be both cardiovascular and noncardiovascular.
- Anaphylaxis occurs when the immune system reacts violently to a substance to which it has already been sensitized.
- Although shock itself cannot be seen, you can see its signs and symptoms progress.
- First aiders should automatically treat victims for shock.

▶ Vital Vocabulary

anaphylaxis A life-threatening allergic reaction.

epinephrine auto-injector Prescribed device used to administer an emergency dose of epinephrine to a victim experiencing anaphylaxis.

shock Inadequate tissue oxygenation resulting from serious injury or illness.

▶ Assessment in Action

Your neighbor was working in her garden on a warm summer day. She unintentionally disturbed a nest of yellow jackets and was stung several times on her face and neck. She has begun coughing and wheezing. She complains that she is dizzy and having difficulty breathing. You notice that her face is swelling.

Directions: Circle Yes if you agree with the statement, circle No if you disagree.

Yes No 1. Breathing difficulty and swelling can be signs of a severe allergic reaction.

Yes No 2. This victim is likely experiencing a type of shock known as anaphylaxis.

Yes No 3. The condition this victim is experiencing is life threatening, and medical care is needed.

Yes No 4. If the victim has a prescribed epinephrine auto-injector, help her use it.

Yes No 5. You should place this victim in the usual shock position—lying down with the legs raised.

Answers: 1. Yes; 2. Yes; 3. Yes; 4. Yes; 5. No

▶ Check Your Knowledge

Directions: Circle Yes if you agree with the statement, circle No if you disagree.

Yes No 1. Raise the legs of *all* severely injured victims.

Yes No 2. Prevent body heat loss by putting blankets under and over the victim.

Yes No 3. A shock victim with possible spinal injuries should be placed in a seated position.

Yes No 4. A shock victim with breathing difficulty or chest injury should be placed on his or her back with the legs raised.

Yes No 5. Anxiety and restlessness are signs of shock.

Yes No 6. An epinephrine auto-injector requires a doctor's prescription.

Yes No 7. All severely injured or ill victims should be treated for shock.

Yes No 8. Treat severely injured victims for shock even though there are no signs of it.

Yes No 9. Anaphylaxis is a life-threatening breathing emergency.

Yes No 10. Victims in shock have hot skin.

Answers: 1. No; 2. Yes; 3. No; 4. No; 5. Yes; 6. Yes; 7. Yes; 8. Yes; 9. Yes; 10. No

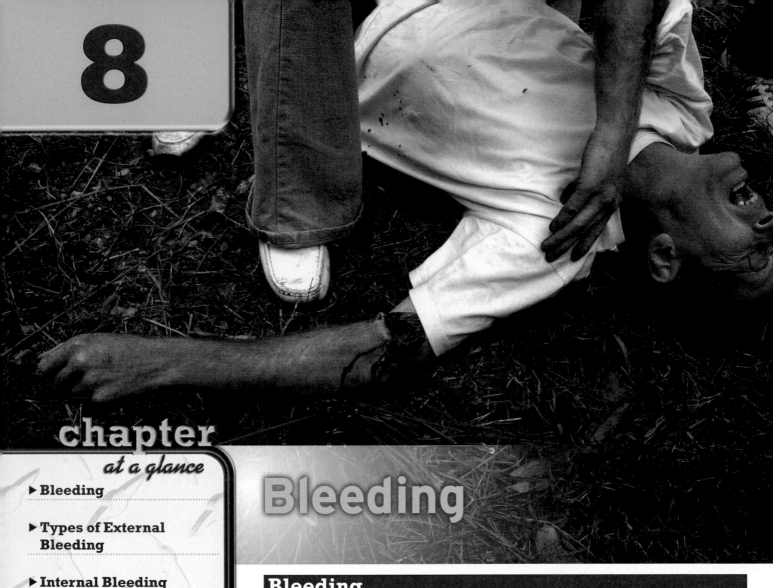

Bleeding

Bleeding

The average-size adult has 5 to 6 quarts (10–12 pints) of blood and can safely donate a pint. However, rapid blood loss of 1 quart or more can lead to shock and death. A child who loses 1 pint of blood is in extreme danger.

▶ Types of External Bleeding

External bleeding refers to blood coming from an open wound. The term __hemorrhage__ refers to a large amount of bleeding in a short time. External bleeding can be classified into three types according to the type of blood vessel that is damaged: an artery, vein, or capillary Figure 8-1 . In arterial bleeding, blood spurts (up to several feet) from the wound. __Arterial bleeding__ is the most serious type of bleeding because a large amount of blood can be lost in a very short period of time. Arterial bleeding also is less likely to clot because blood can clot only when it is flowing slowly or not at all. However, unless a very large artery has been cut, it is unlikely that a person will bleed to death before the flow can be controlled. Nevertheless, arterial bleeding is dangerous and must be controlled.

In __venous bleeding__, blood from a vein flows steadily or gushes. Venous bleeding is easier to control than arterial bleeding. Most veins collapse when cut. Bleeding from deep veins, however, can be as massive and as hard to control as arterial bleeding. In __capillary bleeding__, the most common type of bleeding, blood oozes from capillaries. It usually is not serious and can be controlled easily. Quite often,

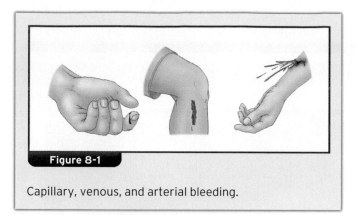

Figure 8-1

Capillary, venous, and arterial bleeding.

this type of bleeding will clot and stop by itself. Each type of blood vessel—artery, vein, or capillary—contains blood of a different shade of red. An inexperienced person may have difficulty detecting the difference but identifying the type of bleeding by its color is not important. The body naturally responds to bleeding in the following way:

- *Blood vessel spasm.* Arteries contain small amounts of muscle tissue in their walls. If a blood vessel is completely severed, it draws back into the tissue, constricts its diameter, and slows the bleeding dramatically. If an artery is only partially cut across its diameter, however, constriction is incomplete. The vessel may not contract and the loss of blood may not slow as dramatically.

- *Clotting.* Special elements (*platelets*) in blood form a clot. Clotting serves as a protective covering for a wound until the tissues underneath can repair themselves. In a healthy person, initial clot formation normally takes about 10 minutes. Clotting time is longer in people who have lost a great deal of blood over a prolonged period of time, are taking aspirin or anticoagulants, are anemic, or have hemophilia or severe liver disease.

CAUTION

DO NOT come in contact with blood with your bare hands. Protect yourself with medical exam gloves, extra gauze pads, or clean cloths, or have the victim apply the direct pressure. If you must use your bare hands, do so only as a last resort. After the bleeding has stopped and the wound has been cared for, vigorously wash your hands with soap and water.

DO NOT use direct pressure on an eye injury, a wound with an embedded object, or a skull fracture.

DO NOT remove a blood-soaked dressing because this can pull off clots that have already formed. Apply another dressing on top and continue putting pressure over the wound.

Care for External Bleeding

Regardless of the type of bleeding or the type of wound, the first aid is the same. First, and most important, you must control the bleeding **Skill Drill 8-1** :

1. Protect yourself against disease by wearing medical exam gloves. If they are not available, use several layers of gauze pads, clean cloths, plastic wrap, a plastic bag, or waterproof material. If those are unavailable, you can have the victim apply pressure on the wound with his or her hand.

2. Expose the wound by removing or cutting the victim's clothing to find the source of the bleeding (**Step ❶**).

3. Place a sterile gauze pad or a clean cloth such as a handkerchief, washcloth, or towel over the entire wound and apply direct pressure with your fingers or the palm of your hand (**Step ❷**). Hold steady, firm, and uninterrupted pressure on the wound for at least 5 minutes. The gauze or cloth allows you to apply even pressure. Direct pressure stops most bleeding. Applying direct pressure to the wound compresses the sides of the torn vessel and helps the body's natural clotting mechanisms to work. Be sure the pressure remains constant, is not too light, and is applied to the bleeding source. Do not remove blood-soaked dressings; simply add new dressings over the old ones.

4. If the bleeding is from an arm or leg, elevate the injured area above the level of the heart to reduce blood flow as you continue to apply pressure (**Step ❸**). Elevation allows gravity to make it more difficult for the body to pump blood to the affected extremity. Elevation alone, however, will not stop bleeding and must be used in combination with direct pressure over the wound.

5. To free you to attend to other injuries or victims, use a pressure bandage to hold the dressing on the wound. Wrap a roller gauze bandage tightly over the dressing and above and below the wound site (**Step ❹**). Do not wrap it so tightly that it cuts off circulation.

6. If the bleeding continues, apply pressure at a pressure point to slow the flow of blood as you continue putting direct pressure over the wound (**Step ❺**).

7. A *pressure point* is where an artery near the skin's surface passes close to a bone, against which it can be compressed. The most accessible pressure points on both sides of the body are the brachial point on the inside of the upper arm and the femoral point in the groin. Using pressure points requires skill, because unless the exact location of the pulse point is used, the pressure-point

skill drill

| 8-1 | Care for External Bleeding |

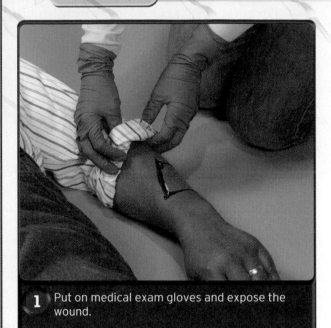

1 Put on medical exam gloves and expose the wound.

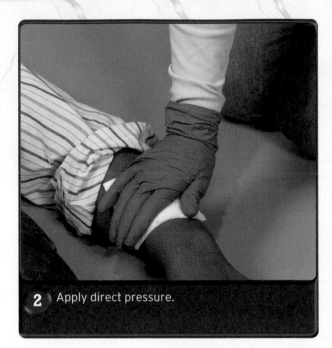

2 Apply direct pressure.

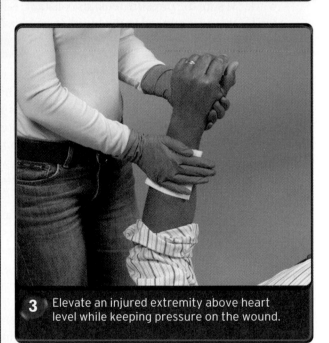

3 Elevate an injured extremity above heart level while keeping pressure on the wound.

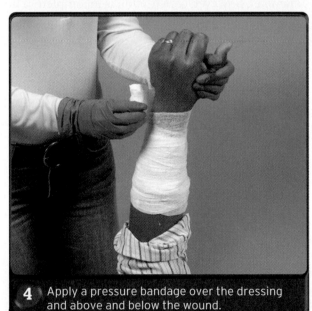

4 Apply a pressure bandage over the dressing and above and below the wound.

5 If bleeding cannot be controlled, use the brachial or femoral pressure point.

technique is useless. Many first aiders have difficulty finding the precise pressure-point location. Remember, however, that direct pressure stops most bleeding.

8. When direct pressure cannot be applied, such as in the case of a protruding bone, skull fracture, or embedded object, use a doughnut-shaped (ring) pad to control bleeding. To make a ring pad, wrap one end of a narrow bandage (roller or cravat) several times around your four fingers to form a loop. Pass the other end of the bandage through the loop and wrap it around and around until the entire bandage is used and a ring has been made.

9. When bleeding stops, use procedures found in Chapter 9 for wound care.

10. Some people panic when they see even the smallest amount of blood. The sight of more than a couple of tablespoonfuls of blood generally is enough to frighten victims and bystanders. Take time to reassure the victim that everything possible is being done. Do not belittle the victim's concerns.

CAUTION

DO NOT apply a pressure bandage so tightly that it cuts off circulation. Check the radial pulse if the bandage is on an arm; for a leg, check the pulse between the inside ankle bone knob and the Achilles tendon (posterior tibial). Pulses are hard to feel. Other signs that the dressing is too tight are increasing pain, numbness or tingling, loss of color in the skin, loss of muscle function.

DO NOT use a tourniquet. They are rarely needed and can damage nerves and blood vessels. The use of a tourniquet may cause the loss of an arm or a leg. If you must use one, apply wide, flat materials—never rope or wire—and do not loosen it.

▶ Internal Bleeding

Internal bleeding occurs when the skin is not broken and blood is not seen. It can be difficult to detect and can be life threatening. A person with bleeding stomach ulcers, a lacerated liver, or a ruptured spleen may lose a considerable amount of blood into the abdomen with no outward sign of bleeding other than the presence of shock. Broken bones can also cause serious internal blood loss. A broken femur can easily result in a loss of 1 or more quarts of blood.

Recognizing Internal Bleeding

The signs of internal bleeding may be seen in either injured or suddenly ill victims:

- Bright red blood from the mouth or rectum or blood in the urine
- Nonmenstrual vaginal bleeding
- Vomited blood; may be bright red, dark red, or look like coffee grounds
- Black, foul-smelling, tarry stools
- Pain, tenderness, bruising, or swelling
- Broken ribs, bruises over the lower chest, or a rigid abdomen

Care for Internal Bleeding

For severe internal bleeding, follow these steps:

1. Monitor breathing.
2. Expect vomiting. If vomiting occurs, keep the victim lying on his or her left side to allow drainage and to prevent inhalation (aspiration) of vomitus.
3. Treat for shock by raising the victim's legs 6 to 12 inches and covering the victim with a coat or blanket for warmth. See Chapter 7 for when to use other body positions.
4. Treat suspected internal bleeding in an extremity by applying a splint.
5. Seek immediate medical care.

CAUTION

DO NOT give a victim anything to eat or drink. It could cause nausea and vomiting, which could result in aspiration. Food or liquids could cause complications if surgery is needed.

Bruises are a form of internal bleeding, but they are not life threatening. To treat bruises:

1. Apply an ice pack over the injury for 20 minutes.
2. If the bruise is on an arm or leg, raise the limb if it is not broken.
3. If an arm or a leg is involved, apply an elastic bandage for compression.

Bleeding

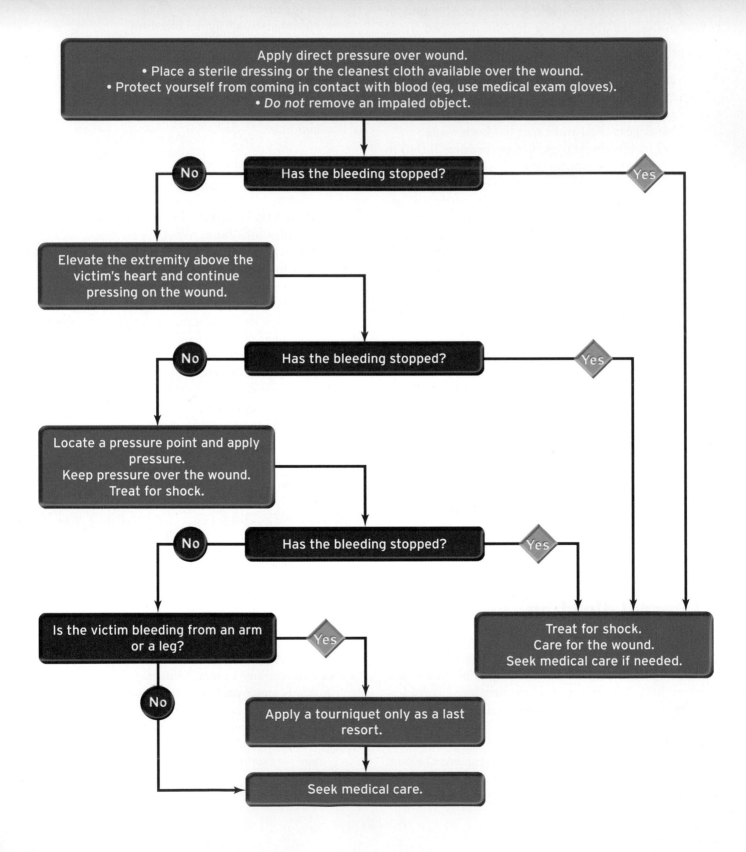

Apply direct pressure over wound.
- Place a sterile dressing or the cleanest cloth available over the wound.
- Protect yourself from coming in contact with blood (eg, use medical exam gloves).
- *Do not* remove an impaled object.

No ← Has the bleeding stopped? → Yes

Elevate the extremity above the victim's heart and continue pressing on the wound.

No ← Has the bleeding stopped? → Yes

Locate a pressure point and apply pressure.
Keep pressure over the wound.
Treat for shock.

No ← Has the bleeding stopped? → Yes

Is the victim bleeding from an arm or a leg? → Yes

No

Treat for shock.
Care for the wound.
Seek medical care if needed.

Apply a tourniquet only as a last resort.

Seek medical care.

▶ Bleeding

What to Look For	What to Do
External bleeding	1. Protect against blood contact. 2. Place sterile dressing over wound and apply pressure. 3. Elevate the injured area if possible. 4. Apply a pressure bandage. 5. If bleeding cannot be controlled, apply pressure to a pressure point.

Internal bleeding	Minor internal bleeding (bruise):
	    Use RICE procedures:
	      R = Rest
	      I = Ice
	      C = Compress the area with elastic bandage
	      E = Elevate the injured extremity.
	Serious internal bleeding:
	    Call 9-1-1
	    Care for shock.
	    If vomiting occurs, roll the victim onto the side.

prep kit

▶ Ready for Review

- Rapid blood loss of 1 quart or more can lead to shock and death.
- External bleeding can be classified into three types according to the type of blood vessel that is damaged: an artery, vein, or capillary.
- Regardless of the type of bleeding or the type of wound, the first aid is the same. First, and most important, you must control the bleeding.

▶ Vital Vocabulary

arterial bleeding Bleeding from an artery; this type of bleeding tends to spurt with each heartbeat.

capillary bleeding Bleeding that oozes from a wound steadily but slowly.

hemorrhage A large amount of bleeding in a short time.

venous bleeding Bleeding from a vein; this type of bleeding tends to flow steadily.

▶ Assessment in Action

A 25-year-old construction worker has been badly cut on his thigh by a circular power saw. The cut is approximately 5 inches long, and blood is spurting from the wound.

Directions: Circle Yes if you agree with the statement, circle No if you disagree.

Yes   No   1. This victim is experiencing venous bleeding.

Yes   No   2. You should be certain to wash this wound with soap and water.

Yes   No   3. Direct pressure should stop the bleeding.

Yes   No   4. Treat the victim for shock.

Yes   No   5. The type of bleeding experienced by this man is the most common type.

Answers: 1. No; 2. No; 3. Yes; 4. Yes; 5. No

▶ Check Your Knowledge

Directions: Circle Yes if you agree with the statement, circle No if you disagree.

Yes   No   1. Most cases of bleeding require more than direct pressure to stop the bleeding.

Yes   No   2. Remove any blood-soaked dressings before applying additional ones.

Yes   No   3. Whenever elevating an arm or leg to control the bleeding, you should also keep applying pressure on the wound.

Yes   No   4. If a bleeding arm wound is not controlled through direct pressure, elevation, and pressure bandaging, apply pressure to the brachial artery.

Yes   No   5. Dressings are placed directly on a wound.

Yes   No   6. Internal bleeding is normal.

Yes   No   7. Dressings should be sterile or as clean as possible.

Yes   No   8. Clotting is the body's way of stopping bleeding.

Yes   No   9. If the victim feels sick to the stomach and may vomit, roll her onto the left side.

Yes   No   10. It is important to remove impaled objects because they could be driven in deeper.

Answers: 1. No; 2. No; 3. Yes; 4. Yes; 5. Yes; 6. No; 7. Yes; 8. Yes; 9. Yes; 10. No

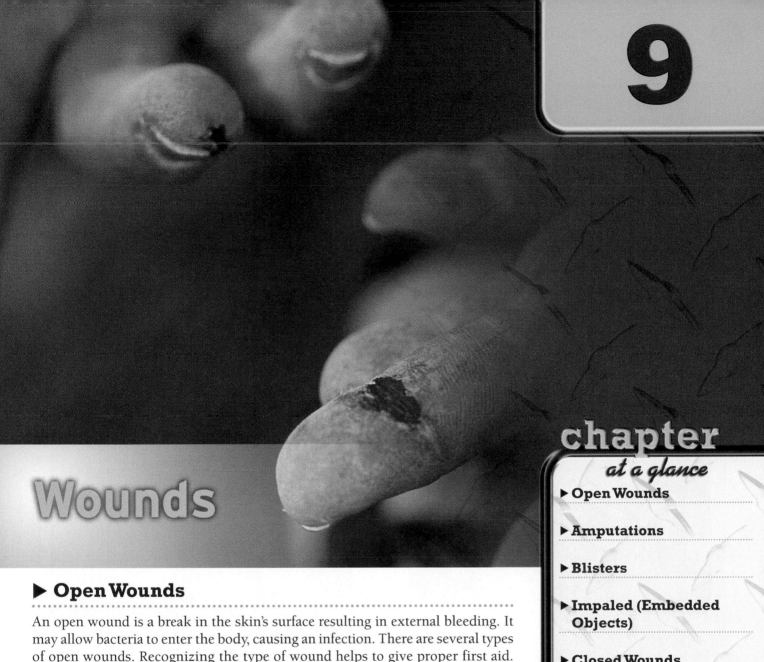

Wounds

chapter
at a glance

▶ Open Wounds

An open wound is a break in the skin's surface resulting in external bleeding. It may allow bacteria to enter the body, causing an infection. There are several types of open wounds. Recognizing the type of wound helps to give proper first aid. With an <u>abrasion</u>, the top layer of skin is removed, with little or no blood loss **Figure 9-1** . Abrasions tend to be painful because the nerve endings often are abraded along with the skin. Ground-in debris may be present. This type of wound can be serious if it covers a large area or becomes embedded with foreign matter. Other names for an abrasion are *scrape, road rash,* and *rug burn.*

A <u>laceration</u> is cut skin with jagged, irregular edges **Figure 9-2** . This type of wound is usually caused by a forceful tearing away of skin tissue. <u>Incisions</u> tend to have smooth edges and resemble a surgical or paper cut **Figure 9-3** . The amount of bleeding depends on the depth, the location, and the size of the wound. <u>Punctures</u> are usually deep, narrow wounds in the skin and underlying organs such as a stab wound from a nail or a knife **Figure 9-4** . The entrance is usually small, and the risk of infection is high. The object causing the injury may remain impaled in the wound.

With an <u>avulsion</u>, a piece of skin is torn loose and is hanging from the body or completely removed. This type of wound can bleed heavily. If the flap is still attached, lay it flat and realign it into its normal position. Avulsions most often involve ears, fingers, and hands **Figure 9-5** . An <u>amputation</u> involves the cutting or tearing off of a body part, such as a finger, toe, hand, foot, arm, or leg.

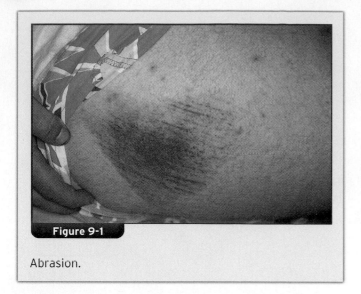

Figure 9-1

Abrasion.

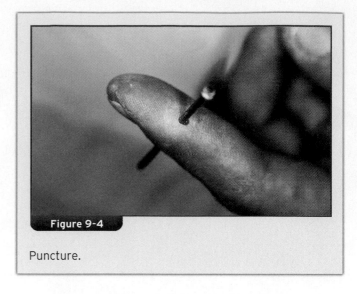

Figure 9-4

Puncture.

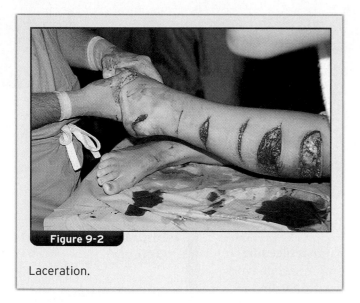

Figure 9-2

Laceration.

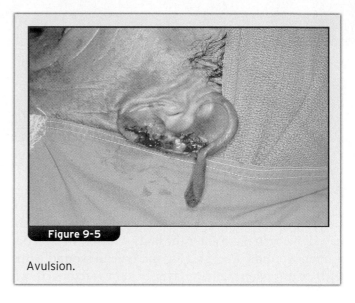

Figure 9-5

Avulsion.

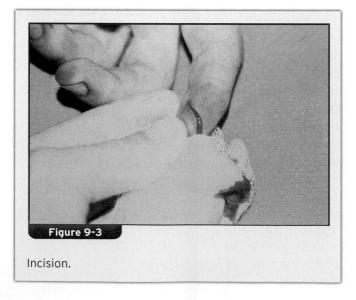

Figure 9-3

Incision.

Care for Open Wounds

1. Protect yourself against disease by wearing medical exam gloves. If they are not available, use several layers of gauze pads, clean cloths, plastic wrap or bags, or waterproof material. If none of these area available, you can have the victim apply pressure with his or her hand. Your bare hand should be used only as a last resort.
2. Expose the wound by removing or cutting away the clothing to find the source of the bleeding.
3. Control the bleeding by using direct pressure and, if needed, other methods described in Chapter 8.

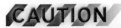

CAUTION

DO NOT clean large, extremely dirty, or life-threatening wounds. Let the hospital emergency department personnel do the cleaning.

DO NOT scrub a wound. The benefit of scrubbing a wound is debatable, and it can bruise the tissue.

Cleaning a Wound

A victim's wound should be cleaned to help prevent infection. Wound cleaning usually restarts the bleeding by disturbing the clot, but it should be done anyway for shallow wounds. For wounds with a high risk for infection, leave the pressure bandage in place because medical personnel will clean the wound.

1. Scrub your hands vigorously with soap and water. Put on medical exam gloves, if available.
2. Expose the wound.
3. Clean the wound.
   - *For a shallow wound:*
     - Wash inside the wound with soap and water.
     - Flush the wound with water (use water that is clean enough to drink) **Figure 9-6**. Run water directly into the wound and allow the water to run over the wound and out, thus carrying the dirty particles away from the wound. Flushing with water needs pressure (at least 5 to 8 psi) to adequately cleanse the tissue. Water from a faucet provides sufficient pressure and quantity. Pouring water on the wound

or using a bulb syringe will not generate enough force for adequate cleaning.
   - *For a wound with a high risk for infection* (such as an animal bite, a very dirty or ragged wound, or a puncture), seek medical care for wound cleaning. If you are in a remote setting (more than 1 hour from medical care), clean the wound as best you can.
4. Remove small objects not flushed out with sterile tweezers. A dirty abrasion or other wound that is not properly cleaned will leave a "tattoo" on the victim's skin.
5. If bleeding restarts, apply direct pressure over the wound.

FYI

Wound Irrigation

This study compared the effectiveness of tap water with saline solution for irrigating simple skin lacerations to remove bacteria. The results showed no significant difference between bacterial counts in wounds irrigated with normal saline and those irrigated with tap water. The removal of bacteria from a wound depends more on the mechanical effects (speed and pressure) than on the type of solution. Tap water has these advantages over saline—it is readily available; it is more continuous and, therefore, takes less time; it is less expensive; and it does not require other materials such as sterile syringes or splash guards. Other irrigation solutions with bactericidal properties and detergents have an anticellular effect that impairs wound healing and/or resistance to infection. Irrigation pressures more than the 20 to 30 psi range are discouraged because the higher pressure can damage tissue.

Source: Moscati R, Mayrose J, Fincher L, Jehle D: Comparison of normal saline with tap water for wound irrigation. Am J Emerg Med 164(4):379-381.

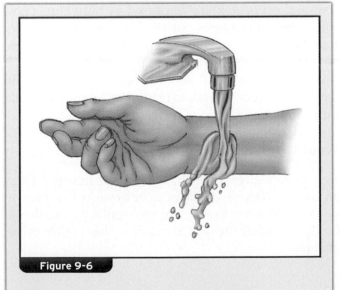

Figure 9-6

Irrigate a wound with water under pressure.

FYI

High-Risk Wounds

These types of wounds have a high potential for infection:

- Bite wounds
- Very dirty, contaminated wounds
- Crushing, ragged wounds
- Wounds over injured bone, joint, or tendon
- Puncture wounds

Covering a Wound

For a small wound that does not require sutures:

1. Cover it with a thin layer of antibiotic ointment. These ointments can kill many bacteria and rarely cause allergic reactions. No physician prescription is needed.

2. Cover the wound with a sterile dressing. Do not close the wound with tape or butterfly bandages. Bacteria may remain, leading to a greater chance of infection than if the wound were left open and covered by a sterile dressing. Closing a wound should be left to a physician.

3. If a wound bleeds after a dressing has been applied and the dressing becomes stuck, leave it on as long as the wound is healing. Pulling the scab loose to change the dressing retards healing and increases the chance of infection. If you must remove a dressing that is sticking, soak it in warm water to help soften the scab and make removal easier.

4. If a dressing becomes wet or dirty, change it. Dirt and moisture are both breeding grounds for bacteria.

Dressings and bandages are two different kinds of first aid supplies. A **dressing** is applied over a wound to control bleeding and prevent contamination. A **bandage** holds the dressing in place. Dressings should be sterile or as clean as possible; bandages need not be.

When to Seek Medical Care

High-risk wounds should receive medical care. Examples of high-risk wounds include those with embedded foreign material (such as gravel), animal and human bites, puncture wounds, and ragged wounds. Large or deep wounds should receive medical care. Any wound where edges do not come together spontaneously should receive medical care. Any wounds that have visible bone, joint, muscle, fat, or tendons and wounds that may have entered a joint or body cavity should receive medical care. A particularly high-risk wound is the "fight bite," a wound over the knuckle caused by punching a person in the teeth. Sutures, if needed, are best placed within 6 to 8 hours after the injury. Anyone who has not had a tetanus vaccination within 10 years (5 years in the case of a dirty wound) should seek medical attention within 72 hours to update his or her tetanus inoculation status.

Wound Infection

Any wound, large or small, can become infected. Once an infection begins, damage can be extensive, so prevention is the best way to avoid the problem. A wound should be cleaned using the procedures described earlier in this chapter.

It is important to know how to recognize and treat an infected wound. The signs and symptoms of infection include the following:

- Swelling and redness around the wound
- A sensation of warmth
- Throbbing pain
- Pus discharge
- Fever
- Swelling of lymph nodes
- One or more red streaks leading from the wound toward the heart

The appearance of one or more red streaks leading from the wound toward the heart is a serious sign that the infection is spreading and could cause death **Figure 9-7** . If chills and fever develop, the infection has reached the circulatory system (known as *blood poisoning*). Seek immediate medical care.

Factors that increase the likelihood for wound infection include the following:

- Dirty and foreign material left in the wound
- Ragged or crushed tissue
- Injury to an underlying bone, joint, or tendon
- Bite wounds (human or animal)
- Hand and foot wounds
- Puncture wounds or other wounds that cannot drain

In the early stages of an infection, a physician may allow a wound to be treated at home. Such home treatment would include the following:

- Keeping the area clean
- Soaking the wound in warm water or applying warm, wet packs
- Elevating the infected portion of the body
- Applying antibiotic ointment
- Changing the dressings daily
- Seeking medical help if the infection persists or becomes worse

Tetanus

Tetanus is also called *lockjaw* because of its best-known symptom, tightening of the jaw muscles. Tetanus is caused by a toxin produced by a bacterium. The bacterium, which is found throughout the world, forms a spore that can survive for years in a variety of environments. The World Health Organization reports that tetanus causes at least 500,000—perhaps even up to 1 million—deaths each year.

> ### FYI
>
> **Tetanus Prevalence**
>
> Despite the wide availability of immunization against tetanus in the United States, many people are inadequately protected against this uncommon but often lethal disease. Protection was found in only 70% of people studied, with levels of immunity varying widely.
>
> About 50 cases of tetanus occur in the United States each year, principally among elderly people and people who never received a primary series of vaccinations. Adults should have booster shots for tetanus every 10 years.
>
> *Source:* Gergen P J, McQuillan G M, Kiely M, Ezzati-Rice T M, Sutter R W, Virella G: A population-based serologic survey of immunity to tetanus in the United States. *N Engl J Med* 332(12):761-766.

Millions of adults in the United States have let their tetanus immunizations lapse; a smaller number have never been vaccinated. In addition, antibody levels in immunized children decline over time; one fifth of youngsters ages 10 to 16 years do not have protective levels. Tetanus is not communicable from one person to another.

The tetanus bacterium by itself does not cause tetanus. When it enters a wound, such as a puncture wound that contains little oxygen, the bacterium can produce a powerful, poisonous toxin. The toxin travels through the nervous system to the brain and the spinal cord. It then causes contractions of certain muscle groups, particularly in the jaw. There is no known antidote to the toxin once it enters the nervous system. It is not just stepping on a rusty nail that can bring on the disease. Tetanus bacteria are commonly found in soil, street dust, organic garden fertilizers, and pet feces, and even minor cuts can introduce them into the bloodstream.

A tetanus vaccination can completely prevent the disease. Everyone needs an initial series of vaccinations to prepare the immune system to defend against the toxin

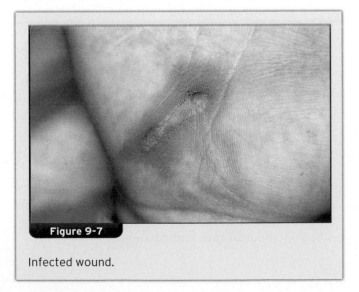

Figure 9-7

Infected wound.

but then only a booster shot every 5 to 10 years is sufficient to maintain immunity.

The guidelines for tetanus immunization boosters are as follows:

- Anyone with a wound who has never been immunized against tetanus should be given a tetanus vaccine and booster immediately.
- A victim who was once immunized but has not received a tetanus booster within the last 10 years should receive a booster.
- A victim with a dirty wound who has not had a booster within the past 5 years should receive a booster.
- Tetanus immunization shots must be given within 72 hours of the injury to be effective.

▶ Amputations

In many cases, an amputated extremity can be successfully replanted (reattached). It is generally only attempted for upper extremities.

Types of Amputations

Amputations usually involve fingers, hands, and arms rather than legs. Amputations are classified according to the type of injury:

- A **guillotine amputation** is a clean-cut, complete detachment. Examples would include a finger cut off with an ax or an arm severed with a power tool.
- A **crushing amputation** occurs when an extremity separates by being crushed or mashed off, such as when a hand is caught in a roller machine.
- **Degloving** is when the skin is peeled off, much as you would take off a glove **Figure 9-8**.

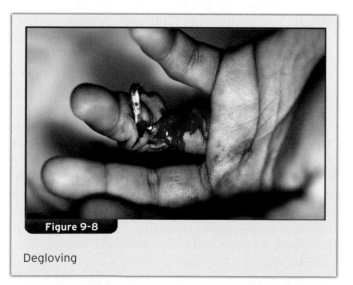

Figure 9-8

Degloving

In a crushing amputation, the most common type, the chance of reattachment is poor. In a guillotine type, the chance of reattachment is much better because it is clean cut. Many amputations can be replanted by an experienced surgeon, and time is a critical element in success. Function may be nearly normal in some cases.

A complete amputation may not involve heavy blood loss because blood vessels tend to go into spasms, recede

---

FYI

NEWS: Amputations

Ronald Malt, MD, performed the first successful replantation in 1962 on a young boy's severed arm. In the 1960s, the replantation success rate ranged from 25% to 39%, compared with the current 80% to 90% success rate when appropriate actions are taken.

Source: R. Malt, et. al, Journal of the American Medical Association 189(6):716-722.

---

into the injured body parts, and shrink in diameter, resulting in a surprisingly small blood loss. More blood is seen in a partial amputation.

Care for Amputation

1. Control the bleeding with direct pressure and elevate the extremity. Apply a dry dressing or bulky cloths. Be sure to protect yourself against disease. Tourniquets are rarely needed and, if used, will destroy tissue, blood vessels, and nerves necessary for replantation.
2. Treat the victim for shock.
3. Recover the amputated part and, whenever possible, take it with the victim to the hospital. However, in multicasualty cases, in reduced lighting conditions, or when untrained people transport the victim, someone may be requested to locate and take the severed body part to the hospital after the victim's departure.
4. To care for the amputated body part **Figure 9-9**:
   - Do not clean the amputated portion.
   - Wrap the amputated part with dry, sterile gauze or other clean cloth.
   - Put the wrapped amputated part in a plastic bag or other waterproof container.
   - Place the bag or container with the wrapped part on a bed of ice. Keep the amputated part cool, but do not freeze.
5. Seek medical care immediately.

Amputations

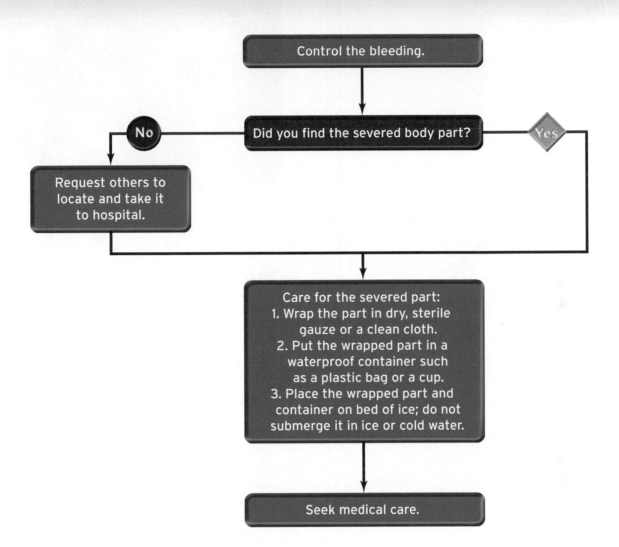

Control the bleeding.

Did you find the severed body part?

No → Request others to locate and take it to hospital.

Yes

Care for the severed part:
1. Wrap the part in dry, sterile gauze or a clean cloth.
2. Put the wrapped part in a waterproof container such as a plastic bag or a cup.
3. Place the wrapped part and container on bed of ice; do not submerge it in ice or cold water.

Seek medical care.

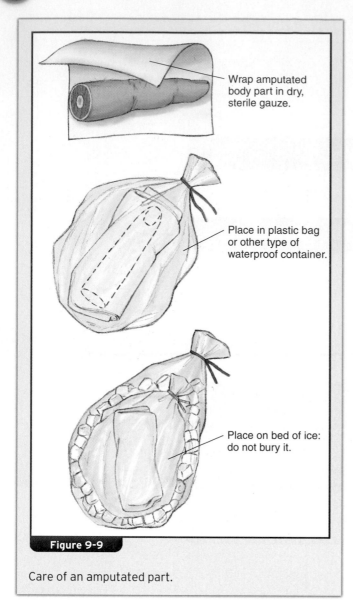

Wrap amputated body part in dry, sterile gauze.

Place in plastic bag or other type of waterproof container.

Place on bed of ice: do not bury it.

Figure 9-9

Care of an amputated part.

CAUTION

DO NOT try to decide whether a body part is salvageable or too small to save—leave that decision to a physician.

DO NOT wrap an amputated part in a wet dressing or cloth. Using a wet wrap on the part can cause waterlogging and tissue softening, which will make reattachment more difficult.

DO NOT bury an amputated part in ice—place it on ice. Reattaching frostbitten parts is usually unsuccessful.

DO NOT use dry ice.

DO NOT cut a skin "bridge," a tendon, or other structure that is connecting a partially attached part to the rest of the body. Instead, reposition the part in the normal position, wrap the part in a dry, sterile dressing or clean cloth, and place an ice pack on it.

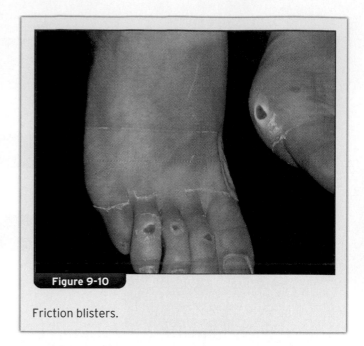

Figure 9-10

Friction blisters.

▶ Blisters

A blister is a collection of fluid in a "bubble" under the outer layer of skin. (Note: This section applies only to friction blisters and does not apply to blisters from burns, frostbite, drug reactions, insect or snake bites, or contact with a poisonous plant.)

Repeated rubbing of a small area of the skin will produce a blister **Figure 9-10**. Blisters are so common that many people assume they are a fact of life. However, blisters are avoidable, and life for many people could be more comfortable if they knew how to treat and prevent blisters.

Rubbing—as between a sock and a foot—causes stress on the skin's surface because the underlying supporting tissue remains stationary. The stress separates the skin into two layers, and the resulting space fills with fluid. The fluid may collect under or within the skin's outer layer, the epidermis. Because of differences in skin, blister formation varies considerably from person to person.

Care for Blisters

When caring for a friction blister, try to (1) avoid the risk of infection, (2) minimize the victim's pain and discomfort, (3) limit the blister's development, and (4) promote a fast recovery. The best care for a particular blister is determined mainly by its size and location.

If an area on the skin becomes a "hot spot" (painful, red area), snugly apply a piece of tape (adhesive or duct). You could also cut a hole in several pieces of moleskin or molefoam in layered stacks around the blister, make a doughnut-shaped pad, and apply it over the blister.

If a blister on a foot is closed and not very painful, a conservative approach is to tape the blister with duct tape or waterproof adhesive tape. The tape must remain on the blister for several days; removing it may tear off the blister's "roof" and expose unprotected skin. Unfortunately, the tape may become damp and contaminated and have to be replaced, risking a tear. Small blisters, especially on weight-bearing areas, generally respond better if left intact.

With a few exceptions, the blister's roof (which is the best and most comfortable "dressing") should be removed only when an infection is present. Once a blister has been opened, the area should be washed with soap to prevent further infection. For 10 to 14 days, or until new skin forms, a protective bandage or other cover should be used.

Even with no evidence of infection, consider removing the blister's roof when a partially torn blister roof may tear skin adjacent to the blister site, resulting in an even larger open wound. In such cases, use sterilized scissors to remove the loose skin of the blister's roof up to the edge of the normal tissue. Treat it the same as for an open blister. Rubbing alcohol is effective for sterilizing instruments such as needles or scissors.

If a blister on the foot is open or a very painful closed blister affects walking or running:

1. Clean the area with soap and water.

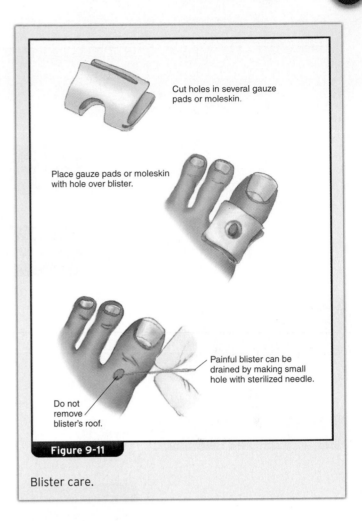

Cut holes in several gauze pads or moleskin.

Place gauze pads or moleskin with hole over blister.

Painful blister can be drained by making small hole with sterilized needle.

Do not remove blister's roof.

Figure 9-11

Blister care.

2. Drain all fluid out of the blister by making several small holes at the base of the blister with a sterilized needle. Press the fluid out. Do not remove the roof of a blister unless it is torn and it may tear adjacent skin, or if there is an infection.

3. Apply several layers of moleskin or molefoam cut in a doughnut shape on top of each other **Figure 9-11**

4. Apply antibiotic ointment in the hole and cover it securely with tape. The pressure dressing ensures that the blister's roof sticks to the underlying skin and that the blister does not refill with fluid after it has been drained.

▶ Impaled (Embedded) Objects

Impaled objects come in all shapes and sizes, from pencils and screwdrivers to knives, glass, steel rods, and fence posts **Figure 9-12**. Proper first aid requires that the impaled object be stabilized because there can be significant internal damage.

Blisters

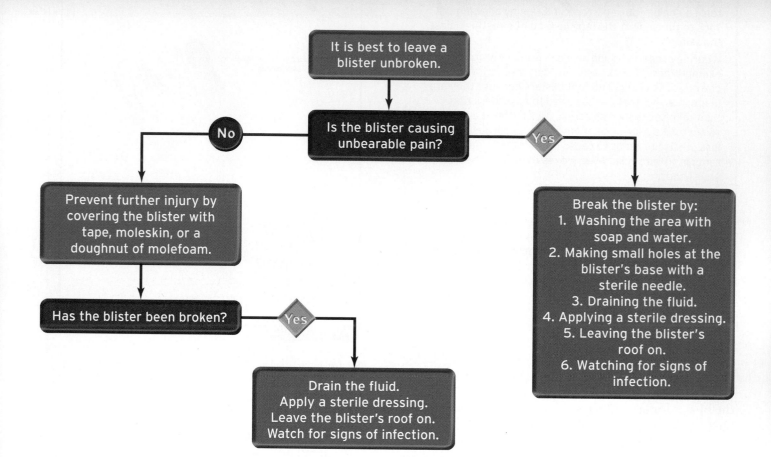

It is best to leave a blister unbroken.

Is the blister causing unbearable pain?

No

Yes

Prevent further injury by covering the blister with tape, moleskin, or a doughnut of molefoam.

Has the blister been broken?

Yes

Drain the fluid.
Apply a sterile dressing.
Leave the blister's roof on.
Watch for signs of infection.

Break the blister by:
1. Washing the area with soap and water.
2. Making small holes at the blister's base with a sterile needle.
3. Draining the fluid.
4. Applying a sterile dressing.
5. Leaving the blister's roof on.
6. Watching for signs of infection.

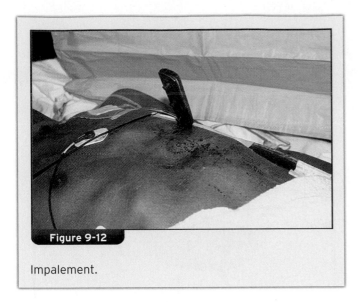

Figure 9-12

Impalement.

Care for Impaled Objects

1. Expose the area. Remove or cut away any clothing surrounding the injury. If clothes cover the object, leave them in place; removing them could cause the object to move.
2. Do not remove or move the object. Movement of any kind could produce additional bleeding and tissue damage. Cheeks are one exception because the object or the bleeding could cause an airway obstruction. See the following section on impaled object in the cheek for more information. Small objects such as slivers can be safely removed.
3. Control any bleeding with pressure around the impaled object. Straddle the object with gauze. Do not press directly on the object or along the wound next to the cutting edge, especially if the object has sharp edges.
4. Stabilize the object with bulky dressings or clean cloths around the object. Some experts suggest securing 75% of the object with bulky dressings or cloths to reduce motion.
5. Shorten the object only if necessary. In most cases, do not shorten the object by cutting or breaking it. There are times, however, when cutting or shortening the object allows for easier transportation. Be sure to stabilize the object before shortening it. Remember that the victim will feel any vibrations from the object being cut away; also the injury could be worsened by this action.

Impaled Object in the Cheek

The only time it is safe to remove an impaled object outside a medical setting is when the object is in the victim's cheek.

Care for Impaled Object in the Cheek

1. Examine the injury inside the mouth. If the object extends through the cheek and you are more than 1 hour from medical help, consider removing it.
2. To remove the object: Place two fingers next to the object, straddling it; then gently pull it in the direction from which it entered. If it cannot be removed easily, leave it in place and secure it with bulky dressings.
3. Control the bleeding. After you have removed the object, place dressings over the wound inside the mouth between the cheek and the teeth. The dressings will help control the bleeding and will not interfere with the victim's airway. Also place a dressing on the outside wound.

Impaled Object in the Eye

If an object is impaled in the eye, it is vital that pressure not be put on the eye. The eyeball consists of two chambers, each filled with fluid. Do not exert any pressure against the eyeball because fluid can be forced out of it, worsening the injury.

Care for Impaled Object in the Eye

1. Stabilize the object. Use bulky dressings or clean cloths to stabilize a long, protruding object. You can place a protective paper cup or cardboard folded into a cone over the affected eye to prevent bumping of the object. For short objects, surround the eye—without touching the object—with a doughnut-shaped (ring) pad held in place with a roller bandage.
2. Cover the undamaged eye. Most experts suggest that the undamaged eye should be covered to prevent sympathetic eye movement (that is, the injured eye moves when the undamaged eye does, thus aggravating the injury). Remember that the victim is unable to see when both eyes are covered and may be anxious. Make sure you explain to the victim everything you are doing.
3. Seek medical care immediately.

Slivers

Small slivers of wood, glass, thorns, or metal can be painful and irritating and they also can cause infection. Because of their size, these slivers can usually be easily removed with tweezers. Sometimes, it is necessary to tease one end of the object with a sterile needle to place it in a better position for removal with tweezers. After you have removed the sliver, clean the area with soap and water and apply an adhesive strip (such as a Band-Aid).

Cactus Spines

Cacti are a part of the desert environment, and they also are used as ornamental plants. Infection from cactus-spine punctures is rare. Removing cactus spines is time consuming because they usually are acquired in groupings, are difficult to see, and are designed by nature to resist removal. Usually spines can easily, yet tediously, be removed with tweezers.

Another method for removing a large number of cactus spines is to coat the area with a thin layer of white woodworking glue or rubber cement and allow it to dry for at least 30 minutes. Slowly roll up the dried glue from the margins. Applying the glue in strips rather than puddles will make the rolling procedure go more smoothly. A single layer of gauze gently pressed onto the still-damp glue helps to remove it after it has dried. The combination of using tweezers and glue will remove most of the spines.

Using adhesive tape, duct tape, or cellophane tape, although quick and easy, removes only about 30% of the spines, even after multiple attempts. Do not use super glue (or other similar products) to remove cactus spines. Not only does it fail to roll up when applied to the skin, but it also welds the spines to the skin. In addition, there is the risk that the skin will permanently bond to anything it touches.

Fishhooks

Tape an embedded fishhook in place and do *not* try to remove it if injury to a nearby body part such as the eye or an underlying structure such as a blood vessel or nerve is possible or if the victim (such as a young child) is uncooperative.

If the point of a fishhook has penetrated the skin but the barb has not, remove the fishhook by backing it out. Then treat the wound like a puncture wound. Seek medical advice for a possible tetanus shot.

If the hook's barb has entered the skin, follow these procedures:

1. If medical care is near, transport the victim and have a physician remove the hook.
2. If you are in a remote area, far from medical care, remove the hook using either the pliers method or the fishline method.

Care for Fishhooks

Use extreme care with the pliers method of fishhook removal because it can produce further severe injury if the hook is pushed into blood vessels, nerves, or tendons. Use pliers with tempered jaws that can cut through a hook **Figure 9-13** . The proper kind of pliers is often unavailable, or sometimes the barb is buried too deep to be

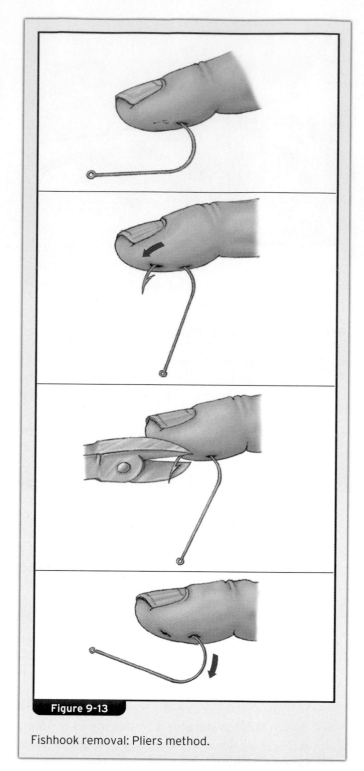

Figure 9-13

Fishhook removal: Pliers method.

pushed through. Test the pliers by first cutting a similar fishhook.

1. Use cold or hard pressure around the hook to provide temporary numbness.
2. Push the embedded hook further in, in a shallow curve, until the point and the barb come out through the skin.

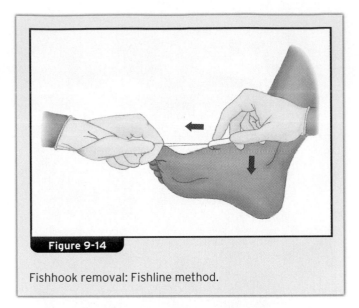

Figure 9-14

Fishhook removal: Fishline method.

3. Cut the barb off, then back the hook out the way it came in.
4. After removing the hook, treat the wound and seek medical attention for a possible tetanus shot.

Another method to remove a fishhook is the fishline method.

1. Loop a piece of fishline over the bend or curve of the embedded hook **Figure 9-14** .
2. Stabilize the part of the victim's body in which the hook is embedded.
3. Use cold or hard pressure around the hook to provide temporary numbness.
4. With one hand, press down on the hook's shank and eye while the other hand sharply jerks the fishline that is over the hook's bend or curve. The jerk movement should be parallel to the skin's surface. The hook will neatly come out of the same hole it entered, causing little pain.
5. After removing the hook, care for the wound and seek medical attention for a possible tetanus shot.

▶ Closed Wounds

A closed wound happens when a blunt object strikes the body. In other words, the skin is not broken, but tissue and blood vessels beneath the skin's surface are crushed, causing bleeding within a confined area. There are three types of closed wounds:

1. *Bruises and contusions* occur when blood collects under the skin in the injured area. The victim will experience pain and swelling (immediately or within 24 to 48 hours). As blood accumulates, a black-and-blue mark may appear.

2. A *hematoma* is a clot of blood under the skin. There may be a lump or bluish discoloration.
3. *Crush injuries* are caused by extreme forces, which can injure vital organs and bones without breaking open the skin. Crush injuries may indicate an underlying problem such as a fracture. Signs and symptoms include discoloration, swelling, pain, and loss of use.

Care for Closed Wounds

1. Control bleeding by applying an ice pack over the area for no more than 20 minutes.
2. If the injury involves a limb, apply an elastic bandage for compression. A splint may help make the victim more comfortable. See Chapter 10.
3. Check for a possible fracture.
4. Elevate an injured extremity above the victim's heart level to decrease the pain and swelling.

▶ Wounds That Require Medical Care

At some point, you will probably have to decide whether medical care is needed for a wounded victim. As a guideline, seek medical care for the following conditions as offered by the American College of Emergency Physicians:

- Wounds that will not stop bleeding after 5 minutes of applying direct pressure
- Long or deep cuts that need stitches
- Cuts over a joint
- Cuts that may impair function of a body area such as an eyelid or lip
- Cuts that remove all of the layers of the skin; such as those from slicing off the tip of a finger
- Cuts from an animal or human bite
- Cuts that have damaged or may have damaged underlying nerves, tendons, or joints
- Cuts over a possible broken bone
- Cuts caused by a crushing injury
- Cuts with an object embedded in them
- Cuts caused by metal object or a puncture wound

Call 9-1-1 immediately if:

- Bleeding from a cut does not slow during the first 15 minutes of steady pressure
- Signs of shock occur
- Breathing is difficult because of a cut to the neck or chest
- A deep cut to the abdomen causes moderate to severe pain
- A cut occurs to the eyeball
- A cut amputates or partially amputates an extremity

Sutures

If sutures (stitches) are needed, they usually should be placed by a physician within 6 to 8 hours of the injury. Suturing wounds allows faster healing, reduces infection, and lessens scarring. Some wounds do not usually require sutures:

- Wounds in which the skin's cut edges tend to fall together
- Shallow cuts less than 1 inch long

Rather than close a gaping wound with butterfly bandages or elastic skin closures, cover the wound with sterile gauze. Closing the wound might trap bacteria inside, resulting in an infection. In most cases, a physician can be reached in time for sutures to be placed; if not, a wound without sutures will still heal but with scars. Scar tissue can be attended to later by a plastic surgeon.

▶ Gunshot Wounds

Guns are abundant in the United States; it is estimated that about one half of all American homes have a firearm. There are two general types of firearms: low velocity, such as most civilian firearms, and high velocity, such as military weapons. Shotguns have low velocity but create severe tissue damage.

A bullet causes injury in the following ways, depending on its velocity, or speed:

- *Laceration and crushing.* When the bullet penetrates the body, it crushes tissue and forces it apart. That is the main effect of low-velocity bullets. The crushing and laceration caused by the passage of the bullet usually are not serious unless vital organs or major blood vessels are injured. The bullet damages only the tissues that it contacts directly, and the wound is comparable to that caused by weapons such as knives.
- *Shock waves and temporary cavitation.* When a bullet penetrates the body, a shock wave exerts outward pressure from the bullet's path. The shock wave pushes tissues away and creates a temporary cavity that can be as much as 30 times the diameter of the bullet. As the cavity forms, a negative pressure develops inside, creating a vacuum. The vacuum then draws debris in with it. Temporary cavitation occurs only with high-velocity bullets and is the main reason for their immensely destructive effect. The cavitation lasts only a millisecond but can damage muscles, nerves, blood vessels, and bone.

In a *penetrating* wound, there is a bullet entry point but no exit. In a *perforating* wound, there are both entry

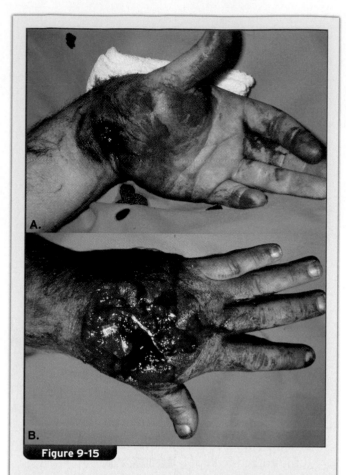

Figure 9-15

Gunshot wounds. **A.** An entrance wound from a gunshot may have burns around the edges. **B.** An exit wound is sometimes larger and results in greater damage to soft tissues.

and exit points. The exit wound of a high-velocity bullet is larger than the entrance wound; the exit wound from a low-velocity bullet is about the same size as the entry wound **Figure 9-15**. If the bullet was fired at very close range, the entrance wound may be larger than the exit wound because the gases from the gun's muzzle contribute to the surface-tissue damage.

Bullets sometimes hit hard tissue such as bones and may bounce around in the body cavities, causing a great deal of damage to tissue and organs. Moreover, bone chips can ricochet to other body areas and cause damage. Because a split or misshapen bullet tumbles and exerts its force over a larger area, it does more damage than a smooth bullet going in a straight line.

Care for Gunshot Wounds

Regardless of the type of gunshot wound, initial care is roughly the same as for any other wound.

1. Monitor the victim's breathing.
2. Expose the wound(s). Look for entrance and exit wounds.
3. Control the bleeding with direct pressure.
4. Apply dry, sterile dressings to the wound(s) and bandage them securely in place.
5. Treat the victim for shock.
6. Keep the victim calm and quiet.
7. Seek immediate medical care.

CAUTION

DO NOT try to remove material from a gunshot wound. The hospital emergency department personnel will clean the wound.

Legal Aspects

Because interactions with victims of gunshot wounds will involve contact with law enforcement agencies and possibly have you testifying in court, carefully observe the scene and the victim. Keep an accurate record of your observations. Preserve possible evidence, such as cartridge casings or shells, for the police. Do not touch or move anything unless absolutely necessary to treat the victim. All gunshot wounds must be reported to the police regardless of whether they are intentional (suicide, assault, murder, self-defense) or unintentional.

What to Look For | What to Do

Open wound care

1. Wash with soap and water.
2. Flush with running water under pressure.
3. Remove remaining small object(s).
4. If the bleeding restarts, apply pressure on the wound.
5. Apply antibiotic ointment.
6. Cover with sterile or clean dressing.
7. For wounds with a high risk for infection, seek medical care for cleaning, possible tetanus booster, and closing.

Amputation

Call 9-1-1
Control bleeding.
Care for shock.
Recover amputated part(s) and wrap in sterile or clean dressing.
Place wrapped part(s) in a plastic bag or waterproof container.
Keep part(s) cool.

Embedded (impaled) object

Do not remove object.
Control bleeding with pressure around the object.
Stabilize the object with bulky dressings or clean clothes.

prep kit

▶ Ready for Review

- An open wound is a break in the skin's surface resulting in external bleeding.
- Knowing what type of open wound the victim has will help you in providing first aid.
- In many cases, an amputated extremity can be successfully replanted.
- A blister is a collection of fluid in a bubble under the outer layer of skin.
- Proper first aid of an impaled object requires that the object be stabilized because significant internal damage can occur.
- A closed wound happens when a blunt object strikes the body and while the skin remains unbroken, the tissue and blood vessels beneath the skin's surface are crushed, causing bleeding within a confined area.
- Wounds that require medical care include:
  - Wounds that will not stop bleeding after 5 minutes of applying direct pressure
  - Long or deep cuts that need stitches
  - Cuts over a joint
  - Cuts that may impair function of a body area such as an eyelid or lip
  - Cuts that remove all of the layers of the skin such as those from slicing off the tip of a finger
  - Cuts from an animal or human bite
  - Cuts that have damaged or may have damaged underlying nerves, tendons, or joints
  - Cuts over a possible broken bone
  - Cuts caused by a crushing injury
  - Cuts with an object embedded in them
  - Cuts caused by metal object or a puncture wound
- Call 9-1-1 immediately if:
  - Bleeding from a cut does not slow during the first 15 minutes of steady pressure.
  - Signs of shock occur
  - Breathing is difficult because of a cut to the neck or chest
  - A deep cut to the abdomen causes moderate to severe pain

- A cut occurs to the eyeball
- A cut amputates or partially amputates an extremity
- Guns are abundant in the United States, thus raising the risk of an accidental gunshot wound.

▶ Vital Vocabulary

abrasion An injury consisting of the loss of the partial thickness of skin from rubbing or scraping on a hard, rough surface; also called brush burn, friction burn, or rug burn.

amputation Complete removal of an appendage.

avulsion An injury that leaves a piece of skin or other tissue either partially or completely torn away from the body.

bandage Used to cover a dressing to keep it in place on the wound and to apply pressure to help control bleeding.

crushing amputation An extremity separates by being crushed or mashed off.

degloving The skin is peeled off of the extremity.

dressing A sterile gauze pad or clean cloth covering that is placed over an open wound.

guillotine amputation A clean-cut, complete detachment of an extremity.

incisions A wound usually made deliberately in connection with surgery; clean cut as opposed to a laceration.

laceration A wound made by the tearing or cutting of body tissues.

punctures Deep, narrow wounds in the skin and underlying organs.

▶ Assessment in Action

While taking your morning walk, you hear a yelp from behind a fence. You stop and peer over to find your neighbor rubbing her hand. "Darn cat," she mutters. She was trying to coax her old tabby inside with a can of tuna when the cat jumped up and knocked the tuna can out of her hand. As she bent down to pick up the can that the cat was now eating out of, the cat bit her hand between the thumb and forefinger.

Directions: Circle Yes if you agree with the statement, circle No if you disagree.

Yes   No   **1.** This wound is not more likely to become infected.

Yes No 2. The next morning, your neighbor wakes up with a fever and a throbbing pain in her hand. Is her hand infected?

Yes No 3. You advise your neighbor to soak the wound in warm water.

Yes No 4. Your neighbor should not apply antibiotic ointment.

Yes No. 5. She does not need to seek medical help.

Answers: 1. No; 2. Yes; 3. Yes; 4. No; 5. No

▶ Check Your Knowledge

Directions: Circle Yes if you agree with the statement, circle No if you disagree.

Yes No 1. An open wound may allow bacteria to enter the body, causing an infection.

Yes No 2. A laceration is cut skin with smooth, straight edges.

Yes No 3. A dressing is applied over a wound to control bleeding and prevent contamination.

Yes No 4. A bandage is also applied over a wound to hold a dressing in place.

Yes No 5. Any wound can become infected.

Yes No 6. The signs and symptoms of an infection include swelling and redness around the wound, throbbing pain, and a lack of fever.

Yes No 7. A bite wound is more likely to become infected.

Yes No 8. Impaled objects should be removed immediately.

Yes No 9. Tetanus is communicable from one person to another.

Yes No 10. In many cases, an amputated extremity can be successfully reattached.

Answers: 1. Yes; 2. No; 3. Yes; 4. Yes; 5. Yes; 6. No; 7. Yes; 8. No; 9. No; 10. Yes

10

Bandaging Wounds

Dressings

A dressing covers an open wound; it touches the wound. Whenever possible, a dressing should be:

- Sterile. If a sterile dressing is not available, use a clean cloth, handkerchief, washcloth, or towel.
- Larger than the wound.
- Thick, soft, and compressible so pressure is evenly distributed over the wound.
- Lint free.

The purposes of using a dressing are to:

- Control bleeding
- Prevent infection and contamination
- Absorb blood and wound drainage
- Protect the wound from further injury

▶ Types of Dressings

Use commercial dressings whenever possible. Dressings used in most first aid situations are commercially prepared, but dressings may need to be improvised.

- <u>Gauze pads</u> are used for small wounds. They come in separately wrapped packages of various sizes (for example, 2 inches by 2 inches; 4 inches by 4 inches) and are sterile, unless the package is broken. Some gauze pads

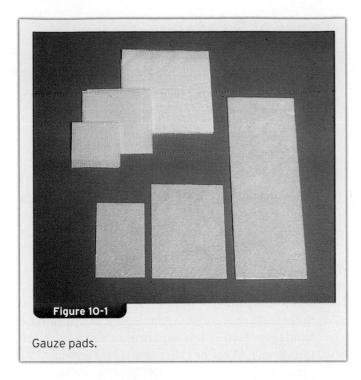

Figure 10-1

Gauze pads.

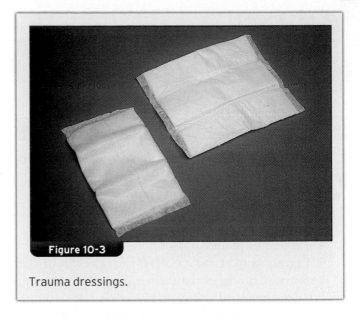

Figure 10-3

Trauma dressings.

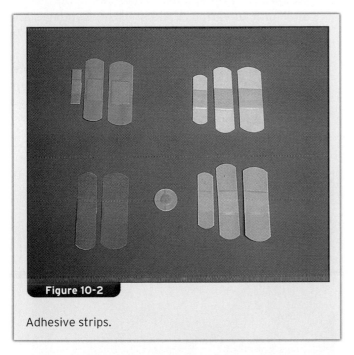

Figure 10-2

Adhesive strips.

have a special coating to keep them from sticking to the wound and are especially helpful for burns or wounds secreting fluids **Figure 10-1**.

- **Adhesive strips** (for example, Band-Aids) are used for small cuts and abrasions and are a combination of a sterile dressing and a bandage **Figure 10-2**.

- **Trauma dressings** are made of large, thick, absorbent, sterile materials. Individually wrapped sanitary napkins can serve because of their bulk

and absorbency, but they usually are not sterile **Figure 10-3**.

- When commercial sterile dressings are not available, an improvised dressing should be as clean, absorbent, soft, and free of lint as possible (for example, a handkerchief or a towel). Use the cleanest cloth available, or, in some conditions and if time allows, sterilize a cloth by boiling it and allowing it to dry, by ironing it for several minutes, or by soaking it in rubbing alcohol and allowing it to dry.

CAUTION

DO NOT use fluffy cotton or cotton balls as a dressing. Cotton fibers can get in the wound and be difficult to remove.

DO NOT remove a blood-soaked dressing until the bleeding stops. Cover it with a new dressing.

DO NOT pull off a dressing stuck to a wound. If it needs to be removed, soak it off in warm water.

Applying a Sterile Dressing

1. If possible, wash your hands and wear medical examination gloves.

2. Use a dressing large enough to extend beyond the edges of the wound. Hold the dressing by a corner. Place the dressing directly over the wound. Do not slide it on.

3. Cover the dressing with one of the types of bandages.

Bandages

A bandage should be clean but need not be sterile. A bandage can be used to:

- Hold a dressing in place over an open wound
- Apply direct pressure over a dressing to control bleeding
- Prevent or reduce swelling
- Provide support and stability for an extremity or joint

Remember, bandages should be applied firmly enough to keep dressings and splints in place but not so tightly that they will reinjure the body part or impede blood circulation. The signs that a bandage is too tight include:

- Blue tinge of the fingernails or toenails
- Blue or pale skin
- Tingling or loss of sensation
- Coldness of the extremity
- Inability to move the fingers or toes
- A pulse could be felt before bandaging, but not after

A square knot is preferred because it is neat, holds well, and can be easily untied. However, the type of knot is not important. If the knot or the bandage is likely to cause the victim discomfort, a pad should be placed between the knot or bandage and the body.

▶ Types of Bandages

These are the basic types of bandages:

- **Roller bandages** come in various widths, lengths, and types of material. For best results, use different widths for different body areas:
  - 1-inch width for fingers
  - 2-inch width for wrists, hands, and feet
  - 3-inch width for ankles, elbows, and arms
  - 4-inch width for knees and legs
- **Self-adhering, conforming bandages** **Figure 10-4** come as rolls of slightly elastic, gauzelike material in various widths. Their self-adherent quality makes them easy to use.
- **Gauze rollers** are cotton, rigid, and nonelastic. They come in various widths (1, 2, and 3 inches) and usually are 10 yards long. When commercial roller bandages are unavailable, you can improvise bandages from belts, neckties, or strips of cloth torn from a sheet or other similar material.
- **Elastic roller bandages** **Figure 10-5** are used for compression on sprains, strains, and contusions and come in various widths. Elastic bandages are not usually applied over dressings covering a wound.
- **Triangular bandages** **Figure 10-6** are available commercially or can be made from a 36- to 40-inch square of preshrunk cotton muslin. Cut the mate-

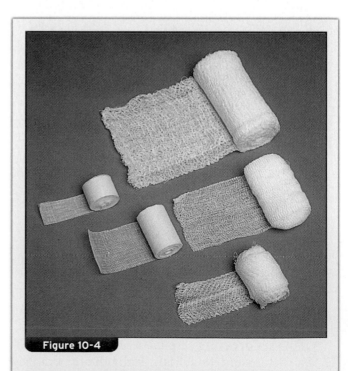

Figure 10-4

Self-adhering conforming bandages and gauze bandages of various sizes.

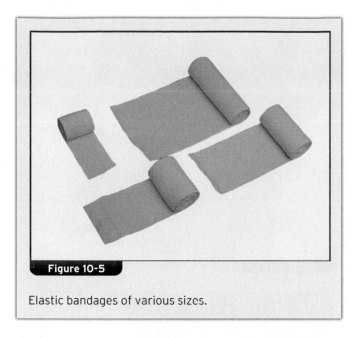

Figure 10-5

Elastic bandages of various sizes.

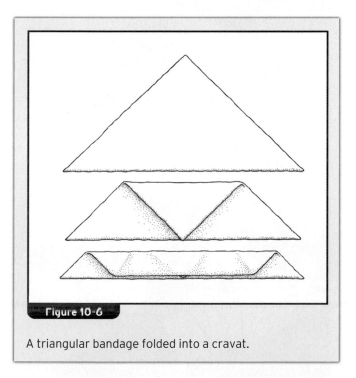

Figure 10-6

A triangular bandage folded into a cravat.

• As a *cravat* (folded triangular bandage). The point is folded to the center of the base and then the fabric is folded in half again from the top to the base to form a cravat. It is used to hold splints in place, to hold dressings in place, to apply pressure evenly over a dressing, or as a swathe (binder) around the victim's body to stabilize an injured arm in an arm sling.

• <u>Adhesive tape</u> comes in rolls and in a variety of widths. It is often used to secure roller bandages and small dressings in place. For people allergic to adhesive tape, use paper tape or special dermatologic tape.

• Adhesive strips are used for small cuts and abrasions and are a combination of a dressing and a bandage.

FYI

Removing Adhesive Tape

• When you first apply the tape, fold over one end (sticky sides together) to make a tab. Then when it comes time to remove the tape, you can grasp the starter tab. No need to pick at the tape (and the victim's skin) to get the strip started.

• To remove adhesive tape from the skin, gently lift the tape with one hand as you gently push the skin down and away from the tape with the other hand.

• Save time and reduce frustration by leaving a tab on the end of the roll of tape for quick access the next time you need it.

CAUTION

Adhesive tape should only be applied directly to the skin.

rial diagonally from corner to corner to produce two triangular pieces of cloth. The longest side is called the *base*; the corner directly across from the base is the *point*; and the other two corners are called *ends*. A triangular bandage may be applied two ways:

• Fully opened (not folded). Best used for an arm sling. When used to hold dressings in place, fully opened triangular bandages do not apply sufficient pressure on the wound.

Applying a Cravat Bandage

This method employs a cravat bandage (Figure 10-6). The bandage can be applied on the head, forehead, ear, eyes, arm, leg, or hand **Skill Drill 10-1**. For an injured eye, cover both eyes to prevent the injured eye from moving.

1. Place the middle of the bandage over the dressing covering the wound (or eyes) and wrap the bandage around the head (**Step ❶**).

2. Cross the two ends snugly over each other (**Step ❷**).

3. Bring the ends back around to where the dressing is and tie the ends in a knot (Step ❸). When wrapping a roller bandage around the head, keep the bandage near the eyebrows and low on the back of the head to prevent the bandage from slipping.

To apply a cravat bandage to the arm or leg using the cravat method, follow the steps in **Skill Drill 10-2**.

1. Wrap the center of the bandage over the dressing (Step ❶).
2. With one end, make one turn going up the extremity and another turn going down (Step ❷).
3. Tie the bandage off over the dressing (Step ❸).

To apply a bandage to the palm of the hand using the cravat method, follow the steps in **Skill Drill 10-3**.

1. Fill the palm with a bulky dressing or pad and close fingers over it (Step ❶).
2. Wrap the bandage crossing over the fingers and around the wrist (Step ❷).
3. Tie the bandage off at the wrist (Step ❸).

Applying a Roller Bandage

With a little ingenuity, you can apply a roller bandage to almost any body part. Self-adhering, conforming roller bandages eliminate the need for many of the complicated bandaging techniques that standard gauze roller, cravat, and triangular bandages require.

The Spiral Method

This method employs a 2- or 3-inch bandage roller for the arm or a 4-inch bandage for the leg. To apply a bandage to the arm or leg using the spiral method, follow the steps here:

1. Start at the narrow part of an arm or leg and wrap upward toward the wider part to make the bandage more secure. Start below and at the edge of the dressing **Figure 10-7**.
2. Make two straight anchoring turns with the bandage.
3. Make a series of turns, progressing up the arm or leg. Each turn should overlap the previous wrap. Wrap with criss-cross (figure-of-eight) turns.
4. Finish with two straight turns, and secure the bandage.

The Figure-of-Eight Method

Use this method of applying a roller bandage to hold dressings or to provide compression at or near a joint such as the ankle. The figure-of-eight method involves continuous spiral loops of bandage, one up and one down,

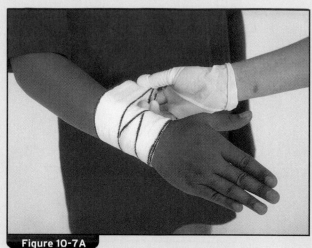

Figure 10-7A

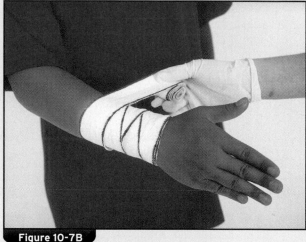

Figure 10-7B

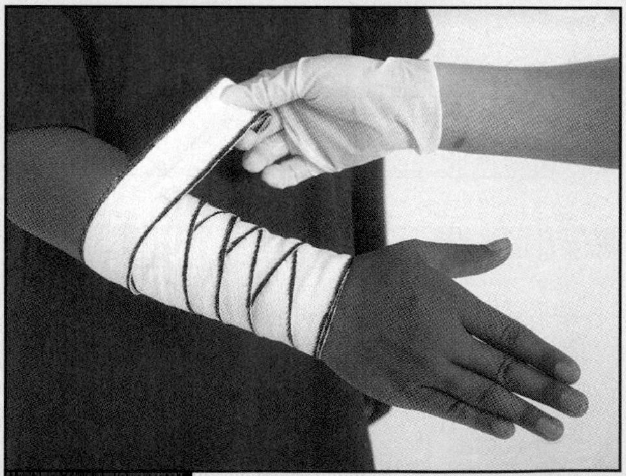

Figure 10-7C

Spiral method. **A.** Make two straight anchoring turns with the bandage. **B.** Wrap with criss-cross (figure-eight) turns. **C.** Finish with two straight turns and secure the bandage.

skill drill

10-1 Cravat Method of Bandaging the Head, Forehead, Ear, or Eyes

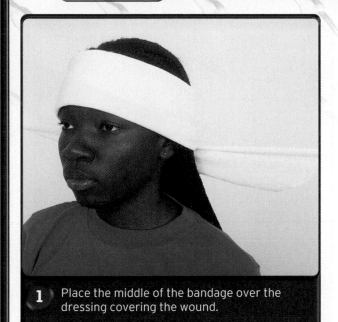

1 Place the middle of the bandage over the dressing covering the wound.

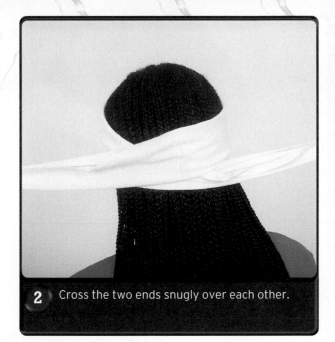

2 Cross the two ends snugly over each other.

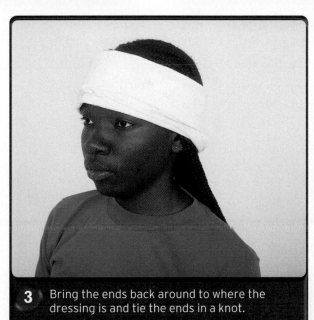

3 Bring the ends back around to where the dressing is and tie the ends in a knot.

skill drill

10-2 Cravat Method of Bandaging the Arm or Leg

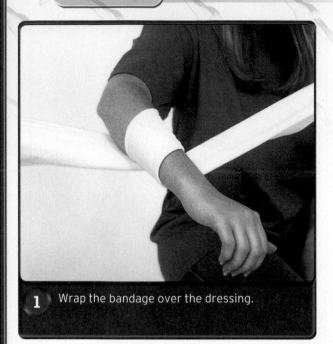

1 Wrap the bandage over the dressing.

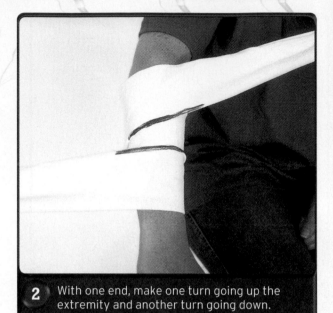

2 With one end, make one turn going up the extremity and another turn going down.

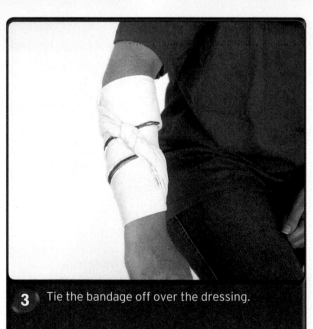

3 Tie the bandage off over the dressing.

skill drill

10-3   Cravat Method for Applying a Bandage to the Palm of the Hand

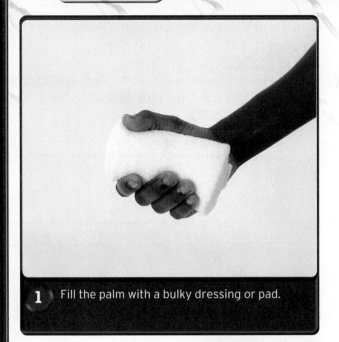

1 Fill the palm with a bulky dressing or pad.

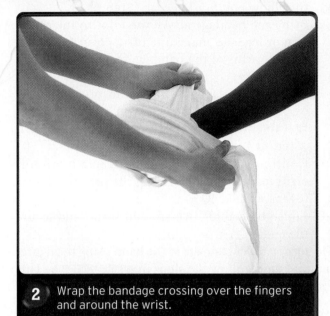

2 Wrap the bandage crossing over the fingers and around the wrist.

3 Tie the bandage off at the wrist.

crossing each other to form an "8." To apply a 4- or 6-inch roller bandage to the elbow or knee using the figure-of-eight method, follow the steps in **Skill Drill 10-4** :

1. Bend the elbow or knee slightly and make two straight anchoring turns with the bandage over the elbow point or kneecap (**Step ❶**).
2. Bring the bandage above the joint to the upper arm or leg, and make one turn, covering half to three fourths of the bandage from the first turn (**Step ❷**).
3. Bring the bandage just under the joint and make one turn around the lower arm or leg, covering half to three fourths of the first straight turn (**Step ❸**).
4. Continue alternating the turns in a figure-of-eight maneuver by covering the previous layers (**Steps ❹ₐ and ❹ᵦ**).
5. Finish by making two straight turns, and secure the end.

To apply a roller bandage to the hand using the figure-of-eight method, follow the steps in **Skill Drill 10-5** . This method uses a 2- or 3-inch roller bandage.

1. Make two straight anchoring turns with the bandage around the palm of the hand (**Step ❶**).
2. Carry the bandage diagonally across the back of the hand and then around the wrist and back across the palm (**Step ❷**).
3. Complete several figure-of-eight turns, overlapping each by about three fourths of the previous bandage width. Repeat this figure-of-eight maneuver as many times as necessary to cover the dressing, overlapping wraps to "stair-step" up the hand (**Step ❸**).
4. Make two straight turns around the wrist, and secure the bandage.

To wrap an ankle or foot using the figure-of-eight method, follow the steps in **Skill Drill 10-6** . This wrapping will hold a dressing or apply pressure to treat a sprained ankle. It should not be used to support the ankle and foot during sports activity; that type of bandaging involves additional maneuvers. Either 2- or 3-inch roller bandages can be used.

1. Make two straight anchoring turns with the bandage around the foot's instep (**Step ❶**).
2. Make a figure-of-eight turn by taking the bandage diagonally across the front of the foot, around the ankle, and again diagonally across the foot and under the arch (**Step ❷**).

3. Make several of these figure-of-eight turns, each time overlapping the previous one by about three fourths the width of the bandage. The bandage advances up the leg (**Step ❸**).
4. Finish with two straight turns around the leg, and secure the bandage.

To securely fasten a roller bandage, you can:

- Apply adhesive tape to secure the bandage **Figure 10-8** .
- Use safety pins to secure the bandage **Figure 10-9** .
- Use the special clips provided with elastic bandages **Figure 10-10** .

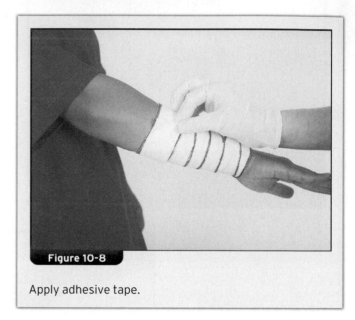

Figure 10-8

Apply adhesive tape.

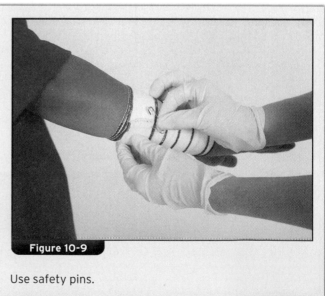

Figure 10-9

Use safety pins.

10-4 | **The Figure-of-Eight Method of Bandaging a Knee or Elbow**

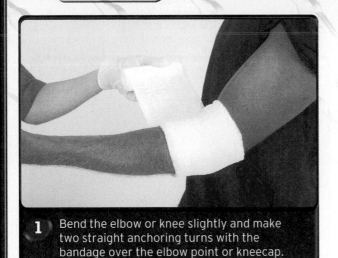

1 Bend the elbow or knee slightly and make two straight anchoring turns with the bandage over the elbow point or kneecap.

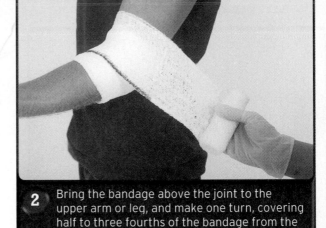

2 Bring the bandage above the joint to the upper arm or leg, and make one turn, covering half to three fourths of the bandage from the first turn.

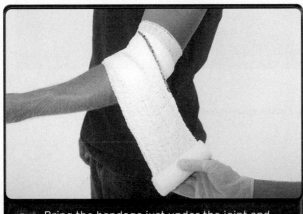

3 Bring the bandage just under the joint and make one turn around the lower arm or leg, covering half to three fourths of the first straight turn.

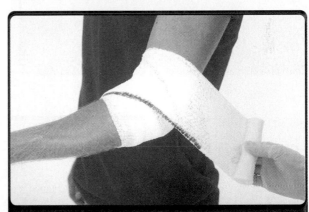

4a Continue alternating the turns in a figure-of-eight maneuver by covering the previous layers.

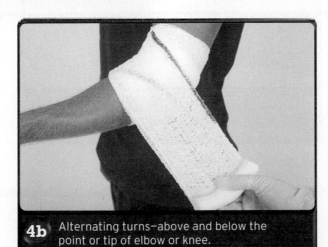

4b Alternating turns—above and below the point or tip of elbow or knee.

skill drill

10-5 Figure-of-Eight Method of Bandaging a Hand

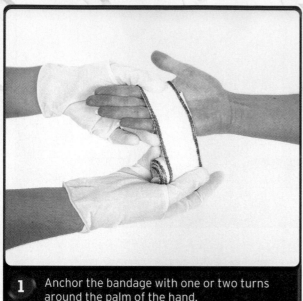

1 Anchor the bandage with one or two turns around the palm of the hand.

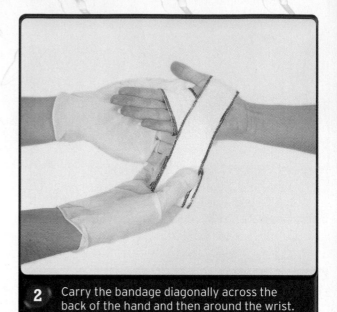

2 Carry the bandage diagonally across the back of the hand and then around the wrist.

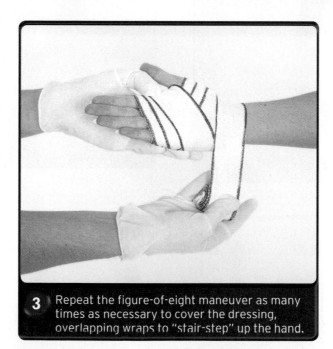

3 Repeat the figure-of-eight maneuver as many times as necessary to cover the dressing, overlapping wraps to "stair-step" up the hand.

skill drill

10-6   Figure-of-Eight Method of Bandaging an Ankle or Foot

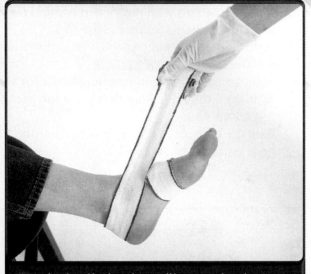

1 Anchor the bandage with one or two turns around the foot. Bring the bandage diagonally across the top of the foot and around the back of the ankle.

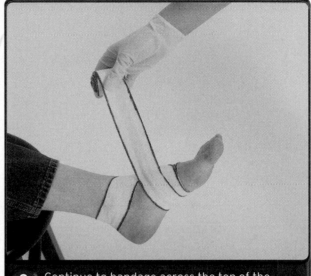

2 Continue to bandage across the top of the foot and underneath the arch of the foot.

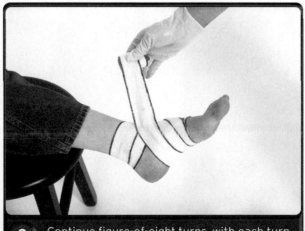

3 Continue figure-of-eight turns, with each turn overlapping the last turn and progressing up the ankle.

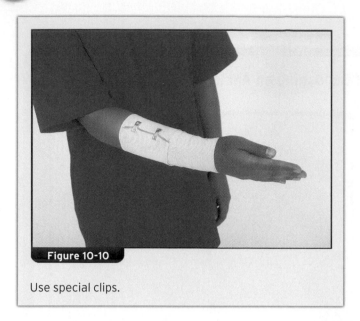

Figure 10-10

Use special clips.

You can also use either the loop or split-tail methods, described in Skill Drills 10-7 and 10-8. To perform the loop method, follow the steps in **Skill Drill 10-7**:

1. Reverse the direction of the bandage by looping it around a thumb or finger and continue back to the opposite side of the body part (**Step ❶**).
2. Encircle the part with the looped end and the free end and tie them together (**Step ❷**).

To perform the split-tail method of securing a bandage, follow the steps in **Skill Drill 10-8**:

1. Split the end of the bandage lengthwise for about 12 inches, then tie a knot to prevent further splitting (**Step ❶**).
2. Pass the ends in opposite directions around the body part and tie (**Step ❷**).

skill drill

10-7 | Loop Method of Securing Bandages

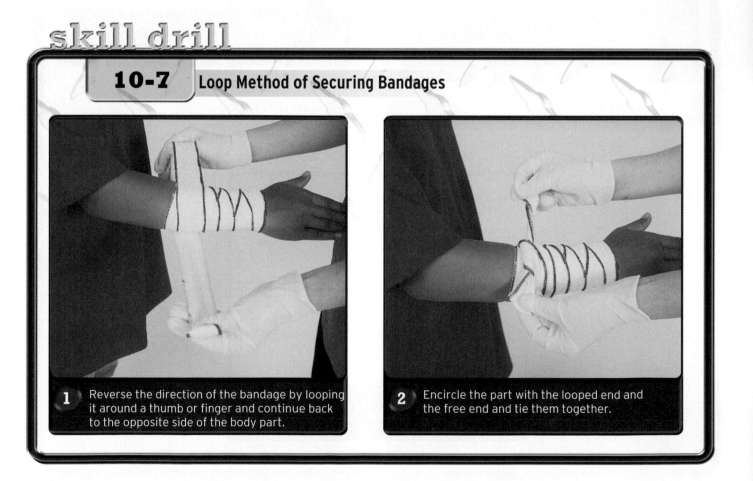

1 Reverse the direction of the bandage by looping it around a thumb or finger and continue back to the opposite side of the body part.

2 Encircle the part with the looped end and the free end and tie them together.

skill drill

10-8 | Split-Tail Method

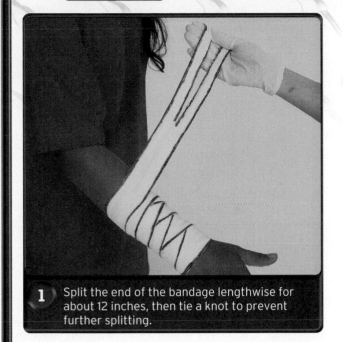

1 Split the end of the bandage lengthwise for about 12 inches, then tie a knot to prevent further splitting.

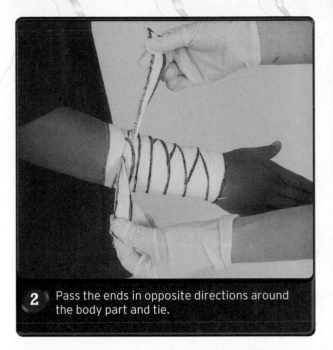

2 Pass the ends in opposite directions around the body part and tie.

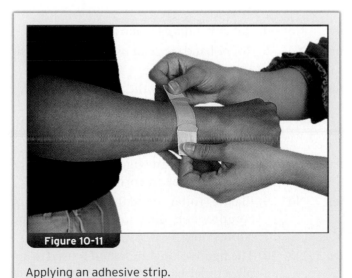

Figure 10-11

Applying an adhesive strip.

Applying an Adhesive Strip

1. Remove the wrapping and hold the dressing, pad-side down, by the protective strips **Figure 10-11** .
2. Peel back, but do not remove, the protective strips. Without touching the dressing pad, place it directly onto the wound.
3. Carefully pull away the protective strips. Press the ends and edges down.

FYI

Adhesive Strip Bandage

To make an adhesive strip bandage snug on a chin, knee, or elbow, first cut the adhesive parts of the bandage lengthwise, but do not cut into the pad. Place the pad horizontally over the cut or wound. Then bring the bottom strips of the adhesive strip up and smooth them on the skin. Bring the top parts of the adhesive strips down and smooth them on the skin. Result: An adhesive bandage that contours to the wound.

prep kit

▶ Ready for Review

- A dressing covers an open wound; it touches the wound.
- Dressing used in most first aid situations are commercially prepared, but dressings may need to be improvised.
- A bandage should be clean but need not be sterile.
- The basic types of bandages are roller bandages; self-adhering, conforming bandages; gauze rollers; elastic roller bandages; triangular bandages; adhesive tape; and adhesive strips.
- With a little ingenuity, you can apply a roller bandage to almost any body part.

▶ Vital Vocabulary

<u>adhesive strips</u> A combination of both a sterile dressing and a bandage.

<u>adhesive tape</u> Come in rolls and in a variety of widths.

<u>elastic roller bandages</u> Used for compression on sprains, strains, and contusions and come in various widths.

<u>gauze pads</u> Used for small wounds, sterile, and available in separately wrapped packages of various sizes. Some have a special coating to keep them from sticking to the wound.

<u>gauze rollers</u> Cotton, rigid, and nonelastic that come in various widths.

<u>roller bandages</u> Come in various widths, lengths, and types of material.

<u>self-adhering, conforming bandages</u> Come as rolls of slightly elastic, gauzelike material in various widths.

<u>trauma dressings</u> Made of large, thick, absorbent, sterile materials.

<u>triangular bandages</u> Available commercially or can be made from a 36- to 40-inch square of preshrunk cotton muslin material.

▶ Assessment in Action

It is a bright and sunny spring day, so you and your friend decide to take a hike in the local nature reserve. You pack a first aid kit, water, and a sweater in your hiking pack. You and your friend have a great time hiking through the forest and climbing rocks. Toward the end of the day, your friend slips while climbing a rock. You hurry over and find her clutching her arm, which is bleeding.

Directions: Circle Yes if you agree with the statement, circle No if you disagree.

Yes No 1. The first thing that you should do is wash your hands in the nearby stream and apply your medical gloves.

Yes No 2. You should place the dressing around the wound, not directly on it.

Yes No 3. After applying the bandage, you see that your friend's fingers are blue. This is a sign that you applied the bandage correctly.

Yes No 4. You can use the spiral method to apply a roller bandage to the arm.

Yes No 5. You should use the slip knot to secure the bandage.

Answers: **1.** Yes; **2.** No; **3.** No; **4.** Yes; **5.** No

▶ Check Your Knowledge

Directions: Circle Yes if you agree with the statement, circle No if you disagree.

Yes No 1. A dressing does not touch an open wound.

Yes No 2. Adhesive strips are used for small cuts and abrasions.

Yes No 3. A bandage should be clean but need not be sterile.

Yes No 4. Roller bandages come in only one size.

Yes No 5. Roller bandages can only be used on the arm.

Yes No 6. A square knot is the preferred knot for bandages.

Yes No 7. Check the lips for signs of a too tight bandage.

Yes No 8. If the victim can wiggle her fingers, the bandage is not on correctly.

Yes No 9. Elastic roller bandages are used for compression on sprains, strains, and contusions.

Yes No 10. The figure-of-eight method is used to apply a roller bandage to hold dressings or to provide compression at or near a joint.

Answers: **1.** No; **2.** Yes; **3.** Yes; **4.** No; **5.** No; **6.** Yes; **7.** No; **8.** No; **9.** Yes; **10.** Yes

Burns

Burns

An estimated 2 million burn injuries occur each year in the United States, resulting in 75,000 hospitalizations and more than 3,000 deaths. <u>Burns</u> occur in every age group, across all socioeconomic levels, at home and in the workplace, and in urban, suburban, and rural settings. It has been estimated that about 70% of all burn injuries occur in the home, with house fires responsible for the majority of fire deaths. Most burn victims are injured as a result of their own actions.

The highest-risk age groups for burn injuries are children younger than 5 years and adults older than 55 years. Both groups may have limited ability to recognize and escape from a fire or burn incident. In addition, their relatively thinner skin predisposes them to more serious injuries. Death and complications increase dramatically for burn victims older than 55 years owing to the likelihood of preexisting health problems and their immune system's decreased ability to fight infection.

Skin death and injury occur as the applied heat exceeds the body's ability to disperse the heat; that point starts at about 113° F. The amount and depth of skin damage depend on the heat's intensity, the duration of contact, and the skin's thickness.

▶ Types of Burns

Burn injuries can be classified as thermal (heat), chemical, or electrical.

- Not all <u>thermal (heat) burns</u> are caused by flames. Contact with hot objects, flammable vapor that ignites and causes a flash or an explosion, and steam and hot liquid are other common causes of burns. Just 3 seconds of exposure to water at 140° F can cause a full-thickness (third-degree) burn in an adult. At 156° F, the same burn occurs in 1 second.

- **Chemical burns.** A wide range of chemical agents can cause tissue damage and death on contact with the skin. As with thermal burns, the amount of tissue damage depends on the duration of contact, the skin thickness in the area of exposure, and the strength of the chemical agent. Chemicals will continue to cause tissue destruction until the chemical agent is removed. Three types of chemicals—acids, alkalis, and organic compounds—are responsible for most chemical burns. Alkalis produce deeper, more extensive burns than acids.
- **Electrical burns.** The injury severity from contact with electric current depends on the type of current (direct or alternating), the voltage, the area of the body exposed, and the duration of contact. Electricity can induce ventricular fibrillation (a type of cardiac arrest), cause respiratory arrest, or "freeze" the victim to the electrical contact point with powerful muscle spasms that increase the length of exposure. Victims of low-voltage electrical injuries may have no skin burns at all but might still have cardiac or respiratory arrest.

Thermal Burns

Evaluate a thermal burn using the following steps. These steps form the basis for treatment of thermal burns.

1. Determine the depth (degree) of the burn. Historically, burns have been described as first-degree, second-degree, and third-degree injuries. The terms *superficial, partial thickness,* and *full thickness* are often used by burn-care professionals because they are more descriptive of the tissue damage.
   - **First-degree (superficial) burns** affect the skin's outer layer (epidermis) **Figure 11-1** . Characteristics include redness, mild swelling, tenderness, and pain. Healing occurs without scarring, usually within a week. The outer edges of deeper burns often are first-degree burns.
   - **Second-degree (partial-thickness) burns** extend through the entire outer layer and into the inner skin layer **Figure 11-2** . Blisters, swelling, weeping of fluids, and severe pain characterize these burns, which occur because the capillary blood vessels in the dermis are damaged and give up fluid into surrounding tissues. Intact blisters provide a sterile, waterproof covering.

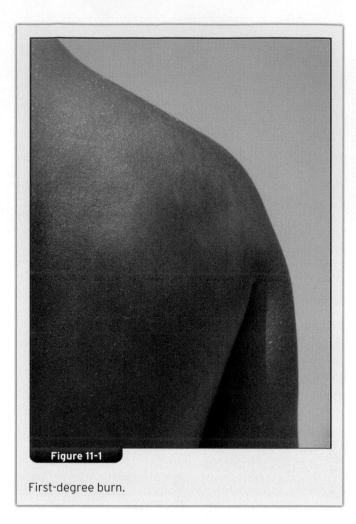

Figure 11-1

First-degree burn.

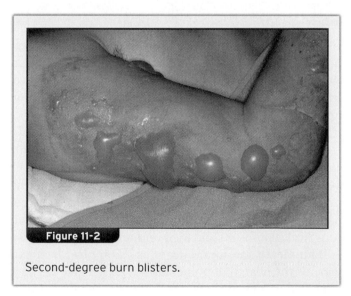

Figure 11-2

Second-degree burn blisters.

Once a blister breaks, a weeping wound results, and the risk of infection increases.
   - **Third-degree (full-thickness) burns** are severe burns that penetrate all the skin layers into the

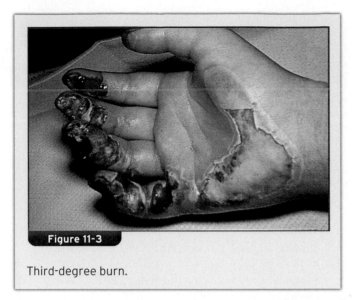

Figure 11-3

Third-degree burn.

underlying fat and muscle **Figure 11-3** . The skin looks leathery, waxy, or pearly gray and sometimes charred. It has a dry appearance because capillary blood vessels have been destroyed and no more fluid is brought to the area. The skin does not blanch after being pressed because the area is dead. The victim feels no pain from a third-degree burn because the nerve endings have been damaged or destroyed. Any pain felt is from surrounding burns of lesser degrees. A third-degree burn requires medical care and the removal of dead tissue and often a skin graft to heal properly.

2. Determine the extent of the burn. Skin will not ignite unless heated to thousands of degrees. However, if clothing ignites or skin is kept in contact with a heat source, such as scalding water, large areas of the skin will be injured. Determining the extent of a burn means estimating how much body surface area the burn covers. A rough guide known as the *Rule of Nines* **Figure 11-4** assigns a percentage value of total body surface area (BSA) to each part of an adult's body. The entire head is 9%, one complete arm is 9%, the front torso is 18%, the complete back is 18%, and each leg is 18%. The Rule of Nines must be modified to take into account the different proportions of a small child. In small children and infants, the head accounts for 18% and each leg is 14%. For small or scattered burns, use the *Rule of the Palm* **Figure 11-5** . The victim's hand, excluding the fingers and the thumb, represents about 1% of his or her total body surface. For a very large burn, estimate the unburned area in number of hands and subtract from 100%.

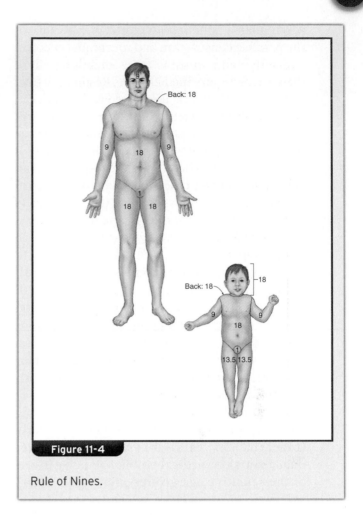

Figure 11-4

Rule of Nines.

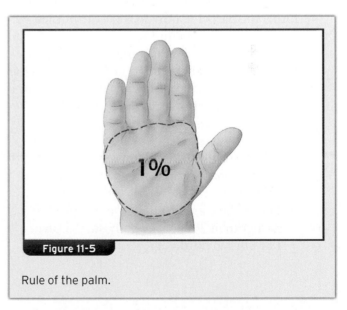

Figure 11-5

Rule of the palm.

3. Determine which parts of the body are burned. Burns on the face, hands, feet, and genitals are more severe than on other body parts. A circumferential burn (one that goes around a finger, toe, arm, leg, neck, or chest) is considered more

severe than a noncircumferential one because of the possible constriction and tourniquet effect on circulation and, in some cases, breathing. All of these burns require medical care. Respiratory tract damage caused by heat associated with a burn can cause death after a victim is hospitalized. Respiratory damage may result from breathing heat or the products of combustion, from being burned by a flame while in a closed space, or from being in an explosion. In these cases, even with no skin burn injury, there may be respiratory damage. Superheated air will be absorbed by the upper respiratory tract (the area from the nose to the trachea), resulting in inflammation. Swelling occurs in 2 to 24 hours, restricting or completely shutting off the airway so that air cannot reach the lungs. All respiratory injuries must receive medical care. Burns can aggravate existing medical conditions such as diabetes, heart disease, and lung disease, as well as other medical problems. Concurrent injuries such as fractures, internal injuries, and open wounds increase the severity of a burn.

4. Determine whether other injuries or preexisting medical problems exist or if the victim is elderly (older than 55 years) or very young (younger than 5 years). A medical problem or being in one of the sensitive age groups increases a burn's severity.

5. Determine the burn's severity (Table 11-1). This forms the basis for how to treat the burned victim. Most burns are minor, occur at home, and can be managed outside a medical setting. Seek medical care for all moderate and severe burns, as classified by the American Burn Association, or if any of the following conditions applies:
   - The victim has difficulty breathing.
   - Other injuries exist.
   - An electrical injury exists.
   - The face, hands, feet, or genitals are burned.
   - Child abuse is suspected.
   - The surface area of a second-degree burn is greater than 20% of the body surface area.
   - The burn is third degree.

CAUTION

DO NOT remove clothing stuck to the skin. Cut around the areas where clothing sticks to the skin.

DO NOT pull on stuck clothing; pulling will further damage the skin.

Table 11-1   Burn Severity

Minor Burns
- First-degree burn covering less than 50% BSA* in adults (face, hands, feet, and genitals not burned)†
- Second-degree burn covering less than 15% BSA in adults
- Second-degree burn covering less than 10% BSA in children and elderly persons
- Third-degree burn covering less than 2% BSA in adults (face, hands, feet, and genitals not burned)

Moderate Burns
- First-degree burn covering more than 50% BSA in adults
- Second-degree burn covering 15% to 30% BSA in adults†
- Second-degree burn covering 10% to 20% BSA in children and elderly persons
- Third-degree burn covering 2% to 10% BSA in adults (face, hands, and feet not burned)

Critical Burns
- Second-degree burn covering more than 30% BSA in adults
- Second-degree burn covering more than 20% BSA in children and elderly persons
- Third-degree burn covering more than 10% BSA in adults
- Third-degree burn covering more than 2% BSA in children and elderly persons
- Third-degree burns of hands, face, eyes, feet, or genitalia; also most inhalation injuries, electrical injuries, and burns accompanied by major trauma or significant preexisting conditions

Source: Adapted from the American Burn Association categorization.
†Criteria for children have not been established. If in doubt, consult a medical professional.

Care for Thermal Burns

Burn care aims to reduce pain, protect against infection, and prevent evaporation (Table 11-2). Because burns can continue to injure tissue for a surprisingly long time, it is critical to stop the burning. If clothing is burning, have the victim roll on the ground using the "stop, drop, and roll" method. Smother the flames with a blanket or douse the victim with water. Stop a person whose clothes are on fire from running, which only fans the flames. The victim should not remain standing, because he or she is more apt to inhale flames. Once the fire is extinguished, remove all hot or smoldering clothing because the burning may continue if the clothing is left on. If possible, remove jewelry because heat may be held near the skin and cause more damage and swelling could make jewelry difficult to remove later. Monitor the victim's breathing.

Table 11-2   First Aid for Burns

Type of Burn	Do . . .	Don't . . .
First-degree burn (redness, mild swelling, and pain)	Apply cold water and, after cooled, apply aloe vera gel or a body lotion.	Apply butter, oleomargarine, or similar substances.
Second-degree burn (deeper injury; blisters develop)	Apply cold water. After cooled, apply antibiotic ointment. Treat for shock.	Break blisters. Remove shreds of tissue. Use a home remedy.
Third-degree burn (deeper destruction; skin layers destroyed)	Cover the burn with a sterile cloth to protect it. Treat the victim for shock. Watch for breathing difficulty. Obtain medical attention quickly.	Remove charred clothing that is stuck to the burn. Apply ice. Use a home medication.
Chemical burn	Remove chemical by flushing with large quantities of water for at least 20 minutes or longer. Remove surrounding clothing. Quickly obtain medical care.	Apply water under high pressure. Try to neutralize with other chemicals.

Care of First-Degree Burns

1. Immerse the burned area in cold water **Figure 11-6** or apply a wet, cold cloth to reduce pain. Apply cold until the part is pain free while in and out of the water (usually in 10 minutes, but it may take up to 45 minutes). Cold also stops the progression of the burn into deeper tissue. If cold water is unavailable, use any cold, drinkable liquid to reduce the temperature of the burned skin.

2. Give ibuprofen to relieve pain and inflammation.

3. Have the victim drink as much water as possible without becoming nauseous.

4. After the burn has been cooled, apply an aloe vera gel or an inexpensive skin moisturizer lotion to keep the skin moistened and to reduce itching and peeling. Use a lotion that does not have alcohols or strong fragrances. Lotions with glycerin and mineral oil are best. Aloe vera has antimicrobial and anti-inflammatory properties and is a mild analgesic.

5. Keep a burned arm or leg raised to reduce swelling and pain.

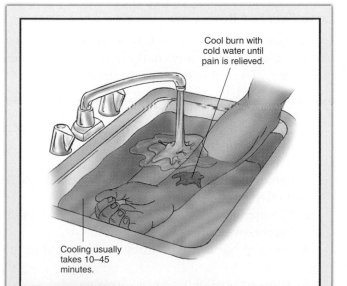

Cool burn with cold water until pain is relieved.

Cooling usually takes 10–45 minutes.

Figure 11-6

Immerse the burn. Cool burn with cold water until pain is relieved. Cooling usually takes 10–45 minutes.

CAUTION

DO NOT apply cold to more than 20% of an adult's body surface (10% for children). Widespread cooling can cause hypothermia. Burn victims lose large amounts of heat and water.

DO NOT use an ice pack unless it is the only source of cold. If you must use one, apply it for only 10 to 15 minutes.

DO NOT apply grease, butter, cream, or a home remedy. Such coatings are unsterile and can lead to infection. They also can seal in heat, causing further damage.

DO NOT cover a first-degree burn.

DO NOT use anesthetic sprays because they may sensitize the skin to "-caine" anesthetics.

Care of Small Second-Degree Burns (<20% BSA)

1. Immerse the burned area in cold water or apply a wet, cold cloth to reduce pain. Apply cold until the part is pain free while in and out of the water (usually in 10 minutes, but it may take up to 45 minutes). Cold also stops the progression of the burn into deeper tissue. If cold water is unavailable, use any cold, drinkable liquid to reduce the temperature of the burned skin.
2. Give ibuprofen to relieve pain and inflammation.
3. Have the victim drink as much water as possible without becoming nauseated.
4. After a burn has been cooled, apply a thin layer of an antibiotic ointment. Topical antibiotic therapy does not sterilize a wound, but it decreases the number of bacteria to a level that can be controlled by the body's defense mechanisms and prevents the entrance of bacteria. Physicians may prescribe a silver-based antibiotic, which is the agent of choice for burn wounds.
5. Cover the burn with a dry, nonsticking, sterile dressing or a clean cloth. Covering the burn reduces the amount of pain by keeping air from the exposed nerve endings. The main purpose of a dressing over a burn is to keep the burn clean, prevent evaporative moisture loss, and reduce pain. If fingers or toes have been burned, place dry dressings between them.
6. Seek medical care for second-degree burns covering more than 20% of the BSA in adults or 10% to 20% in children or elderly victims.

Care for Large Second-Degree Burns (>20% BSA)

1. Do not apply cold because it could cause hypothermia.
2. Follow steps 2 and 3 for first-degree and small second-degree burn care.

FYI

Burned Tongue

A few grains of sugar sprinkled on the tongue can relieve the misery of a tongue burned by hot food or drink. Repeat as often as needed. Sucking on ice chips or a popsicle can cool the burn.

CAUTION

DO NOT cool more than 20% of an adult's body surface area (10% for a child) except to extinguish flames.

---

3. Cover the burn with a dry, nonstick, sterile, or clean dressing.
4. Care for shock.
5. Seek medical care.

Care for Third-Degree Burns

1. It usually is not necessary to apply cold to third-degree burns because pain is absent. Any pain felt with a third-degree burn comes from accompanying first- and second-degree burns, for which cold applications can be helpful.
2. Cover the burn with a dry, nonsticking, sterile dressing or a clean cloth.
3. Treat the victim for shock by elevating the legs and keeping the victim warm with a clean sheet or blanket.
4. Seek medical care.

CAUTION

DO NOT break any blisters. Intact blisters serve as excellent burn dressings. Cover a ruptured blister with an antibiotic ointment and a dry, sterile dressing.

DO NOT apply cold over a large area because it can induce hypothermia.

DO NOT use plastic as a dressing because it will trap moisture and provide a good place for bacteria to grow (its only advantage is that it will not stick to the burn).

Later Thermal Burn Care

For after-thermal burn care, follow a physician's recommendations, if there are any (many burns are never seen by a doctor). The following suggestions may apply:

- Wash hands thoroughly before changing any dressing.
- Leave unbroken blisters intact.
- Change dressings once or twice a day unless a physician instructs otherwise.

To change a dressing:

1. Remove the old dressing. If a dressing sticks, soak it off with cool, clean water.
2. Cleanse the area gently with mild soap and water.
3. Pat the area dry with a clean cloth.
4. Apply a thin layer of antibiotic ointment to the burn.
5. Apply a nonsticking sterile dressing.

Watch for signs of infection. Call a physician if any of these appear:

- Increased redness, pain, tenderness, swelling, or red streaks near the burn

• Pus
• Elevated temperature (fever)

Keep the area and dressing as clean and dry as possible. Elevate the burned area, if possible, for the first 24 hours. Give pain medication, if necessary.

Scald Burns

Scald burns are the result of contact with hot liquids. Scald burns can be divided into two types: immersion burns and spill burns. An *immersion burn* results when an area of the body is fully immersed in a hot liquid. It generally has definite demarcations between healthy and injured tissue. This type of burn tends to be deep and is often full thickness. This type of injury is generally caused by abuse and is seen most often in children.

A *spill burn* occurs when a liquid spills, drops, or is thrown on a person. The pattern of this type of burn generally is irregular and may be scattered across large body areas. A spill burn usually is not as deep as an immersion burn.

Neglect and lack of supervision of children in the kitchen and the bathtub are frequent causes of spill burns. Scalds in adults occur more often in the elderly population, who generally have decreased sensation. As a result, many elderly victims are scalded in the bath.

Sunburn

Sunburn is the skin's response to the trauma of ultraviolet (UV) radiation that results mainly from exposure to UVB radiation or, rarely, to UVA radiation. Sunburn may be the most common burn suffered by humans, and probably all persons have had one at some time **Figure 11-7**. True sunburn reaction begins 2 to 8 hours after UV radiation exposure. The amount of UV light the skin has received is difficult to gauge accurately. Not until after exposure (4 to 12 hours later) does the redness, tenderness, and discomfort of sunburned skin confirm the overexposure. Painful blistering and swelling peak about 24 hours later.

Sunburn results in first- or second-degree burns. A third-degree burn can occur from a sunburn, but it is rare. The redness of a sunburn is caused by the dilation of the small blood vessels. Blister formation comes from plasma leakage.

Human skin displays marked differences in its response to UV radiation exposure. Some individuals always burn and never tan, while others rarely experience a painful sunburn. The variability is largely attributed to the degree of pigmentation (melanin) that the skin contains. Darker-hued individuals generally are more resistant to the sun's rays than are those with light complexions, but all human beings eventually will burn if exposed to enough UVB. Other variables that contribute to individual sensitivity include the area of the body exposed, the underlying condition of the skin, the degree of tanning, and the role of various photosensitizing medicines.

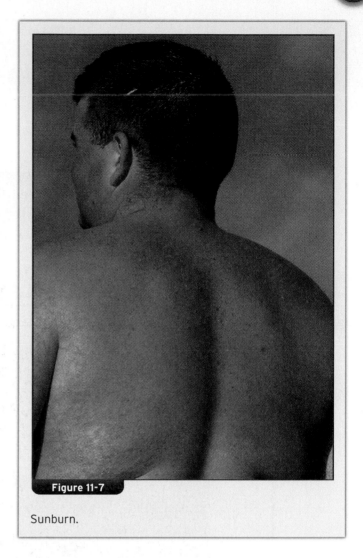

Figure 11-7

Sunburn.

Various skin types respond differently to UV light:
• Type I skin always burns easily and never tans. A type I person normally has blue eyes, red hair, and freckles.
• Type II skin burns easily, tans slightly.
• Type III skin sometimes burns, but always tans gradually and moderately.
• Type IV skin minimally burns and always tans well. Examples of people with type IV skin are people of Hispanic or Asian descent.
• Type V skin rarely burns and tans deeply. Examples of people with type V skin are Middle Easterners and Indians (heavily pigmented).
• Type VI skin does not burn (although it can burn or peel with significant exposure). An example of people with type VI skin is people of African descent (deeply pigmented).

Thermal Burns

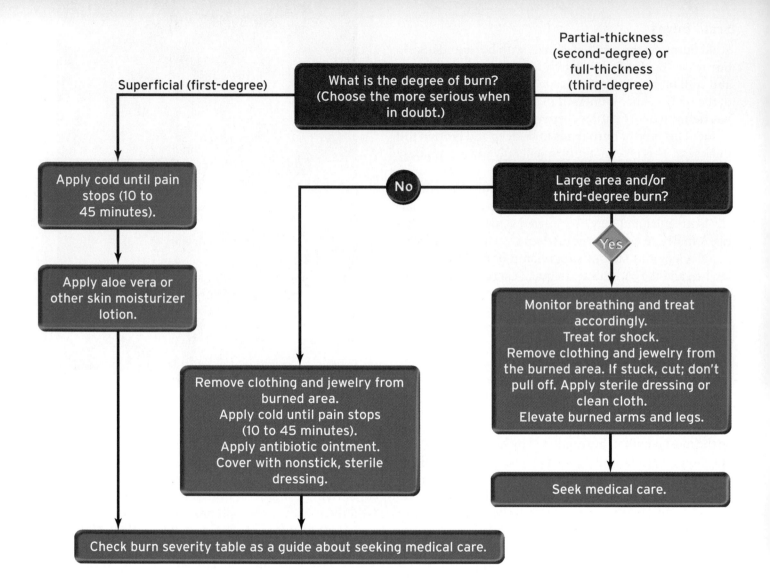

What is the degree of burn? (Choose the more serious when in doubt.)

Superficial (first-degree)

Partial-thickness (second-degree) or full-thickness (third-degree)

Apply cold until pain stops (10 to 45 minutes).

Apply aloe vera or other skin moisturizer lotion.

No

Large area and/or third-degree burn?

Yes

Remove clothing and jewelry from burned area.
Apply cold until pain stops (10 to 45 minutes).
Apply antibiotic ointment.
Cover with nonstick, sterile dressing.

Monitor breathing and treat accordingly.
Treat for shock.
Remove clothing and jewelry from the burned area. If stuck, cut; don't pull off. Apply sterile dressing or clean cloth.
Elevate burned arms and legs.

Seek medical care.

Check burn severity table as a guide about seeking medical care.

Care for Sunburns

1. Cool compresses for up to 45 minutes are quite soothing to sunburned skin. Frequent cool showers or soaking in a tub may provide remarkable relief. Some experts advise against the use of topical analgesics, sprays, or lotions, especially those containing benzocaine. Benzocaine may sensitize the skin, resulting in contact dermatitis that compounds the original problem. Topical anesthetic sprays or lotions may provide temporary relief, but they are expensive and generally ineffective. Over-the-counter (OTC) analgesics such as ibuprofen should suffice in most cases because they reduce pain and inflammation. Drinking lots of water is also suggested.
2. First- and second-degree sunburns can be quite painful. When a large area of skin is involved, the individual may feel ill and have chills and fever. After the pain of a first-degree sunburn has subsided, the use of aloe vera or another body lotion can keep the skin moist. Do not use butter or petroleum jelly.

Sunburn Aftercare

For aftercare of a second-degree sunburn, apply antibiotic (available as an OTC medication) ointment in a thin layer. It is inexpensive, antimicrobial, widely available, easily applied, and adheres even to exposed areas such as the face. If blisters break, gently wash the area twice daily with soap and water and then cover with an antibiotic ointment and sterile gauze to prevent infection. If the burn becomes infected, seek medical care. If the eyes are affected, seek medical care.

FYI

Windburn resembles a first-degree sunburn. A greasy sunscreen can be used to prevent and treat it.

CAUTION

DO NOT use topical OTC burn ointments or sprays or anesthetic sprays because

- Some products may cause allergic reactions.
- Most do not contain enough benzocaine or lidocaine to suppress pain.
- The duration of any possible relief is relatively short (30 to 40 minutes). More than three or four applications per day of products containing local anesthetics is discouraged because toxic effects can occur if the agents are used too frequently.
- They seal in the heat.
- They are expensive.

FYI

Sunburn Prevention

The best protection against the damaging effects of UV radiation is to limit exposure to sunlight. That is done most easily with protective clothing, such as hats, long-sleeved shirts, and long pants. Wet, white cotton will transmit UV radiation light, so persons can be sunburned while wearing such clothing. People should avoid prolonged exposure during times of the day when radiation is most intense (usually between 10 AM and 2 PM) and apply effective sunscreens.

Sunscreens are readily available and offer the best protection against sunburn, skin cancers, and other long-term skin injury. The proper use of sunscreens will protect an individual from the harmful effects of the sun. Sunscreens must be applied correctly, which generally means applying the sunscreen at least 20 minutes before you go out, so it will "bond" to your skin, and reapplying it every few hours. Use waterproof sunscreen if you sweat a lot or if you are will be in and out of the water. It is important to note that sunscreens do not promote tanning; they do, however, allow the user to tan gradually without serious burning.

To help consumers select an effective sunscreen, the system of rating products by the *skin protection factor (SPF)* has been developed. The higher the SPF number, the greater the protection against sunburn. However, a sunscreen that has an SPF of 30 is not twice as good as one with an SPF of 15. An SPF of 15 blocks out 95% of the most harmful rays; a sunscreen with an SPF of 30 gives you only another 3% of protection. Because most people usually use only half the amount of sunscreen that is effective, using a sunscreen with an SPF of 15 probably affords protection equivalent to a sunscreen with an SPF of 7.5. If they use a sunscreen with a 30 SPF, they are probably getting the protection of a 15 SPF sunscreen.

Many "suntan lotions" have no sunscreen effect and serve only to keep the skin moist. Products such as baby oil and cocoa butter offer little protection against serious sunburn and may actually enhance burning.

Chemical Burns

A *chemical burn* is the result of a caustic or corrosive substance touching the skin **Figure 11-8**. Because chemicals continue to "burn" as long as they are in contact with the skin, they should be removed from the victim as rapidly as possible.

First aid is the same for all chemical burns. Alkalis such as drain cleaners cause more serious burns than acids such as battery acid because they penetrate deeper and remain active longer. Organic compounds such as petroleum products are also capable of burning.

Care for Chemical Burns

1. Immediately remove the chemical by flushing the body portion with water **Figure 11-9**. If available, use a hose or a shower. Brush dry powder chemicals from the skin before flushing. Water may activate a dry chemical and cause more damage to the skin. Take precautions to protect yourself from exposure to the chemical.
2. Remove the victim's contaminated clothing and jewelry while flushing with water. Clothing can hold chemicals, allowing them to continue to burn as long as they are in contact with the skin.
3. Flush for 20 minutes or longer. Let the victim wash with a mild soap before a final rinse. Washing with large amounts of water dilutes the chemical concentration and washes it away.
4. Cover the burned area with a dry, sterile dressing or, for large areas, a clean lint-free cloth, such as a pillowcase.
5. If the chemical is in an eye, flood it for at least 20 minutes, using low pressure.
6. Seek medical care immediately for all chemical burns.

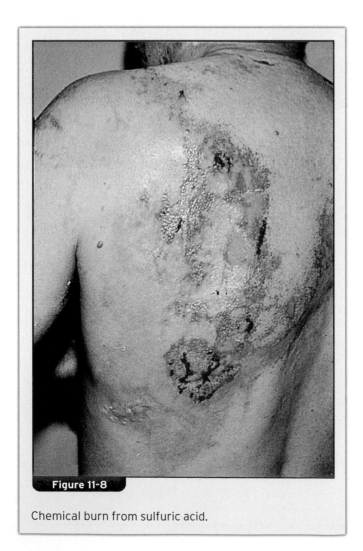

Figure 11-8

Chemical burn from sulfuric acid.

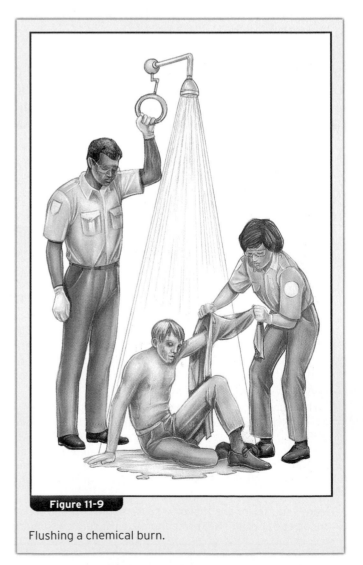

Figure 11-9

Flushing a chemical burn.

Chemical Burns

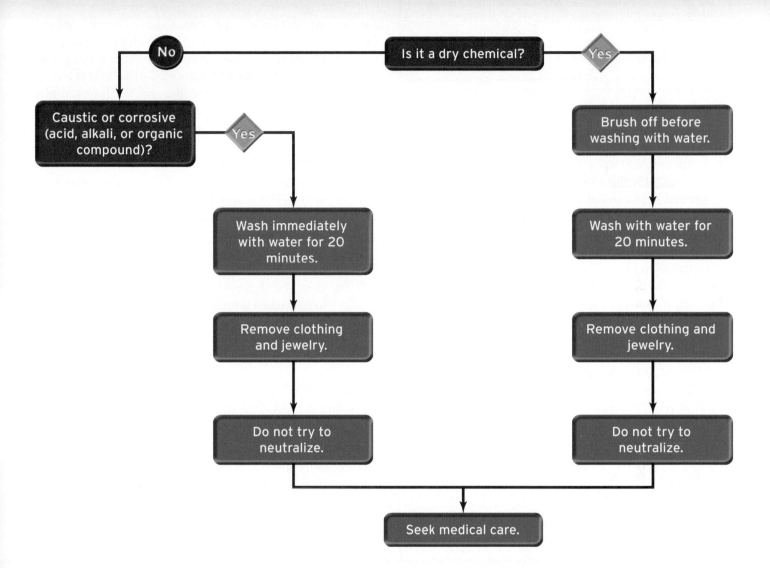

Is it a dry chemical?

No → Caustic or corrosive (acid, alkali, or organic compound)?

Yes (from Caustic or corrosive) → Wash immediately with water for 20 minutes. → Remove clothing and jewelry. → Do not try to neutralize.

Yes (Is it a dry chemical?) → Brush off before washing with water. → Wash with water for 20 minutes. → Remove clothing and jewelry. → Do not try to neutralize.

Seek medical care.

CAUTION

DO NOT waste time! A chemical burn is an emergency!

DO NOT apply water under high pressure; it will drive the chemical deeper into the tissue.

DO NOT try to neutralize a chemical even if you know which chemical is involved; heat may be produced, resulting in more damage. Some product labels for neutralizing may be wrong. Save the container or the label for the chemical's name.

Electrical Burns

Even a mild electrical shock can cause serious internal injuries **Figure 11-10**. A current of 1,000 volts or more is considered high voltage, but even the 110 volts found in ordinary household current can be deadly. There are three types of electrical injuries: thermal burn (flame), arc burn (flash), and true electrical injury (contact). A *thermal burn* (flame) results when clothing or objects in direct contact with the skin are ignited by an electric current. These injuries are caused by the flames produced by the electric current and not by the passage of the electric current or arc.

An *arc burn* (flash) occurs when electricity jumps, or arcs, from one spot to another and not from the passage of an electric current through the body. Although the duration of the flash may be brief, it usually causes extensive superficial injuries.

A true *electrical injury* (contact) happens when an electric current passes directly through the body. This type of injury is characterized by an entrance wound and an exit wound. The important factor with this type

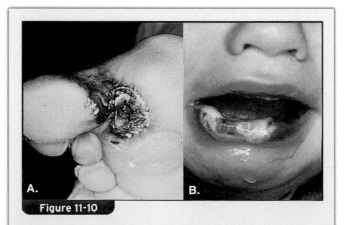

Figure 11-10

Electrical burns. **A.** Exit wound on a toe. **B.** Electrical burn caused by chewing through an electrical cord.

of injury is that the surface injury may be just the tip of the iceberg. High-voltage electric currents passing through the body may disrupt the normal heart rhythm and cause cardiac arrest, internal burns, and other injuries.

During an electrical shock, electricity enters the body at the point of contact and travels along the path of least resistance (nerves and blood vessels). The major damage occurs inside the body—the outside burn may appear small. Usually, the electricity exits where the body is touching a surface or is in contact with a ground (for example, a metal object). Sometimes, a victim has more than one exit site.

Care for Electrical Burns

1. Make sure the area is safe. Unplug, disconnect, or turn off the power. If that is impossible, call 9-1-1 for help. Never touch an energized wire, object, or victim yourself.
2. Monitor breathing and treat accordingly.
3. If the victim fell, check for a spinal injury.
4. Treat the victim for shock by elevating the legs 6 to 12 inches if no spinal injury is suspected.
5. Place blankets under and over the victim.
6. Seek medical care immediately. Electrical injuries may require treatment in a burn center.

Contact With an Outdoor Power Line

If the electrical shock is from contact with a downed power line, the power must be turned off before a rescuer approaches anyone who may be in contact with the wire. If a power line falls across a car containing a person, tell the person to stay in the car until the power can be shut off. The only exception is if fire threatens the car. In that case, tell the victim to jump out of the car without making contact with the car or the wire.

If you feel a tingling sensation in your legs and lower body as you approach a victim, stop. The sensation signals that you are on energized ground and that an electric current is entering through one foot, passing through your lower body, and leaving through the other foot. Raise one foot off the ground, turn around, and hop to a safe place.

If you can safely reach the victim, do not attempt to move any wires, even with wooden poles, tools with wood handles, or tree branches. Wood can conduct electricity and the rescuer will be electrocuted. Do *not* attempt to move downed wires unless you are trained and are equipped with tools able to handle the high voltage. Wait until trained personnel with the proper equipment can cut the wires or disconnect them. Prevent bystanders from entering the danger area.

Contact Inside Buildings

Most electrical burns that occur indoors are caused by faulty electrical equipment or careless use of electrical appliances. Turn off the electricity at the circuit breaker, fuse box, or outside switch box, or unplug the appliance if the plug is undamaged. Do not touch the appliance or the victim until the current is off.

Once there is no danger to rescuers, first aid can begin. Electric current flows quickly into the body's tissues and then exits. The surface injuries of the skin involve small surface areas (entrance and exit points); the major damage occurs deep under the skin **Figure 11-11** . See Chapter 24 for lightning burns and their care.

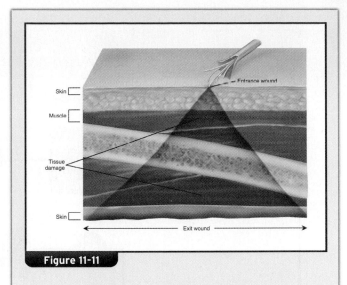

Figure 11-11

The external signs of an electrical burn may be deceiving. The entrance wound may be a small burn, while the damage to the deeper tissue may be massive.

Electrical Burns

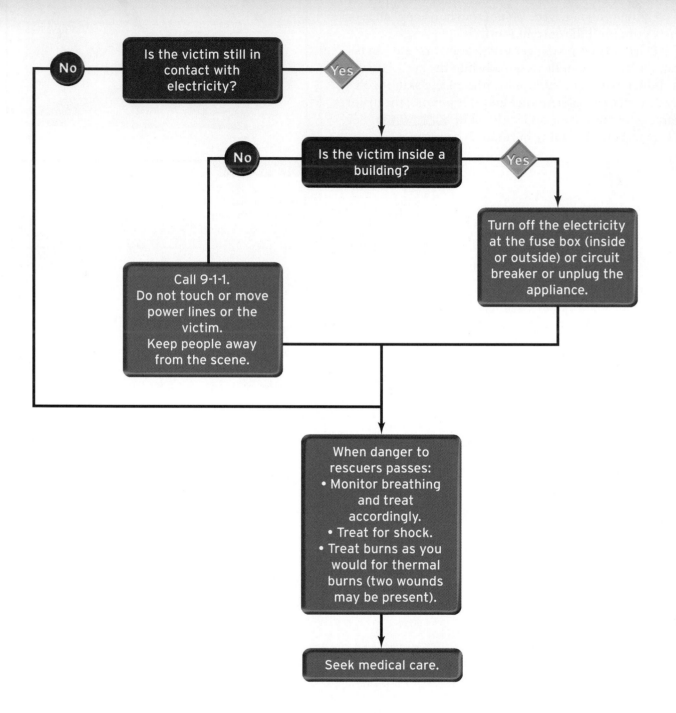

Is the victim still in contact with electricity?

No → Yes →

Is the victim inside a building?

No → Yes →

Turn off the electricity at the fuse box (inside or outside) or circuit breaker or unplug the appliance.

Call 9-1-1.
Do not touch or move power lines or the victim.
Keep people away from the scene.

When danger to rescuers passes:
• Monitor breathing and treat accordingly.
• Treat for shock.
• Treat burns as you would for thermal burns (two wounds may be present).

Seek medical care.

▶ Thermal (Heat) Burns

What to Look For	What to Do

First-degree burn (superficial)

• Redness	Cool the burn with cold water.
• Mild swelling	Apply aloe vera gel or a skin moisturizer.
• Pain	If available, give an OTC medication to reduce pain and swelling.

Second-degree (partial thickness)

• Blisters	If burn is small (<20% of body surface area):
• Swelling	Cool burn with cold water.
• Pain	Apply antibiotic ointment.
• Weeping of fluid	Cover with a dry, nonstick sterile dressing.
	If available, give an OTC medication to reduce pain and swelling.

Third-degree (full thickness)

• Dry, leathery skin	Monitor breathing and provide care as needed.
• Gray or charred skin	Cover burn with a dry, nonstick sterile or clean dressing.
	Care for shock.
	Seek medical care.

▶ Chemical Burns

What to Look For	What to Do
Stinging pain	Brush dry chemicals off skin.
	Flush with a large amount of water for 20 minutes (gentle water flow).
	Remove the victim's contaminated clothing and jewelry while flushing.
	Cover the area with a dry, sterile, or clean dressing.
	Seek medical care.

▶ Electrical Burns

What to Look For	What to Do
Possible third-degree burn with entrance and exit wounds	Safety first! Unplug, disconnect, or turn off the electricity.
	Open the airway, check breathing, and provide care as needed.
	Care for burns as you would a third-degree burn.
	Seek medical care.

prep kit

▶ Ready for Review

- Burns occur in every age group, across all socio-economic levels, at home and in the workplace, and in urban, suburban, and rural settings.
- Burn injuries can be classified as thermal, chemical, or electrical.
- Treatment depends on the depth of thermal burns.
- A chemical burn is the result of a caustic or corrosive substance touching the skin.
- There are three types of electrical injuries: thermal burn (flame), arc burn (flash), and true electrical injury (contact).

▶ Vital Vocabulary

burns Injuries in which soft tissue receives more energy than it can absorb from thermal heat, chemicals, or electricity.

chemical burns Damage caused to the skin by chemicals.

electrical burns Injury caused from contact with electric current.

first-degree (superficial) burns A burn affecting only the epidermis, characterized by skin that is red but not blistered or burned through.

second-degree (partial-thickness) burns Burns affecting the epidermis and some portion of the dermis but not the subcutaneous tissue. Characterized by blisters and skin that is white to red and moist.

thermal (heat) burns Damage to the skin caused by contact with hot objects, flammable vapor, steam, hot liquid, or flames.

third-degree (full-thickness) burns Burns that affects all skin layers and may affect the subcutaneous layers, muscle, bone, and internal organs, leaving the area dry, leathery, and white, dark brown, or charred.

▶ Assessment in Action

At a fast-food restaurant, a worker is burned on his forearm after bumping into a hot pan on the stove. The burned area is about the width of a tennis ball. Blisters are forming and the worker complains about the pain.

Directions: Circle Yes if you agree with the statement, circle No if you disagree.

Yes   No   1. The size of the burn is probably about 1% of the worker's body surface area.

Yes   No   2. The blisters and pain are signs that the burn is a third-degree burn.

Yes   No   3. Reduce the pain and damage by running cold water over the burned area.

Yes   No   4. An antibiotic ointment can be applied to this burn only after cooling the area.

Yes   No   5. This victim needs medical care.

Answers: 1. Yes; 2. No; 3. Yes; 4. Yes; 5. No

▶ Check Your Knowledge

Directions: Circle Yes if you agree with the statement, circle No if you disagree.

Yes   No   1. Victims of a burn should immediately drink water.

Yes   No   2. Petroleum jelly can be applied over a burn.

Yes   No   3. The rule of the palm determines the size of a burned area.

Yes   No   4. Neutralize an acid on the skin by using baking soda.

Yes   No   5. Use a large amount of water to flush chemicals off the body.

Yes   No   6. Brush a dry chemical off the skin before flushing with water.

Yes   No   7. When someone gets electrocuted, there can be two burn wounds: entrance and exit.

Yes   No   8. When a victim is in contact with a power line, use a tree branch to remove the wires.

Yes   No   9. Ibuprofen helps relieve pain and swelling.

Yes   No   10. Cold water can be used on any burn of any size.

Answers: 1. No; 2. No; 3. Yes; 4. No; 5. Yes; 6. Yes; 7. Yes; 8. No; 9. Yes; 10. No

Head and Spinal Injuries

Head Injuries

Any head injury is potentially serious. If not properly treated, injuries that seem minor could become life threatening. Head injuries include scalp wounds, skull fractures, and brain injuries. Spinal injuries (that is, neck and back injuries) can also be present in head-injured victims.

▶ Scalp Wounds

Scalp wounds bleed profusely because the scalp has a rich blood supply and the blood vessels there do not constrict. A bleeding scalp wound does not affect the blood supply to the brain. The brain obtains its blood supply from arteries in the neck, not the scalp. A severe scalp wound may have an accompanying concussion, skull fracture, an impaled object, or a spinal injury.

Care for Scalp Wounds

1. Control the bleeding by gently applying direct pressure with a dry, sterile or clean dressing. If the dressing becomes blood filled, do not remove it. Add another dressing on top of the first one **Figure 12-1**.
2. If you suspect a skull fracture, apply pressure around the edges of the wound and over a broad area rather than on the center of the wound **Figure 12-2**.

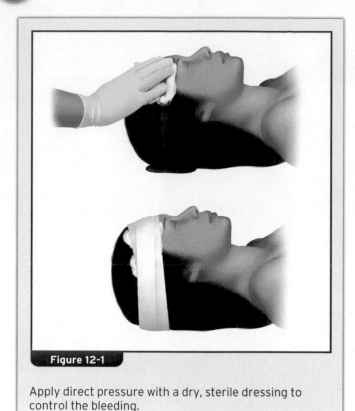

Figure 12-1

Apply direct pressure with a dry, sterile dressing to control the bleeding.

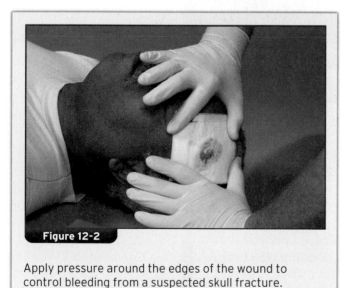

Figure 12-2

Apply pressure around the edges of the wound to control bleeding from a suspected skull fracture.

3. Keep the head and shoulders slightly elevated to help control the bleeding if no spinal injury is suspected.
4. Seek medical care.

▶ Skull Fracture

A **skull fracture** is a break or a crack in the cranium (bony case surrounding the brain). Skull fractures may be open

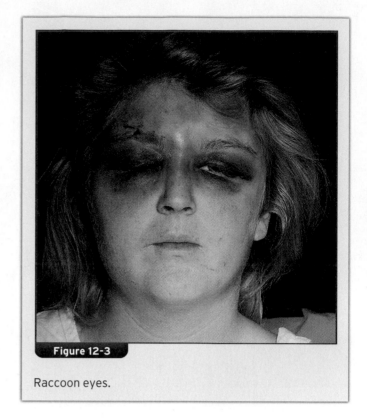

Figure 12-3

Raccoon eyes.

(with an accompanying scalp wound) or closed (without an accompanying scalp wound).

Recognizing Skull Fracture

It is difficult to determine a skull fracture except by X-ray unless the skull deformity is severe. Signs and symptoms of a skull fracture include the following:

- Pain at the point of injury
- Deformity of the skull
- Bleeding from the ears or nose
- Clear, pink, watery cerebrospinal fluid (CSF) leaking from an ear or the nose. A drop of CSF on a handkerchief, pillowcase, or other white or light-colored cloth will form a pink ring around a slightly blood-tinged center, resembling a target; this is called the *halo sign (ring sign)*.
- Discoloration around the eyes ("raccoon eyes") appearing several hours after the injury **Figure 12-3** .
- Discoloration behind an ear (known as **Battle's sign**), appearing several hours after the injury **Figure 12-4** .
- Heavy scalp bleeding if the skin is broken. A scalp wound may expose the skull or brain tissue.
- Penetrating wound such as from a bullet or an impaled object.

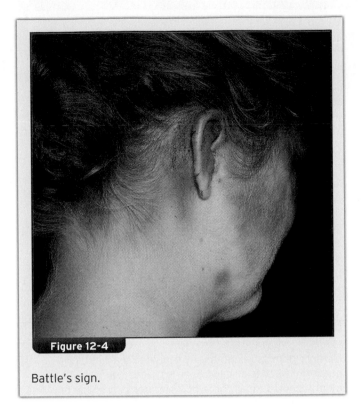

Figure 12-4

Battle's sign.

Care for Skull Fracture

1. Monitor the victim's breathing and provide appropriate care.
2. Stabilize the victim's neck to prevent movement.
3. Slightly elevate the victim's head and shoulders to help control bleeding.
4. Cover the wounds with a sterile dressing.
5. To control bleeding, apply pressure around the edges of the wound, not directly on it.

CAUTION

DO NOT stop the flow of blood or CSF from an ear or nose. Blocking the flow could increase pressure within the skull.

DO NOT remove an impaled object from the head. Stabilize it in place with bulky dressings.

DO NOT clean an open skull fracture; infection of the brain could result.

DO NOT press on the fractured area.

▶ Brain Injuries

It is not injury specifically to the head that causes most short- and long-term problems, but injuries to the brain itself. Most head injuries are a result of motor vehicle crashes and falls. Many of these injuries are minor—shallow lacerations or localized bruising and swelling. However, about 50,000 people die each year in the United States of head trauma, and twice that many have brain injuries that leave them with permanent damage.

The brain is a delicate organ. When the head is struck with sufficient force, the brain bounces against the inside of the skull. Brain injuries can be serious and difficult first aid emergencies to handle. The victim is often confused or unresponsive, making assessment difficult. Many brain injuries are life threatening. Mishandling a victim with a brain injury could result in permanent damage or death.

The brain, like other body tissues, will swell from bleeding when it is injured. Unlike other tissues, however, the brain is confined in the skull where there is little room for swelling. Any swelling of brain tissue or accumulation of blood inside the skull compresses the brain and increases the pressure inside the skull, which interferes with brain functioning. Furthermore, because the skull is hard, the brain and its surface blood vessels may be damaged if they strike the inside of the skull, which can occur when the head is struck directly or is rapidly accelerated or decelerated (such as in a vehicle accident). The phenomenon of a person "seeing stars" when struck on the back of the head results because the occipital lobe of the brain (the part that controls vision) strikes the back of the skull.

The nerve cells of the brain and the spinal cord, unlike most other cells in the body, are unable to regenerate. When those cells die, they are lost forever and cannot be replaced, even by transplantation. Injuries to the brain can be caused by a penetrating foreign object, by bony fragments from a skull fracture, or by the brain striking the inside of the skull after a person's head has hit a stationary object (such as the ground)—a *deceleration injury*—or has been hit by something like a baseball bat or a teammate's knee—an *acceleration injury*. Sometimes there will be two points of injury: one at the point of impact and one where the brain rebounds off the skull on the opposite side.

There are three types of commonly occurring brain injuries. A <u>concussion</u> is temporary loss of brain function, usually without permanent damage Table 12-1 . No bleeding in the brain occurs, and there may not be any external cut or swelling. A person with a concussion can be "knocked out" (unconscious) or have memory loss (amnesia). A concussion can be dangerous even if the person is not knocked out because it affects the brain. The longer the victim is unconscious or the longer the memory loss lasts, the more serious the concussion. Concussions usually are not serious, but occasionally they can result in permanent damage to the brain and even cause death.

Table 12-1   Management of Concussion in Sports

Grades of Concussion
Grade 1
1. Transient confusion (inattention, inability to maintain a coherent stream of thought and carry out goal-directed movements)
2. No loss of consciousness
3. Concussion symptoms or mental status abnormalities resolve in less than 15 minutes.

Grade 2
1. Transient confusion
2. No loss of consciousness
3. Concussion symptoms or mental status abnormalities (including amnesia) last more than 15 minutes.

Grade 3
1. Any loss of consciousness
   a. Brief (seconds)
   b. Prolonged (minutes)

Management Recommendations
Grade 1
1. Remove from contest.
2. Examine immediately and at 5-minute intervals for the development of mental status abnormalities or postconcussive symptoms at rest and with exertion.
3. The person may return to contest if mental status abnormalities and postconcussive symptoms clear within 15 minutes.

Grade 2
1. Remove from contest and disallow return that day.
2. Examine on site frequently for signs of evolving intracranial (within the cranium) abnormalities.
3. A trained person should reexamine the athlete the following day.
4. A physician should perform a neurologic examination to clear the athlete for return to play after 1 week without symptoms at rest and with exertion.

Grade 3
1. Transport the athlete from the field to the nearest emergency department by ambulance if still unconscious or if worrisome signs are detected (with cervical spine immobilization, if indicated).
2. A thorough neurologic evaluation should be performed on an emergency basis, including appropriate evaluation procedures when indicated.
3. Hospital admission is indicated if any abnormal signs are detected or if the mental status of the athlete remains abnormal.

When to Return to Play
Grade of Concussion: Return to play only after being asymptomatic with normal neurologic assessment at rest and with exercise

Grade 1 concussion:	15 minutes or less
Multiple grade-1 concussions:	1 week
Grade 2 concussion:	1 week
Multiple grade-2 concussions:	2 weeks

Grade 3
Brief loss of consciousness (seconds):	1 week
Prolonged loss of consciousness (minutes):	2 weeks

Multiple grade-3 concussions: 1 month or longer, based on decision of evaluating physician

Frequently Observed Features of Concussion
1. Vacant stare (befuddled facial expression)
2. Delayed verbal and motor responses (slow to answer questions or follow instructions)
3. Confusion and inability to focus attention (easily distracted and unable to follow through with normal activities)
4. Disorientation (walking in the wrong direction; unaware of time, date, and place)
5. Slurred or incoherent speech (making disjointed or incomprehensible statements)
6. Gross, observable uncoordination (stumbling, inability to walk in tandem or in a straight line)
7. Emotions out of proportion to circumstances (distraught, crying for no apparent reason)
8. Memory deficits (exhibited by repeatedly asking a question that has already been answered or inability to memorize and recall three of three words or three of three objects in 5 minutes)
9. Any period of loss of consciousness (unresponsiveness to arousal)

Sideline Evaluation
Mental Status Testing
Orientation: Time, place, person, and situation (circumstances of injury)

Concentration: Digits backward (for example, 3-1-7, 4-6-8-2, 5-3-0-7-4)

Months of the year in reverse order

Memory: Names of teams in previous contests

Recall of three words and three objects immediately and at 5 minutes

Recall of recent newsworthy events

Details of the contest (for example, plays, moves, and strategies)

Exertional Provocative Tests
40-yard sprint

5 push-ups

5 sit-ups

5 knee-bends

Neurological Tests
Strength
Coordination and Agility
Sensation
Any appearance of associated symptoms is abnormal; for example, headache, dizziness, nausea, unsteadiness, photophobia (increased sensitivity to light), blurred or double vision, emotional lability (easily changing emotions), or mental status changes.

Source: Quality Standards Subcommittee of the American Academy of Neurology. The management of concussion in sports [practice parameter]. *Neurology* 48(3):581-585.

A <u>contusion</u> is bruising of brain tissue. A <u>hematoma</u> is a localized collection of blood as a result of a broken blood vessel. A hematoma is a very serious type of brain injury.

Brain injuries produce varying degrees of local or generalized <u>edema</u> (swelling). As swelling increases or a hematoma expands, intracranial pressure increases. As pressure rises, it can compress swollen vessels and shut off the blood supply, thus depriving the brain tissue of oxygen. The brain stem can be compressed or crushed by the pressure, affecting heart and lung function.

Children are especially vulnerable to brain injuries. A young child has a relatively large head, supported by a weak neck and positioned on a small trunk. A child's brain tissues are thinner, softer, and more flexible than an adult's. The flexibility of the tissues diffuses the impact of an injury, but because the tissues are fragile, they damage easily. Small children, overbalanced by their large heads, tend to run leaning forward and often run into things or fall over. Their immature motor development makes toddlers clumsy and liable to stumble over their own feet. Unattended infants can tumble from beds, high chairs, and changing tables.

Recognizing Brain Injury

The following are frequently observed initial signs and symptoms of a concussion, according to the American Academy of Neurology and the Brain Injury Association:

- Confused facial expression
- Slow to answer questions or follow instructions
- Easily distracted and unable to follow through with normal activities
- Walking in the wrong direction; unaware of time, date, and place
- Making disjointed or incomprehensible statements
- Stumbling, inability to walk a straight line
- Distraught, crying for no apparent reason
- Asking a question that has already been answered or inability to memorize and recall a series of three words or objects 5 minutes later
- Coma, unresponsiveness

Ask a responsive victim for his or her name and current location. If the victim cannot answer those questions, there may be a significant problem. Another useful test is having the victim recite the months of the year backward. Inability to do so could indicate a concussion.

Care for Brain Injury

1. Seek immediate medical care.
2. Suspect a spinal injury in an unresponsive victim until proven otherwise. Stabilize the victim's head and neck using one of the following methods:
   - Grasp the victim's head over the ears and hold the head and neck still until emergency medical services (EMS) personnel arrive.
   - If you anticipate a long wait for EMS or you are tired from holding the victim's head in place, kneel with the victim's head between your knees or place objects on each side of the victim's head to prevent it from rolling from side to side.
3. Monitor the victim's breathing and provide appropriate care.
4. Control scalp bleeding by covering the wounds with sterile dressings as a barrier against infection. If you suspect a skull fracture, apply pressure around the wound edges, not directly on the wound. Do not try to clean a scalp wound if you suspect a skull fracture. Stabilize impaled objects in place. Do not try to stop blood or CSF draining from the ears or nose. Blocking the flow of either could increase pressure within the skull.
5. Brain-injury victims tend to vomit. Rolling the victim onto his or her side while stabilizing the neck and preventing movement will help drain vomit and keep the airway open.
6. If a spinal injury is not suspected, keep the victim in a slightly head-elevated position to prevent increased blood pressure on the brain. If the victim is unresponsive, roll him or her onto the left side to keep the airway open.
7. The victim's level of responsiveness or mental status is one of the best indicators of neurologic function. Observations for the first 24 hours may offer clues to problems. Using the mnemonic AVPU to assess and describe a victim's mental status is especially helpful with small children who do not talk.
   - A: The victim is *alert* and can recognize and respond to people.
   - V: The victim responds to *verbal* stimuli. The victim may appear sleepy or drowsy but responds to verbal questions by opening the eyes, moving, or waking up.
   - P: The victim responds to *painful* stimuli. The victim is not awake and does not respond to verbal stimuli but does respond to painful stimuli by moving, opening the eyes, or groaning. To stimulate pain, pinch the victim's skin over the clavicle.
   - U: The victim is *unresponsive* to voices and to painful stimuli.

There is little a first aider can do for a brain injury. The victim must be transported to a trauma center for further evaluation. If the victim is wearing a helmet such

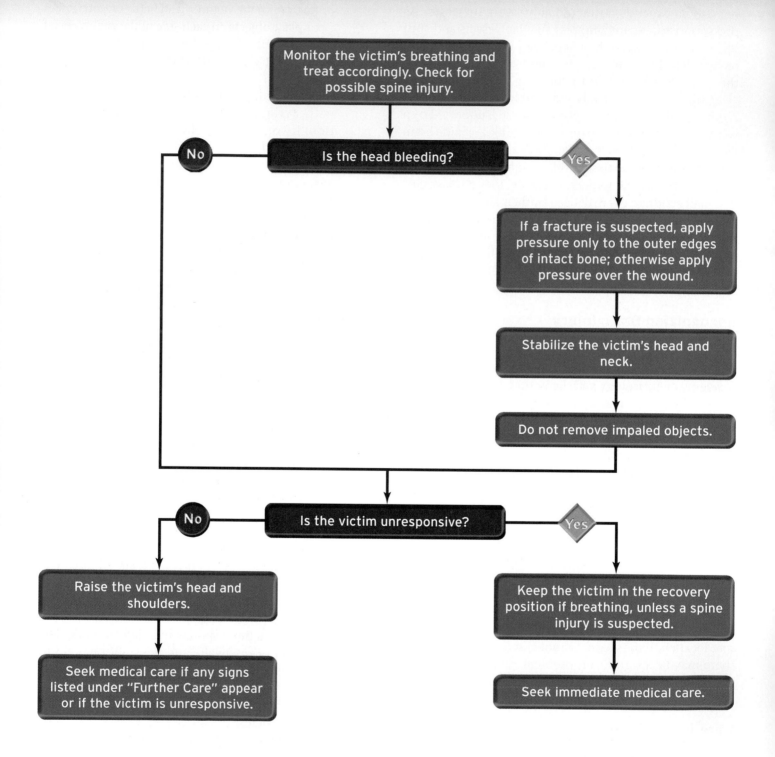

Monitor the victim's breathing and treat accordingly. Check for possible spine injury.

Is the head bleeding?

No

Yes

If a fracture is suspected, apply pressure only to the outer edges of intact bone; otherwise apply pressure over the wound.

Stabilize the victim's head and neck.

Do not remove impaled objects.

Is the victim unresponsive?

No

Yes

Raise the victim's head and shoulders.

Keep the victim in the recovery position if breathing, unless a spine injury is suspected.

Seek medical care if any signs listed under "Further Care" appear or if the victim is unresponsive.

Seek immediate medical care.

as a motorcycle or football helmet, it should not be removed by a first aider unless:

- You suspect an obstructed airway.
- The helmet is so loose that you cannot stabilize the spine.

If the helmet must be removed to provide life-saving care of an airway problem, make sure to stabilize the head and neck as the helmet is carefully removed.

Further Care

Several signs appearing within 48 hours of a head injury indicate a need to seek medical care.

- **Headache:** Expect a headache. If it lasts more than 1 or 2 days or increases in severity, seek medical advice.
- **Nausea, vomiting:** If nausea lasts more than 2 hours, seek medical advice. Vomiting once or twice, especially in children, may be expected after a head injury. Vomiting does not indicate the severity of the injury. However, if vomiting begins again hours after the initial episodes have ceased, seek medical care.
- **Drowsiness:** Allow a victim to sleep, but wake the victim at least every 2 hours to check the state of consciousness and sense of orientation by asking his or her name and to use information-processing skills (for example, "Recite the months of the year backward"). If the victim cannot respond or appears confused or disoriented, call a physician.
- **Vision problems:** If the victim "sees double," if the eyes do not move together, or if one pupil appears to be larger than the other, seek medical advice.
- **Mobility:** If the victim cannot use his or her arms or legs as well as previously or is unsteady when walking, seek medical care.
- **Speech:** If the victim has slurred speech or is unable to talk, consult a doctor.
- **Seizures (convulsions):** If the victim has a violent involuntary contraction (spasm) or series of contractions of the skeletal muscles, seek medical care.

Eye Injuries

Of all the parts of the human body, an injured eye probably causes the most anxiety and concern in a victim. The

---

CAUTION

DO NOT assume that any eye injury is innocent. When in doubt, seek medical care immediately.

DO NOT remove an object stuck in the eye or try to wash out an object with water.

DO NOT exert pressure on an injured eyeball or a penetrating object.

---

eyes—arguably the most important human sense organs—are easily damaged by trauma. A very slight penetration by a metal fragment, for example, means hospitalization. Medical treatment may include surgery; despite technical advances, blindness or the loss of an eye remains a possibility whenever there is an eye injury.

▶ Penetrating Eye Injuries

Penetrating eye injuries are severe injuries that result when a sharp object, such as a knife or a needle, penetrates the eye. Most penetrating injuries are obvious. Suspect penetration any time you see a lid laceration or cut.

Care for Penetrating Eye Injuries

1. Seek immediate medical care. Any penetrating eye injury should be managed in the hospital.
2. Stabilize the object. Stabilize a long, protruding object with bulky dressings or clean cloths. You can place a protective paper cup or cardboard folded into a cone over the affected eye to prevent bumping of the object **Figure 12-5**. For short objects, surround the eye without touching the object with rolled gauze bandage or cloths held in place with a roller bandage.

▶ Blows to the Eye

Blows to the eye can range in severity from minor to sight threatening. One such injury is the common *shiner* or *black eye*, which occurs when some of the many delicate blood vessels around the eye rupture. The bleeding itself is insignificant and will disappear, but it may hide damage to the eyeball **Figure 12-6**. A fist, ball, or other blunt object can break the bone around the eyeball. Symptoms that indicate such a break are double vision and the inability to look upward.

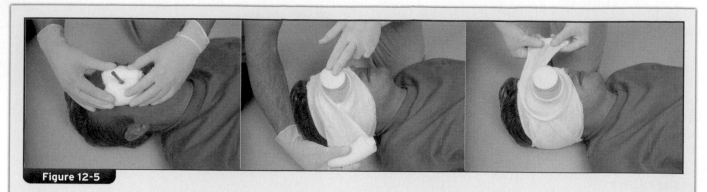

Figure 12-5

Stabilizing a long, penetrating object against movement (using a paper cup to protect object from being hit).

Care for Blows to the Eye

1. Apply an ice or cold pack for about 15 minutes to reduce the pain and swelling. Do not apply any pressure on the eye.
2. Seek medical care immediately if there is double vision, pain, or reduced vision.

▶ Cuts of the Eye or Lid

The signs of a cut eyeball or lid include the following **Figure 12-7** :

- "Cut" appearance of the cornea (clear part of the eye) or sclera (white part of eye).
- Inner liquid filling of the eye may come out through the wound.
- Lid is cut.

Care for Cuts of the Eye or Lid

1. If the eyeball is cut, do not apply pressure. If only the eyelid is cut, apply a sterile or clean dressing with gentle pressure.

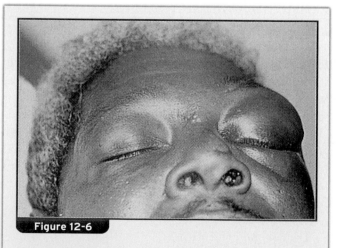

Figure 12-6

Blow to the eye.

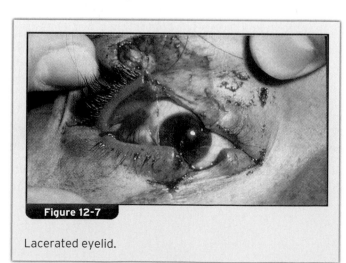

Figure 12-7

Lacerated eyelid.

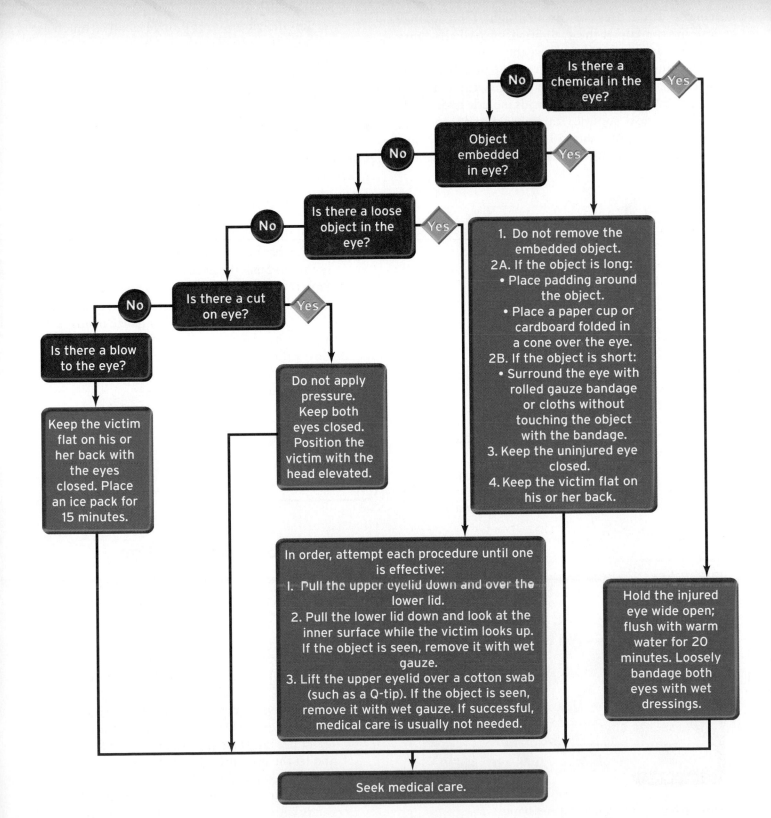

Is there a chemical in the eye? — No / Yes

Object embedded in eye? — No / Yes

Is there a loose object in the eye? — No / Yes

Is there a cut on eye? — No / Yes

Is there a blow to the eye? — No

Keep the victim flat on his or her back with the eyes closed. Place an ice pack for 15 minutes.

Do not apply pressure. Keep both eyes closed. Position the victim with the head elevated.

1. Do not remove the embedded object.
2A. If the object is long:
   • Place padding around the object.
   • Place a paper cup or cardboard folded in a cone over the eye.
2B. If the object is short:
   • Surround the eye with rolled gauze bandage or cloths without touching the object with the bandage.
3. Keep the uninjured eye closed.
4. Keep the victim flat on his or her back.

In order, attempt each procedure until one is effective:
1. Pull the upper eyelid down and over the lower lid.
2. Pull the lower lid down and look at the inner surface while the victim looks up. If the object is seen, remove it with wet gauze.
3. Lift the upper eyelid over a cotton swab (such as a Q-tip). If the object is seen, remove it with wet gauze. If successful, medical care is usually not needed.

Hold the injured eye wide open; flush with warm water for 20 minutes. Loosely bandage both eyes with wet dressings.

Seek medical care.

2. Bandage both eyes lightly.
3. Seek medical care immediately.

▶ Chemical in the Eyes

Chemicals in the eyes can threaten sight. First aid may determine the fate of the eye and vision. Alkalis cause greater damage than acids because they penetrate deeper and continue to burn longer. Common alkalis include drain cleaners, cleaning agents, ammonia, cement, plaster, and caustic soda. Common acids include hydrochloric acid, nitric acid, sulfuric (battery) acid, and acetic acid. Because damage can occur in 1 to 5 minutes, the chemical must be removed immediately **Figure 12-8**.

CAUTION

DO NOT try to neutralize the chemical. Water usually is readily available for eye irrigation.

DO NOT use an eye cup for a chemical burn.

DO NOT bandage the eye tightly.

Care for Chemical in the Eye

1. Use your fingers to keep the eye open as widely as possible.
2. Flush the eye with water immediately. If possible, use warm water. If water is not available, use any nonirritating liquid.
   - Hold the victim's head under a faucet or pour water into the eye from any clean container for at least 20 minutes, continuously and gently. It

is impossible to use too much water on these injuries.
   - Irrigate from the nose side of the eye toward the outside to avoid flushing the material into the other eye.
   - Tell the victim to roll the eyeball as much as possible to help wash out the eye.
3. Loosely bandage both eyes with cold, wet dressings.
4. Seek immediate medical care.

▶ Eye Avulsion

A blow to the eye can *avulse* it (knock it out) from its socket. This is a serious injury.

Care for Eye Avulsion

1. Cover the eye loosely with a sterile or clean dressing that has been moistened with clean water. Do not try to push the eyeball back into the socket.
2. Protect the injured eye with a paper cup, a piece of cardboard folded into a cone, or a doughnut-shaped pad made from a roller gauze bandage or a cravat bandage.
3. Cover the undamaged eye with a patch to stop movement of the damaged eye.
4. Seek medical care immediately.

CAUTION

DO NOT try to remove an object stuck in the eye.

▶ Loose Objects in the Eye

Loose objects in the eye are the most frequent eye injury and can be very painful. Tearing is common because it is the body's way of trying to remove the object.

Care for Objects in the Eye

Try one or more of the following methods to remove the object:

1. Lift the upper lid over the lower lid, so that the lower lashes can brush the object off the inside of the upper lid. Have the victim blink a few times, and let the eye move the object out. If the object remains, keep the eye closed.
2. Try flushing the object out by rinsing the eye gently with warm water. Hold the eyelid open, and tell the victim to move the eye as it is rinsed.

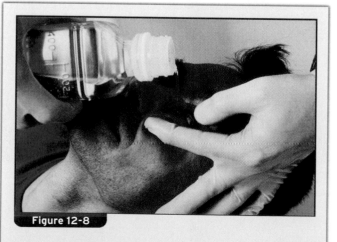
Figure 12-8
Flushing the eye to treat a chemical burn.

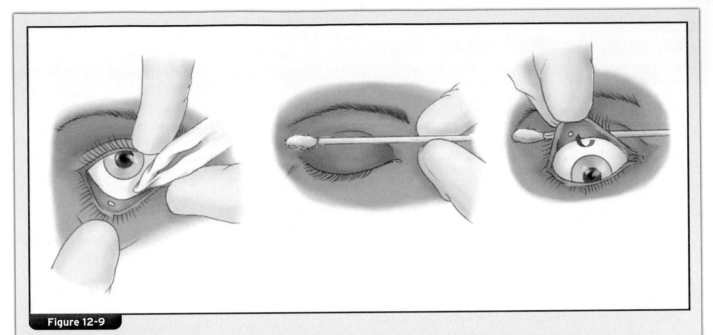

Figure 12-9

Removing loose objects from the eye. Lower lid: If tears or gentle flushing do not remove object, gently pull the lower lid down. Remove an object by gently flushing with lukewarm water or by using wet, sterile gauze. Upper lid 1: Tell the person to look down. Pull gently downward on the upper eyelashes. Lay a swab or matchstick across the top of the lid. Upper lid 2: Fold the lid over the swab or matchstick. Remove an object by gently flushing with lukewarm water or by using wet, sterile gauze.

3. Examine the lower lid by pulling it down gently. If you can see the object, remove it with moistened sterile gauze or a clean cloth **Figure 12-9**.
4. Many foreign bodies lodge under the upper eyelid; however, expertise is required to invert the lid and remove the object. Examine the underside of the upper lid by grasping the lashes of the upper lid, placing a matchstick or cotton-tipped swab across the upper lid and rolling the lid upward over the stick or swab. If you can see the object, remove it with moistened sterile gauze or a clean cloth.

CAUTION

DO NOT allow the victim to rub the eye.
DO NOT try to remove an embedded foreign object.
DO NOT use dry cotton (cotton balls or cotton-tipped swabs) or instruments such as tweezers to remove an object from an eye.

▶ Light Burns to the Eye

Burns can result if a person looks at a source of ultraviolet light such as sunlight, arc welding, bright snow, or tanning lamps. Severe pain occurs 1 to 6 hours after exposure.

Care for Light Burns

1. Cover both eyes with cold, wet packs. Tell the victim not to rub the eyes.
2. Have the victim rest in a darkened room. Do not allow light to reach the victim's eyes.
3. Give pain medication, if needed.
4. Seek medical care.

FYI

An Unresponsive Victim's Eyes
An unconscious victim may lose the reflexes such as blinking that protect the eye. If the eyes do not stay closed, keep them closed by covering them with moist dressings.

▶ Ear Injuries

Most ear problems are not life threatening. Fast action may be needed, however, to relieve pain and to prevent or reverse hearing loss. Head trauma may involve the ear. Foreign bodies in the ear canal usually produce overzealous removal attempts. Except for disk batteries (which damage moist tissue by creating a current) and live insects, few foreign bodies must be extracted immediately. First aiders should seek medical care for the victim because attempts to remove a foreign body from the ear can rupture the eardrum or lacerate the ear canal.

A live insect crawling around in the ear canal can be very uncomfortable for the victim. Shine a small light into the ear. Sometimes the insect will crawl out toward the light. If it will not leave the ear, drown the insect by placing several drops of light mineral oil or vegetable oil (not motor oil) into the ear. Often the insect will crawl out before it dies. When it stops moving and the insect is near the opening, carefully irrigate the ear with warm water. The insect should wash out. If that is unsuccessful, use a bulb syringe to suck the insect out. If the insect cannot be removed, seek medical care.

Children insert all sorts of things into their ears that may be impossible for you to remove safely. If the object is visible near the ear canal opening and you feel it is safe, cautiously try to remove the object with tweezers. Small objects can sometimes be removed by irrigating the ear with warm water. Do not try irrigation if the object is near the eardrum, if it blocks the entire ear canal, or if the object is vegetable matter such as a kernel of corn or a bean, which will swell when wet.

Nose Injuries

▶ Nosebleeds

A severe nosebleed frightens the victim and often challenges the first aider's skill. Most nosebleeds are self-limiting and seldom require medical attention. In cases of accompanying head or neck injuries, stabilize the head and neck for protection. In some cases, loss of blood could cause shock.

There are two types of nosebleeds:

- **Anterior nosebleed** (front of nose) is the most common type (90%). Blood flows from the nose through one nostril.
- The **posterior nosebleed** (back of nose) involves massive bleeding backward into the mouth or down the back of the throat. A posterior nosebleed is serious and requires medical care.

Care for Nosebleeds

To care for an anterior nosebleed, follow these guidelines from the American Academy of Otolaryngology:

1. Pinch the soft parts of the nose together between your thumb and two fingers **Figure 12-10**.
2. Press firmly toward the face, compressing the pinched parts of the nose against the bones of the face.
3. Continue compressing the pinched parts for 5 to 10 minutes.
4. Keep the head higher than the level of the heart. Have the victim sit and lean slightly forward or lie with the head elevated.
5. Apply ice (crushed in a plastic bag or washcloth) to the nose and cheeks.

If bleeding continues:

1. Clear the nose of all blood clots by gently blowing the nose.
2. If available, spray the nose on both sides with decongestant spray (such as Afrin or Neo-Synephrin).
3. Pinch and press the nose toward the face again.
4. If the nosebleed continues, seek medical care.

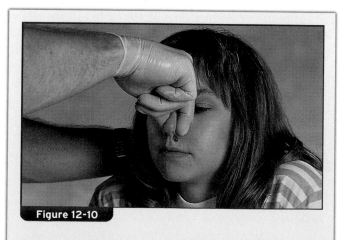

Figure 12-10

Control bleeding from the nose by pinching the nostrils together.

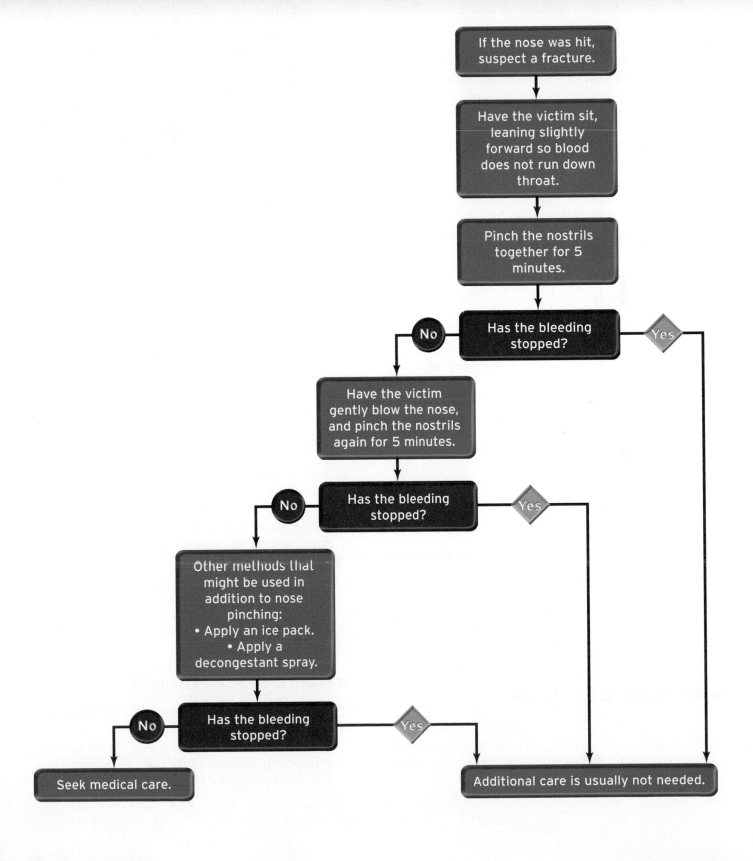

Seek professional medical help if:
- Bleeding cannot be stopped or keeps reappearing.
- Bleeding is rapid or blood loss is large.
- Weakness or fainting is present.
- Blood begins to go down the back of the throat rather than out the front of the nose.

Care After a Nosebleed

After a nosebleed has stopped, suggest that the victim:
- Sneeze through an open mouth, if he or she needs to sneeze.
- Avoid bending over and participating in too much physical exertion.
- Elevate the head with two pillows when lying down.
- Keep the nostrils moist by applying a little petroleum jelly just inside the nostril for 1 week; increase the humidity in the bedroom during the winter months by using a cold-mist humidifier.
- Avoid picking or rubbing the nose.

> **CAUTION**
>
> DO NOT allow the victim to tilt the head backward.
> DO NOT probe the nose with a cotton-tipped swab.
> DO NOT move the victim's head and neck if a spinal injury is suspected.

▶ Broken Nose

The signs of a broken nose include the following:
- Pain, swelling, and a possible crooked appearance
- Bleeding and difficulty breathing through the nostrils
- Black eyes appearing 1 to 2 days after the injury

Care for a Broken Nose

1. Seek medical care.
2. If bleeding is present, give care as for a nosebleed.
3. Apply an ice pack to the nose for 15 minutes.
4. Do not try to straighten a crooked nose.

▶ Objects in the Nose

A foreign object in the nose is a problem mainly among small children, who seem to gain satisfaction from putting peanuts, beans, raisins, and other similar objects into their nostrils.

Care for Objects in the Nose

To remove objects from the nose, try one or more of the following methods:

1. Induce sneezing by having the victim sniff pepper or by tickling the opposite nostril.
2. Have the victim blow gently while you put compression on the opposite nostril.
3. Use tweezers to pull out an object that is visible. Do not probe or push an object deeper.
4. Seek medical care if the object cannot be removed.

Dental Injuries

Because dental emergencies generally cause considerable pain and anxiety, managing them promptly can provide great relief to the victim.

▶ Objects Caught Between the Teeth

The signs of an object caught between teeth include the following:
- Victim says that something is caught between his or her teeth. This is the main method of detecting the problem.
- The object may or may not be seen. Even with the use of a flashlight, it is still difficult to see a small object.

Care for Objects Caught Between the Teeth

1. Try to remove the object with dental floss. Guide the floss carefully to avoid cutting the gums. Do not try to remove the object with a sharp or pointed instrument.
2. If unsuccessful, seek dental care.

▶ Bitten Lip or Tongue

The signs of a bitten lip or tongue include the following:
- Immediate pain when it happens.
- Blood may be seen.

Care for a Bitten Lip or Tongue

1. Apply direct pressure to the bleeding area with sterile gauze or a clean cloth.
2. If swelling is present, apply an ice pack or have the victim suck on an ice pop or ice chips.
3. If the bleeding does not stop, seek medical care.

▶ Loosened Tooth

Trauma can cause teeth to become loosened in their sockets. Applying pressure on either side of each tooth with the fingers can determine looseness. Any tooth movement, even if it is barely felt, indicates a possibly loose tooth.

Care for a Loosened Tooth

1. Have the victim bite down on a piece of gauze to keep the tooth in place.
2. Consult a dentist or an oral surgeon.

▶ Knocked-Out Tooth

A knocked-out tooth is a dental emergency but it is also a common one. A majority of the teeth knocked out each year in the United States could be saved with proper treatment **Figure 12-11**. Emergency care for knocked-out teeth has changed dramatically in recent years. The first question you want to ask when a tooth has been knocked out is, "Where is the tooth?" Time is crucial for successful reimplantation. After a tooth is knocked out, ligament fiber fragments remain attached to the tooth and to the bone in the socket. These ligament fibers begin to die soon after the injury. Therefore, it is important to prevent the tooth from drying and to protect the ligament fibers from damage. Moisture alone is not sufficient to preserve the tooth's ligament fibers. Steps must be taken to prevent the tooth from becoming dehydrated and to protect the ligament fibers from damage.

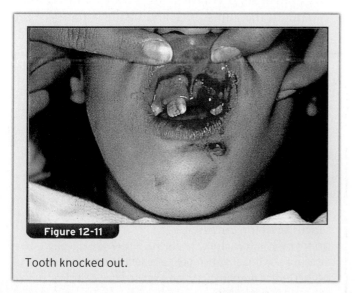

Figure 12-11

Tooth knocked out.

Care for Knocked-Out Tooth

1. Have the victim rinse his or her mouth, and put a rolled gauze pad in the socket to control the bleeding.
2. Find the tooth and handle it by the crown, not the root, to minimize damage to the ligament fibers.
3. A tooth often can be successfully reimplanted if it is replaced in its socket within 30 minutes after the injury; the odds of successful reimplantation decrease about 1% for every minute the tooth is absent from the socket.
   - One of the worst things you can do to a knocked-out tooth is to transport it dry. Consider using saliva for the short term (less than 1 hour). Milk is much better because of its calcium and magnesium concentrations. Ideally, the milk should be whole milk and kept cold to minimize bacterial growth. Do not use reconstituted powdered milk or milk by-products such as yogurt; they can damage the ligaments.
   - The best transport medium is Hank's solution, a balanced-pH cell-culture medium that helps restore the ligament fibers. The use of Hank's solution extends the viability of the ligament fibers for 6 to 12 hours. The solution, which is available commercially as the Save-a-Tooth kit, has been approved by the US Food and Drug Administration for use up to 24 hours after an injury, and there is some evidence that using it enables successful reimplantation, even after 96 hours. A tooth-saving kit is available in drugstores and deserves consideration as a standard item at schools, sporting events, and summer camps.
   - Some experts recommend that the tooth be placed in the victim's mouth to keep it moist until dental treatment is available. Do not use this method for children or others who may swallow the tooth.
4. Take the victim and the tooth immediately to a dentist.
5. If you are in a remote location, try to replace the tooth into the socket, using adjacent teeth as a guide. Apply pressure on the tooth so the top is even with the adjacent teeth. Asking the victim to bite down gently on gauze is helpful. Immediate reinsertion is not always possible, however. The victim may be reluctant to put the knocked-out tooth back into its socket, especially if it has fallen on the ground and is covered with debris—or the

tooth may repeatedly fall out, putting the victim at risk of inhaling or swallowing it. Do not use this method for children or others who may swallow the tooth. In victims with multiple trauma, the presence of more serious injuries may prevent reinsertion.

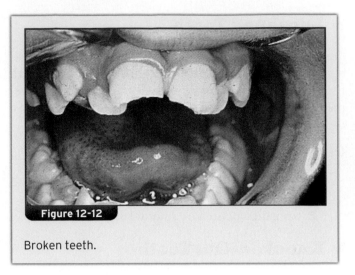

Figure 12-12

Broken teeth.

CAUTION

DO NOT handle a knocked-out tooth roughly.

DO NOT put a knocked-out tooth in water, mouthwash, alcohol, or povidone iodine (Betadine).

DO NOT put a knocked-out tooth in skim milk, reconstituted powdered milk, or milk by-products such as yogurt.

DO NOT rinse a knocked-out tooth unless you are reinserting it in the socket.

DO NOT place a knocked-out tooth in anything that can dry or crush the outside of the tooth.

DO NOT scrub a knocked-out tooth or remove any attached tissue fragments.

DO NOT remove a partially extracted tooth. Push it back into place and seek a dentist so the loose tooth can be stabilized.

▶ Broken Tooth

The front teeth are frequently broken by falls or direct blows **Figure 12-12**. Such damage is not unusual in the victims of violent acts or motor vehicle crashes. It is also common in children, especially those with an overbite.

Care for a Broken Tooth

1. Gently clean dirt and blood from the injured area with a sterile gauze pad or a clean cloth and warm water.
2. Apply an ice pack on the face in the area of the injured tooth to decrease swelling.
3. If you suspect a jaw fracture, stabilize the jaw by wrapping a bandage under the chin and over the top of the head.
4. Seek immediate dental care.

FYI

First Aid

If you are in a remote area with no dentist nearby, you can make a temporary cap from melted candle wax or paraffin and a few strands of cotton. When the wax begins to harden but can still be molded, press a wad of it onto the tooth. Other improvisations include using ski wax or chewing gum (preferably sugarless).

▶ Toothache

The most common reason for toothaches is dental decay. Victims frequently complain of pain limited to one area of the mouth, although it can be more widespread; pain can also affect the ear, eye, neck, or even the opposite side of the jaw. The tooth will be sensitive to heat and cold. Identify the diseased tooth by tapping the area with a spoon handle or similar object. A diseased tooth will hurt.

Care for a Toothache

1. Rinse the mouth with warm water to clean it out.
2. Use dental floss to remove any food that might be trapped between the teeth.
3. If you suspect a cavity, paint the tooth by using a small cotton swab soaked in oil of cloves (eugenol) to help suppress the pain. Take care to keep the oil off the gums, lips, and inside surfaces of the cheeks. If applicable, follow the same procedures as for a broken tooth.
4. Give the victim pain medication—aspirin (adults only), acetaminophen, or ibuprofen.
5. Seek immediate dental care.

CAUTION

DO NOT place pain medication (such as aspirin, acetaminophen, or ibuprofen) on the aching tooth or gum tissues or allow them to dissolve in the mouth. A serious acid burn can result.

DO NOT cover a cavity with cotton if there is any pus discharge or facial swelling. See a dentist immediately.

DO NOT stick anything into an exposed cavity or into a softened exposed root.

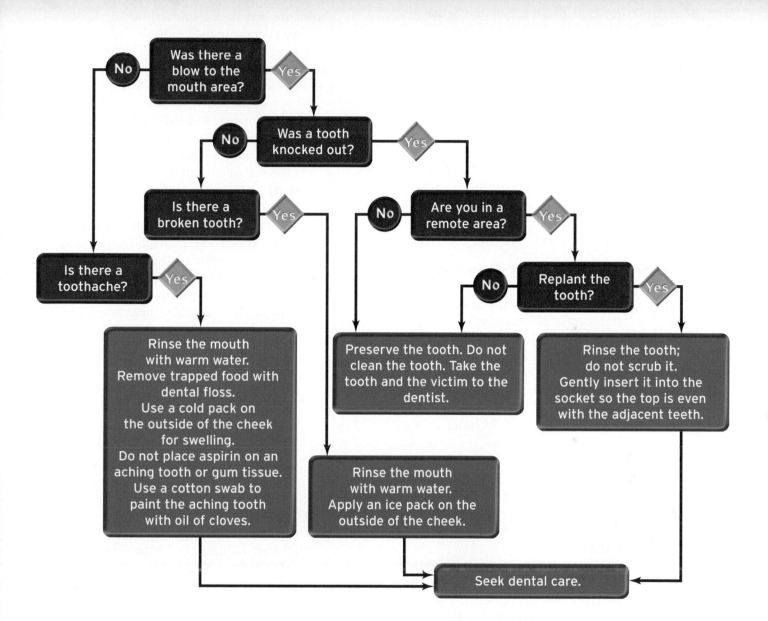

Was there a blow to the mouth area? — No / Yes

Was a tooth knocked out? — No / Yes

Is there a broken tooth? — Yes

Are you in a remote area? — No / Yes

Is there a toothache? — Yes

Replant the tooth? — No / Yes

Rinse the mouth with warm water. Remove trapped food with dental floss. Use a cold pack on the outside of the cheek for swelling. Do not place aspirin on an aching tooth or gum tissue. Use a cotton swab to paint the aching tooth with oil of cloves.

Preserve the tooth. Do not clean the tooth. Take the tooth and the victim to the dentist.

Rinse the tooth; do not scrub it. Gently insert it into the socket so the top is even with the adjacent teeth.

Rinse the mouth with warm water. Apply an ice pack on the outside of the cheek.

Seek dental care.

Spinal Injuries

The *spine* is a column of vertebrae stacked on one another from the tailbone to the base of the skull. Each vertebra has a hollow center through which the spinal cord passes. The spinal cord consists of long tracts of nerves that join the brain with all other body organs and parts.

If a broken vertebra pinches spinal nerves, paralysis can result. All unresponsive victims should be treated as though they have a spinal injury. All responsive victims sustaining injuries from falls, diving accidents, or motor vehicle crashes should be carefully checked for a spinal injury before being moved. Suspect a spinal injury in all head-injury victims.

A mistake in the handling of a spinal injury victim could mean a lifetime of paralysis for the victim. Suspect a spinal injury whenever a significant cause of injury occurs.

▶ Recognizing Spinal Injuries

Because the head may have been snapped suddenly in one or more directions, anytime there is a head injury, there may also be a spinal cord injury. About 15% to 20% of head-injury victims also have a spinal injury. Other signs and symptoms include the following:

- Pain radiating into the arms or legs
- Neck or back pain
- Numbness, tingling, weakness, burning, or lessened sensation in the arms or legs
- Loss of bowel or bladder control
- Paralysis of the arms or legs
- Deformity (odd-looking angle of the victim's head and neck)

Ask a responsive victim these questions and follow these steps **Skill Drill 12-1** :

- Is there pain? Neck (cervical spine) injuries radiate pain to the arms; upper-back (thoracic spine) injuries radiate pain around the ribs; lower-back injuries usually radiate pain down the legs. Often, the victim will describe the pain as "electric."
- Can you wiggle your fingers? Moving the fingers is a sign that nerve pathways are intact (**Step ❶**).
- Can you feel this pressure on your finger? Pinch the tip the victim's finger to check for spinal injury (**Step ❷**).
- Can you squeeze my hand? Ask the victim to grip your hand. A strong grip indicates that an upper spinal injury is unlikely (**Step ❸**).
- Can you wiggle your toes? Moving the toes is a sign that nerve pathways are intact (**Step ❹**).

- Squeeze the victim's toes (**Step ❺**).
- Can you push your foot against my hand? Ask the victim to press a foot against your hand (**Step ❻**). If the victim cannot perform this movement or if the movement is extremely weak against your hand, the victim may have a spinal injury.

If the victim is unresponsive, do the following:

- Look for cuts, bruises, and deformities.
- Test responses by pinching the victim's hand (the palm or back of the hand) and bare foot (the sole or the top of the foot). No reaction could mean spinal cord damage **Skill Drill 12-2** :
  1. Pinch the victim's hand for a response (**Step ❶**).
  2. Pinch the victim's foot for a response (**Step ❷**).
  3. Test the spinal cord by using the *Babinski test* (**Step ❸**): Stroke the bottom of the foot firmly toward the big toe with a key or similar sharp object. The body's normal response is to move the big toe down (except in infants). If the spinal cord or brain is injured, the big toe in an adult and a child will flex upward.
  4. Ask bystanders what happened. If you still are not sure about a possible spinal injury, assume the victim has one until it is proved otherwise.

▶ Care for a Spinal Injury

1. Monitor breathing. For an unresponsive victim, open the airway and check for breathing.
2. Stabilize the victim to prevent movement by using one of the following methods. Whichever method you use, tell the victim not to move.
   - Grasp the victim's head over the ears and hold the head and neck still until the EMS arrives **Figure 12-13** .
   - If you anticipate a long wait for EMS or you are tired from holding the victim's head in place, kneel with the victim's head between your knees or place objects on each side of the victim's head to prevent it from rolling from side to side.

⚠CAUTION

DO NOT move the victim, even if the victim is in water. Wait for EMS personnel to arrive; they have the proper training and equipment. Victims with suspected spinal injury require cervical collars and stabilization on a spine board. It is better to do nothing than to mishandle a victim with a spinal injury.

12-1 Checking for Spinal Injuries in a Responsive Victim

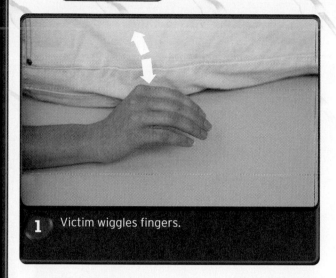

1 Victim wiggles fingers.

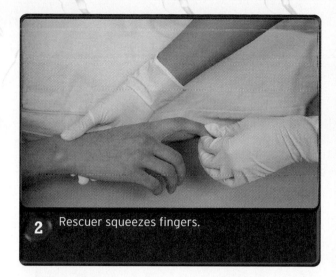

2 Rescuer squeezes fingers.

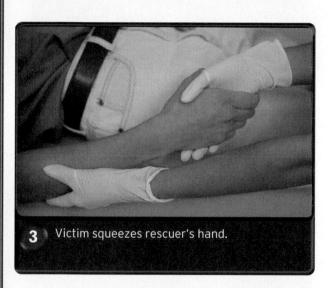

3 Victim squeezes rescuer's hand.

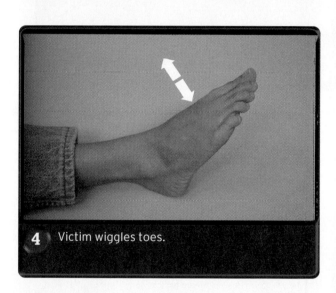

4 Victim wiggles toes.

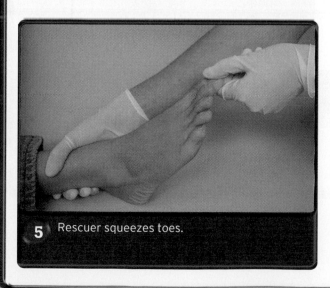

5 Rescuer squeezes toes.

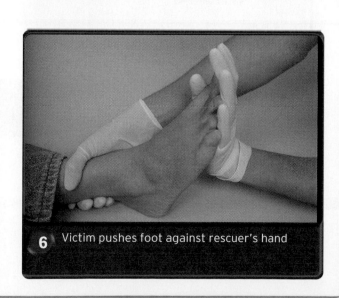

6 Victim pushes foot against rescuer's hand

skill drill

12-2   Checking for Spinal Injuries in an Unresponsive Victim

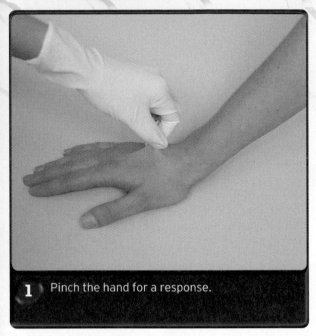

1 Pinch the hand for a response.

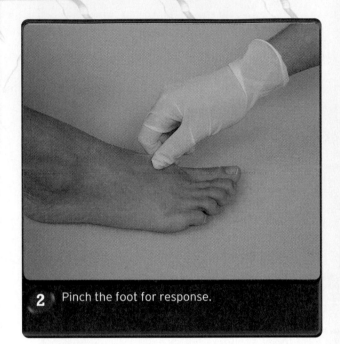

2 Pinch the foot for response.

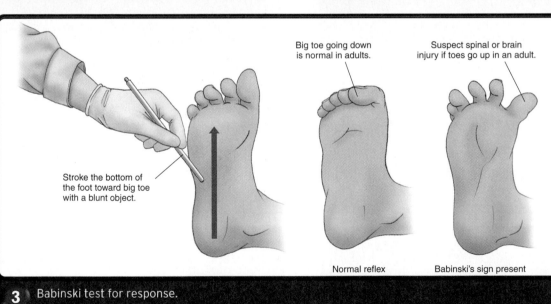

Stroke the bottom of the foot toward big toe with a blunt object.

Big toe going down is normal in adults.

Suspect spinal or brain injury if toes go up in an adult.

Normal reflex

Babinski's sign present

3 Babinski test for response.

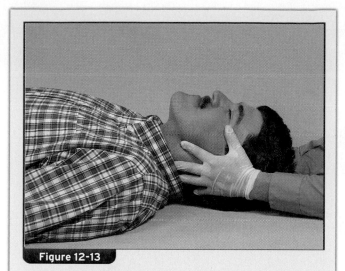

Figure 12-13

Steady and support the victim's head and neck as soon as possible. Have a bystander steady and support the feet. The head and feet should be continuously supported until medical help takes over. Stabilize by holding the head. Keep your arms steady by placing them on your thighs. To free yourself to help others, place heavy objects on each side of the head.

Spinal Injuries

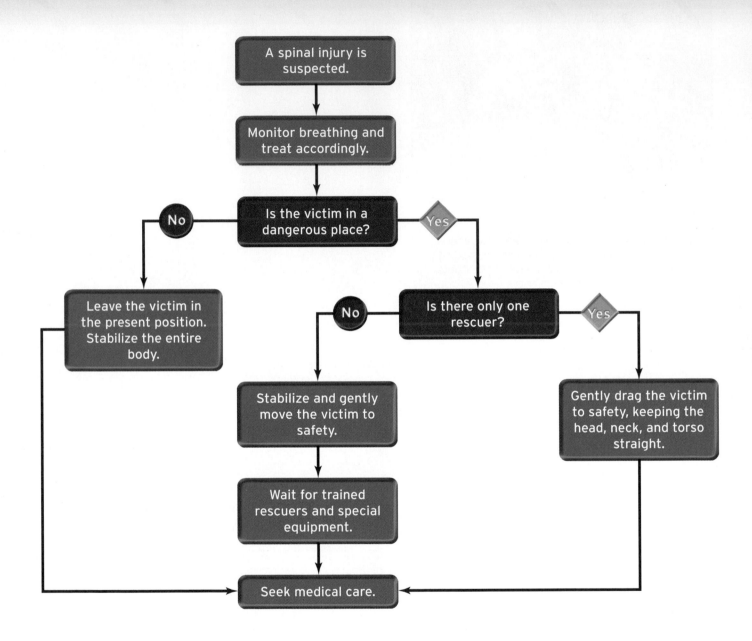

▶ Head Injuries

What to Look For	What to Do
Scalp wound	1. Apply a sterile or clean dressing and direct pressure to control bleeding. 2. Keep the head and shoulders raised. 3. Seek medical care.
Skull fracture	1. Monitor breathing and provide care if needed. 2. Control bleeding by applying pressure around the edges of wound. 3. Stabilize the victim's head and neck against movement. 4. Seek medical care.
Brain injury (concussion)	1. Monitor breathing and provide care if needed. 2. Stabilize the victim's head and neck against movement. 3. Control any scalp bleeding. 4. Seek medical care.

▶ Eye Injuries

What to Look For	What to Do
Loose object in eye	1. Look for object underneath both lids. 2. If seen, remove with wet gauze.
Penetrating eye injury	1. If object is still in eye, protect eye and stabilize long objects. 2. Call 9-1-1.
Blow to the eye area	1. Apply an ice or cold pack. DO NOT place ice or cold pack on eyeball. 2. Seek medical care if vision is affected.
Eye avulsion	1. Cover eye loosely with wet dressing. 2. DO NOT try to put eye back into socket. 3. Call 9-1-1.
Cuts of eye or lid	1. If eyeball is cut, DO NOT apply pressure. 2. If only eyelid is cut, apply dressings with gentle pressure. 3. Call 9-1-1.
Chemical in eye	1. Flush with warm water for 20 minutes. 2. Seek medical care.
Eye burns from light	1. Cover eyes with cold, wet dressings. 2. Seek medical care.

▶ Nose Injuries

What to Look For	What to Do

Nosebleeds	1. Keep the victim sitting up with the head level or tilted forward slightly.
	2. Pinch the soft parts of the nose for 5 to 10 minutes.
	3. Seek medical care if:
	  • Bleeding does not stop
	  • Blood is going down throat
	  • Bleeding is associated with a broken nose

Broken nose	1. Care as for a nosebleed. 2. Apply an ice or cold pack for 15 minutes. 3. Seek medical care.

▶ Dental Injuries

What to Look For	What to Do
Bitten lip or tongue	1. Apply direct pressure. 2. Apply an ice or cold pack.
Knocked-out tooth	1. Control bleeding (place rolled gauze in socket). 2. Find tooth and preserve it in milk or the victim's saliva. Handle the tooth by the crown, not the root. 3. Take the tooth with the victim to a dentist.
Toothache	1. Rinse the mouth and use dental floss to removed trapped food. 2. Give pain medication. 3. Seek dental care.

▶ Spinal Injuries

What to Look For	What to Do
Spinal injury • Inability to move arms and/or legs or painful to move them • Numbness, tingling, weakness, or burning feeling in arms and/or legs • Deformity (head and neck at an odd angle)	1. Stabilize the head and neck against movement. 2. If unresponsive, open the victim's airway and check breathing. 3. Call 9-1-1.

prep kit

▶ Ready for Review

- Any head injury is potentially serious. If not properly treated, injuries that seem minor could become life threatening.
- Scalp wounds bleed profusely because the scalp has a rich supply of blood and the blood vessels do not constrict.
- A skull fracture is a break or crack in the cranium. Skull fractures may be open or closed.
- Injuries to the brain cause short- and long-term problems.
- An injured eye probably causes the most anxiety and concern in a victim.
- Penetrating eye injuries are severe injuries that result when a sharp object penetrates the eye.
- Blows to the eye can range in severity from minor to sight threatening.
- Cuts of the eye or lid require medical care.
- Chemicals in the eyes can threaten sight.
- A blow to the eye can knock it from its socket.
- Loose objects in the eye are the most frequent eye injury and can be very painful.
- Burns to the eye can result if a person looks at a source of ultraviolet light.
- Most ear injuries are not life threatening but fast action may be needed to relieve pain or to prevent or reverse hearing loss.
- Most nosebleeds are self-limiting and seldom require medical attention.
- A foreign object in the nose is a problem mainly among small children who put small objects up their nostrils.
- Because dental emergencies generally cause considerable pain and anxiety, managing them promptly can provide great relief to the victim.
- Trauma can cause teeth to become loosened in their sockets.
- A knocked-out tooth is a dental emergency.
- The front teeth are frequently broken by falls or direct blows.
- The most common reason for toothaches is dental decay.
- A mistake in the handling of a spinal injury victim could mean a lifetime of paralysis for the victim.

▶ Vital Vocabulary

anterior nosebleed Bleeding from the front of the nose.

Battle's sign A contusion on the mastoid area of either ear; sign of a basal skull fracture.

concussion A temporary disturbance of brain activity caused by a blow to the head.

contusion A bruise; an injury that causes a hemorrhage in or beneath the skin but does not break the skin.

edema A condition in which fluid escapes into the body tissues from the vascular or lymphatic spaces and causes local or generalized swelling.

hematoma A localized collection of blood in an organ, tissue, or space as a result of injury or broken blood vessel.

posterior nosebleed Bleeding from the back of the nose into the mouth or down the back of the throat.

skull fracture A break of part of the skull (head bones).

▶ Assessment in Action

You see a middle-aged man walking down the street; suddenly, he is struck by a piece of wood that has fallen 50 feet from a construction site above. The victim collapses and remains on the ground. He is slow to answer questions and cannot remember where he is or the day of the week. He says he feels lightheaded and nauseated. You see a great deal of blood coming from a wound on his head.

Directions: Circle Yes if you agree with the statement, circle No if you disagree.

Yes No 1. Head-injured victims should be checked for possible spinal injury.

Yes No 2. You think the victim may have suffered a skull fracture, so you press around the wound's edges rather than applying hard pressure over the wound to control the bleeding.

Yes No 3. To treat for shock, this victim should be placed flat on his back with his legs elevated.

Yes No 4. You do not suspect a concussion because the victim is still alert.

Yes No 5. Minimize head and neck movement by not touching the victim; leave him as you found him.

Answers: **1.** Yes; **2.** Yes; **3.** No; **4.** No; **5.** Yes

prep kit

▶ Check Your Knowledge

Directions: Circle Yes if you agree with the statement, circle No if you disagree.

Yes   No   **1.** Remove objects embedded in an eyeball.

Yes   No   **2.** Scalp wounds have very little bleeding.

Yes   No   **3.** Scrub and rinse the roots of a knocked-out tooth.

Yes   No   **4.** After a blow to the area around an eye, apply a cold pack.

Yes   No   **5.** Tears are sufficient to flush a chemical from the eye.

Yes   No   **6.** Use clean, damp gauze to remove an object from the eyelid's surface.

Yes   No   **7.** Preserve a knocked-out tooth in mouthwash.

Yes   No   **8.** Do not move a victim with a suspected spinal injury.

Yes   No   **9.** Inability to move the hands or feet, or both, may indicate a spinal injury.

Yes   No   **10.** To care for a nosebleed, have the injured person sit down and tilt his or her head back.

Answers: **1.** No; **2.** No; **3.** No; **4.** Yes; **5.** No; **6.** Yes; **7.** No; **8.** Yes; **9.** Yes; **10.** No

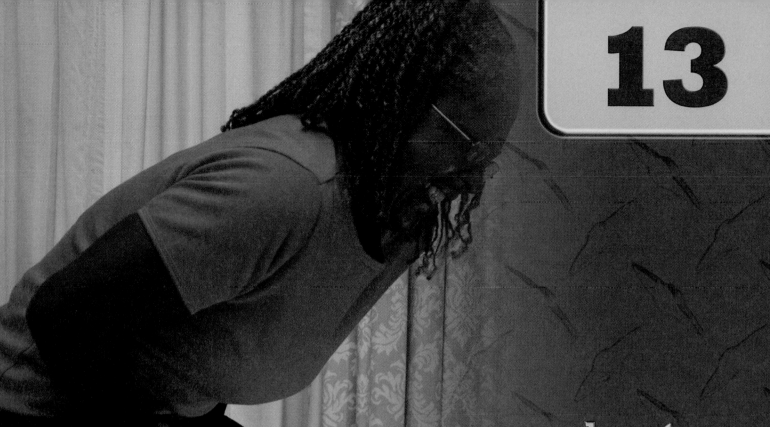

Chest, Abdominal, and Pelvic Injuries

Chest Injuries

Chest injuries fall into two categories: open or closed. In open chest injuries, the chest wall is penetrated by some object (e.g., knife, bullet, or broken end of rib). A closed chest injury is one which the skin is not broken. The injury is caused by blunt trauma (eg, falling object, struck during a fight or assault).

All chest-injury victims should have their airway, breathing, and circulation (ABCs) checked and rechecked. A responsive chest-injury victim should usually sit up or, if the injury is on a side, be placed with the injured side down **Figure 13-1**. This position prevents blood inside the chest cavity from seeping into the uninjured side and allows the uninjured side to expand.

▶ Closed Chest Injuries

In a <u>closed chest injury</u>, the skin is not broken. Closed chest injuries include rib fractures and flail chest.

Rib Fractures

The upper four ribs are rarely fractured because they are protected by the collarbone and the shoulder blades. The upper four ribs are so enmeshed with the muscles that they rarely need to be splinted or realigned like other broken bones. The lower two ribs are difficult to fracture because they are attached on only one end

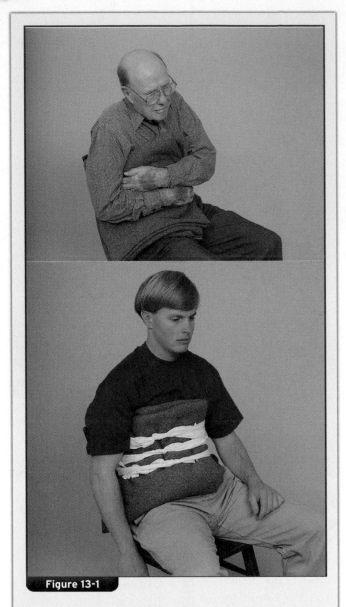

Figure 13-1

Stabilize the chest with a soft object such as a pillow, coat, or blanket (hold or tie). Tell the victim to occasionally take a deep breath and to cough.

and have the freedom to move, which is why they are called *floating ribs*. Broken ribs usually occur along the side of the chest. The main symptom of a rib fracture is pain at the injured rib site or when the victim breathes, coughs, or moves or when the area is touched.

Recognizing Rib Fractures

The signs of rib fracture include:
- Sharp pain, especially when the victim takes a deep breath, coughs, or moves
- Shallow breathing
- Victim holds the injured area, trying to reduce the pain

Care for Rib Fractures

1. Help the victim find a comfortable position.
2. Stabilize the ribs by having the victim hold a pillow or other similar soft object against the injured area or use bandages to hold the pillow in place. You can also tie an arm over the injured area. Do not apply tight bandages around the chest because they will restrict breathing.
3. Give pain medication.
4. Seek medical care.

FYI

Rib Fractures

Fractured ribs are a common injury and most frequently occur between ribs 3 and 10. The location for most fractures is on the sides of the body. The first two pairs of ribs are protected by the clavicles, whereas the last two pairs move freely and give with impact. Little can be done to assist the healing of broken ribs other than binding them to restrict movement. Tightly binding the chest limits breathing, and, because exhalation is inadequate, fluid accumulates in the air sacs (alveoli) and can result in pneumonia. This often explains pneumonia deaths in elderly persons.

Flail Chest

A **flail chest** is a serious injury that involves several ribs in the same area broken in more than one place. The area over the injury may move in a direction opposite to that of the rest of the chest wall during breathing (known as *paradoxical movement*). This injury is very painful and makes breathing difficult.

Recognizing Flail Chest

The signs and symptoms of a flail chest include:
- Paradoxical chest motion takes place. The area over the injury may move in a direction opposite to that of the rest of the chest wall during breathing.
- Breathing is very painful and difficult.
- Bruising of the skin over the injury occurs.

Care for Flail Chest

1. Support the chest by one of several methods:
   - Apply hand pressure. This is useful for a short time.
   - Place the victim on the injured side with a blanket or clothing underneath.
2. Monitor breathing.
3. Seek medical care.

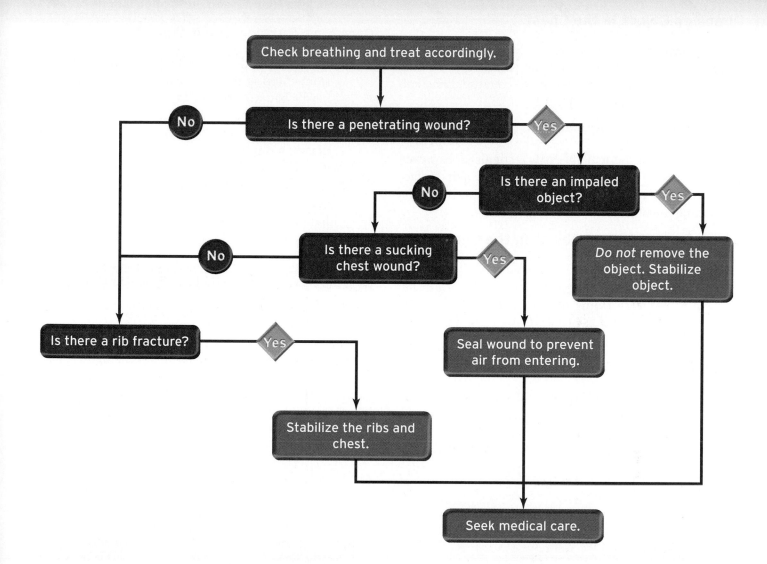

▶ Open Chest Injuries

In an <u>open chest injury</u>, the skin has been broken and the chest wall is penetrated by an object such as a knife or bullet.

Impaled Object in the Chest

If an object penetrates the chest wall, air and blood escape into the space between the lungs and the chest wall. The air and blood cause the lung to collapse. Lung collapse can lead to shock and death.

Recognizing an Impaled Object in the Chest

An impaled object is usually easily recognized. However, in some cases the object may be below the skin surface and is difficult to see. Carefully look at wounds that could be hiding the object that caused the damage.

Care for an Impaled Object in the Chest

1. Stabilize the object in place with bulky dressings or clothes **Figure 13-2** . *Do not try to remove an impaled object*. Doing so can result in bleeding and air in the chest cavity.
2. Call 9-1-1.

Sucking Chest Wound

A <u>sucking chest wound</u> results when a chest wound allows air to pass into and out of the chest with each breath **Figure 13-3** . Bubbles may be seen at the wound during exhalations and a sucking sound heard during inhalations.

Recognizing a Sucking Chest Wound

The signs of a sucking chest wound include:
- Blood bubbling out of a chest wound during exhalation
- Sucking sound heard during inhalations

Care for a Sucking Chest Wound

1. Seal the wound with anything available to stop air from entering the chest cavity. Plastic wrap or a plastic bag works well. Tape it in place, but leave one side untaped to create a flutter valve to prevent air from being trapped in the chest cavity. If plastic wrap is not available, you can use your gloved hand.
2. If the victim has trouble breathing or seems to be getting worse, remove the plastic cover (or your hand) to let air escape, and then reapply.
3. Call 9-1-1.

Abdominal Injuries

Injuries to the abdomen are either open or closed and can involve hollow and/or solid organs. An internal abdominal injury is one of the most frequently unrecognized injuries; when missed, it becomes one of the main causes of death. A hollow-organ rupture (for example, of the stomach or intestines) spills the contents of the organ into the abdominal cavity, causing inflammation. Solid-organ rupture (such as of the liver or pancreas) results in severe bleeding.

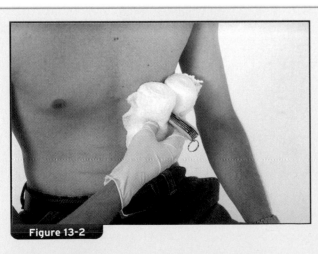

Figure 13-2

Stabilize a penetrating object with bulky padding. Secure the padding and object.

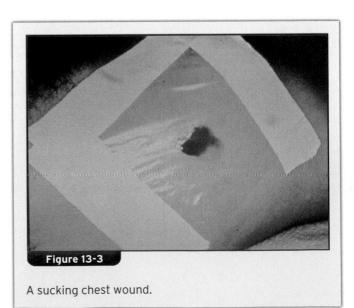

Figure 13-3

A sucking chest wound.

▶ Closed Abdominal Injury

Closed abdominal injuries occur when the internal abdominal tissues are damaged but the skin is unbroken. These are also known as *blunt injuries*. Such an injury might come from striking the handlebar of a bicycle, steering wheel of a car, or when the victim is struck by a board or baseball bat.

A Blow to the Abdomen

Bruising and damage to internal organs can result from a severe blow to the abdomen.

Recognizing a Closed Abdominal Injury

Examine the abdomen by gently pressing all four quadrants of the abdomen with your fingertips. A normal abdomen is soft and not tender when pressed. Signs of a closed abdominal injury include:

- Bruises or other marks
- Pain, tenderness, muscle tightness, or rigidity

Care for a Closed Abdominal Injury

1. Place the victim on one side in a comfortable position with the legs slightly bent. Expect vomiting.
2. Care for shock.
3. Call 9-1-1.

▶ Open Abdominal Injury

Open abdominal injures are those in which the skin has been broken. These injuries are also known as *penetrating injuries*. Examples include stab wounds and gunshot wounds. It is difficult to know whether a penetrating injury involves more than just the abdominal wall. Always assume the worst—that internal organs have been damaged.

A Penetrating Wound

Open abdominal wounds usually result from slashing with a knife or other sharp object and are always serious injuries. Penetrating injuries to the abdomen will cause internal organ damage.

Care for a Penetrating Wound

1. If the penetrating object is still in place, stabilize the object and control the bleeding by placing bulky dressings around it. *Do not try to remove the object.*
2. Call 9-1-1.

Impaled (Embedded) Object

Care is the same as for impaled (embedded) object in the chest.

Protruding Organs

A protruding organ injury refers to a severe injury to the abdomen in which internal organs escape or protrude from the wound.

Care for Protruding Organs

1. Call 9-1-1.
2. Allow the victim to stay in a comfortable position with the legs pulled up toward the abdomen.
3. Cover the protruding organs with a moist sterile dressing or clean cloth **Figure 13-4**.
4. Treat for shock.

CAUTION

DO NOT try to reinsert protruding organs into the abdomen—you could introduce infection or damage the intestines.

DO NOT cover the organs tightly.

DO NOT cover the organs with any material that clings or disintegrates when wet.

DO NOT give anything by mouth.

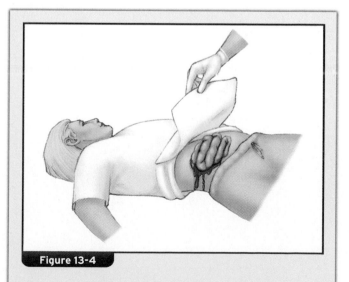

Figure 13-4

Do not reinsert protruding organs. Cover them with a moist, sterile dressing.

Pelvic Injuries

Pelvic fractures are usually caused by falling or a motor vehicle crash.

Recognizing Pelvic Injuries

The signs of a pelvic injury include:
- Pain in the hip, groin, or back that increases with movement.
- Inability to stand or walk.
- Signs of shock.

CAUTION

DO NOT roll the victim—additional internal damage could result.

DO NOT move the victim. Whenever possible, wait for trained EMS personnel with their ambulance, backboard, and other specialized equipment.

Care for Pelvic Injuries

1. Treat the victim for shock.
2. Place padding between the victim's thighs, and then tie the victim's knees and ankles together. If the knees are bent, place padding under them for support.
3. Keep the victim on a firm surface.
4. Call 9-1-1.

FYI

Pelvic Fractures

A pelvic fracture should be suspected in anyone with pelvic pain on movement or with pushing and/or squeezing of the pelvis. Motor vehicle crashes, being struck by a motor vehicle, falls, and bicycle and motorcycle crashes are common causes of pelvic injury. It is important to suspect pelvic injuries because they can result in massive blood loss. Unstable pelvic bones can cause continued arterial and venous bleeding that can go unnoticed. Splinting is necessary. Laypersons should stabilize the victim and wait for trained EMS personnel and their equipment to transport the victim to a hospital emergency department.

Abdominal Injuries

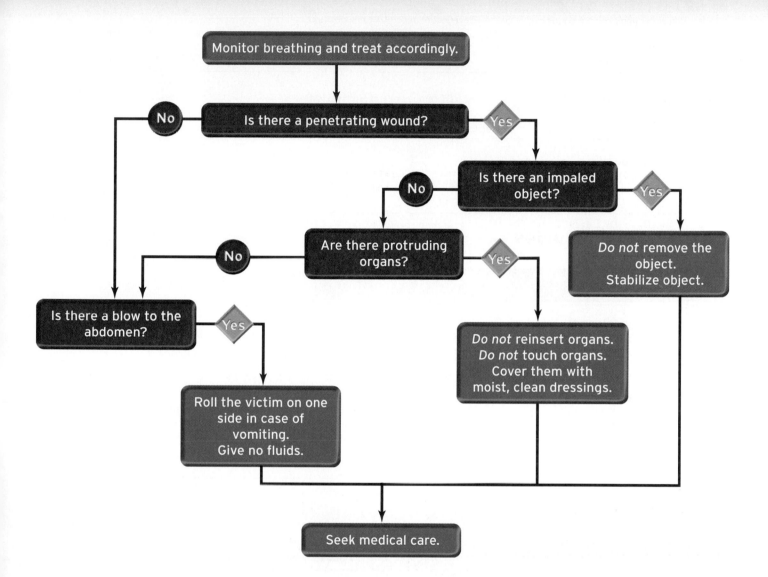

Monitor breathing and treat accordingly.

No — Is there a penetrating wound? — **Yes**

No — Is there an impaled object? — **Yes**

No — Are there protruding organs? — **Yes**

Is there a blow to the abdomen? — **Yes**

Do not remove the object.
Stabilize object.

Do not reinsert organs.
Do not touch organs.
Cover them with moist, clean dressings.

Roll the victim on one side in case of vomiting.
Give no fluids.

Seek medical care.

▶ Chest Injuries

What to Look For	What to Do
Rib fractures • Sharp pain with deep breaths, coughing, or moving • Shallow breathing • Holding of injured area to reduce pain	1. Place victim in comfortable position. 2. Support ribs with a pillow, blanket, or coat (either holding or tying with bandages). 3. Seek medical care.
Embedded (impaled) object • Object remains in wound	1. DO NOT remove object from wound. 2. Use bulky dressings or cloths to stabilize the object. 3. Call 9-1-1.
Sucking chest wound • Blood bubbling out of wound • Sound of air being sucked in and out of wound	1. Seal wound to stop air from entering chest; tape three sides of plastic or use gloved hand. 2. Remove cover to let air escape if victim worsens or has trouble breathing. 3. Call 9-1-1.

▶ Abdominal Injuries

What to Look For	What to Do
Blow to abdomen (closed) • Bruise or other marks • Muscle tightness and rigidity felt while gently pushing on abdomen	1. Place victim in comfortable position with legs pulled up toward the abdomen. 2. Care for shock. 3. Seek medical care.
Protruding organs (open) • Internal organs escaping from abdominal wound	1. Place victim in a comfortable position with the legs pulled up toward the abdomen. 2. DO NOT reinsert organs into the abdomen. 3. Cover organs with a moist, sterile or clean dressing. 4. Care for shock. 5. Call 9-1-1.

▶ Pelvic Injuries

What to Look For	What to Do
Pelvic fractures • Pain in hip, groin, or back that increases with movement • Inability to walk or stand • Signs of shock	1. Keep victim still. 2. Care for shock. 3. Call 9-1-1.

▶ Ready for Review

- Chest injuries fall into two categories: open or closed.
- Closed chest injuries include rib fractures and flail chest.
- In an open chest injury, the skin has been broken and the chest wall is penetrated by an object such as a knife or bullet.
- Injuries to the abdomen are either open or closed and can involve hollow and/or solid organs.
- Closed abdominal injuries occur when the internal abdominal tissues are damaged but the skin is unbroken.
- Open abdominal injuries are those in which the skin has been broken.
- Pelvic fractures are usually caused by falling or motor vehicle crash.

▶ Vital Vocabulary

<u>closed abdominal injuries</u> Injuries to the abdomen that occur as a result of a direct blow from a blunt object and there is no break in the skin.

<u>closed chest injury</u> An injury to the chest in which the skin is not broken; usually due to blunt trauma.

<u>flail chest</u> A condition that occurs when several ribs in the same area are broken in more than one place.

<u>open abdominal injuries</u> Injuries to the abdomen that include penetrating wounds and protruding organs.

<u>open chest injury</u> An injury to the chest in which the chest wall itself is penetrated, either by a fractured rib or, more frequently, by an external object such as a bullet or knife.

<u>protruding organ injury</u> A severe injury to the abdomen in which the internal organs escape or protrude from the wound.

<u>sucking chest wound</u> A chest wound that allows air to pass into and out of the chest cavity with each breath.

▶ Assessment in Action

A 45-year-old repairman falls while carrying replacement glass for a broken window. The new glass breaks into several jagged pieces. You find the repairman lying on his back with a blood-soaked shirt. You see a lacerated abdomen with several loops of intestine protruding from the laceration.

Directions: Circle Yes if you agree with the statement, circle No if you disagree.

Yes No 1. Gently push the protruding intestine back into the wound.
Yes No 2. Place a moist dressing over the protruding intestine.
Yes No 3. Place the victim on his back with the knees bent.
Yes No 4. Cover the victim with a blanket or coat.
Yes No 5. Give the victim something to drink.

Answers: 1. No; 2. Yes; 3. Yes; 4. Yes; 5. No

▶ Check Your Knowledge

Directions: Circle Yes if you agree with the statement, circle No if you disagree.

Yes No 1. Stabilize a broken rib with a soft object such as a pillow or blanket tied to the chest.
Yes No 2. Cover a sucking chest wound with a piece of plastic taped down on three sides.
Yes No 3. Remove a penetrating or impaled object from the chest or the abdomen.
Yes No 4. A flail chest refers to a single broken rib.
Yes No 5. Keep the victim with a broken pelvis still.
Yes No 6. Sharp pain while breathing can be a sign of a rib fracture.
Yes No 7. Rib fractures should be treated by tightly taping the chest.
Yes No 8. Most victims with abdominal injuries are more comfortable with their knees bent.
Yes No 9. Leave a chest wound alone if you hear air being sucked in and out.
Yes No 10. A broken pelvis can threaten life because of the large amount of blood lost.

Answers: 1. Yes; 2. Yes; 3. No; 4. No; 5. Yes; 6. Yes; 7. No; 8. Yes; 9. No; 10. Yes

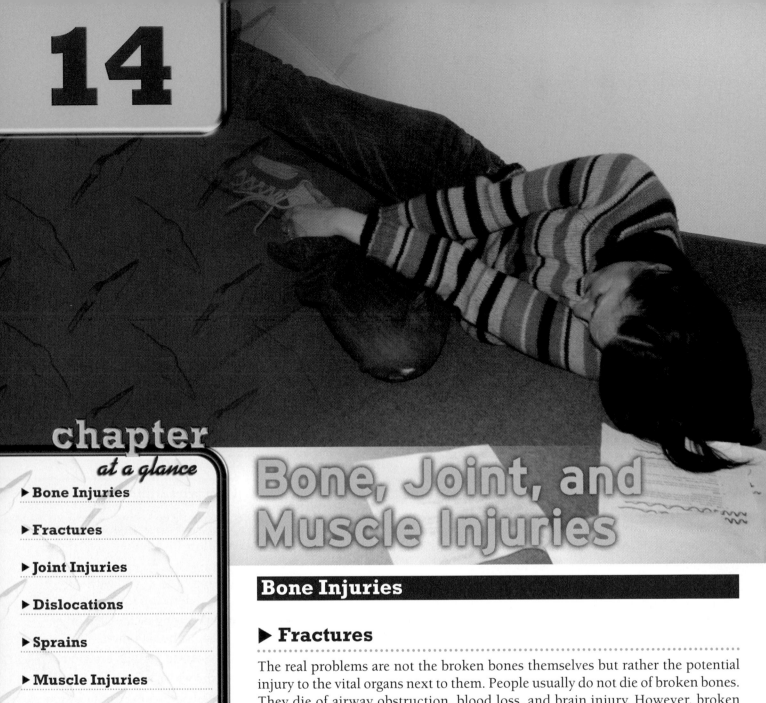

Bone, Joint, and Muscle Injuries

Bone Injuries

▶ Fractures

The real problems are not the broken bones themselves but rather the potential injury to the vital organs next to them. People usually do not die of broken bones. They die of airway obstruction, blood loss, and brain injury. However, broken bones can be painful and debilitating and can cause lifelong aggravation, disability, and deformity.

The terms <u>fracture</u> and broken bone have the same meaning: a break or crack in a bone. There are two categories of fractures:

- <u>Closed fracture</u>. The skin is intact, and no wound exists anywhere near the fracture site **Figure 14-1A** .
- <u>Open fracture</u>. The skin over the fracture has been broken. The wound may result from the bone protruding through the skin or from a direct blow that cut the skin at the time of the fracture. The bone may not always be visible in the wound **Figure 14-1B** .

It is not possible to determine the exact nature of a broken bone outside a medical facility. It may be helpful, however, for first aiders to be familiar with the terminology that physicians use to describe fractures **Figure 14-2** .

A *transverse fracture* cuts across the bone at right angles to its long axis and is often caused by direct injury. *Greenstick fractures* are incomplete fractures that commonly occur in children, whose bones (like green sticks) are pliable. A *spiral fracture* usually results from a twisting injury, and the fracture line has the appearance of a spring. The fracture line of an *oblique fracture* crosses the bone in a slanting direction (or at an oblique angle, thus the name). A comminuted fracture is one in which the bone is fragmented into more than two pieces (that is, splintered or crushed). In an *impacted fracture,* the broken ends of the bone are jammed together and the bone may function as if no fracture were present.

Recognizing Fractures

It may be difficult to tell if a bone is broken **Figure 14-3**. When in doubt, treat the injury as a fracture. Use the mnemonic D-O-T-S to assess for an injury—Deformity, Open wound, Tenderness, Swelling.

- *Deformity* might not be obvious. Compare the injured part with the uninjured part on the other side.
- *Open wound* may indicate an underlying fracture.
- *Tenderness* and pain are commonly found only at the injury site. The victim usually will be able to

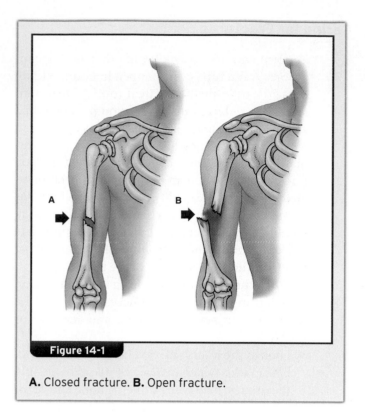

Figure 14-1

A. Closed fracture. **B.** Open fracture.

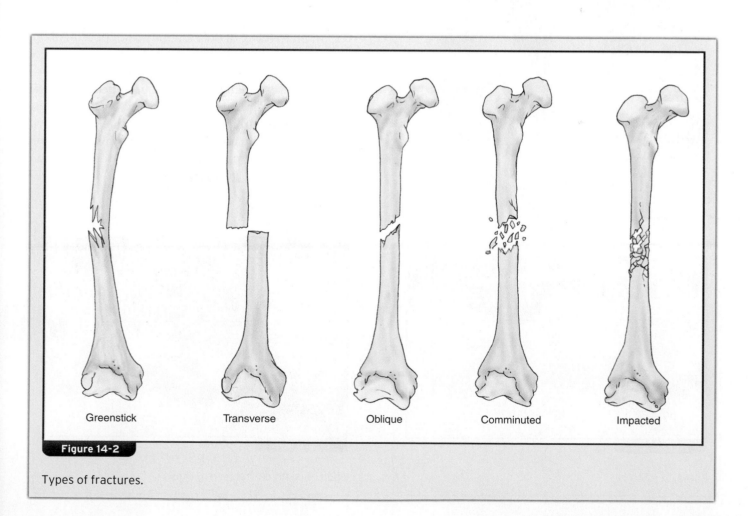

Greenstick   Transverse   Oblique   Comminuted   Impacted

Figure 14-2

Types of fractures.

point to the site of the pain. A useful procedure for detecting a fracture is to gently feel along the bone; a victim's complaint about pain or tenderness serves as a reliable sign of a fracture.

- *Swelling* caused by bleeding happens rapidly after a fracture.

Additional signs and symptoms include the following:

- *Loss of use* may or may not occur. *Guarding* occurs when motion produces pain; the victim refuses to use the injured part. Sometimes, however, the victim is able to move a fractured limb with little or no pain.
- A *grating sensation,* called **crepitus**, can be felt and sometimes even heard when the ends of the broken bone rub together. Do not move the injured limb in an attempt to detect it **Figure 14-4**.
- The *history* of the injury can lead you to suspect a fracture whenever a serious accident has happened. The victim may have heard or felt the bone snap.

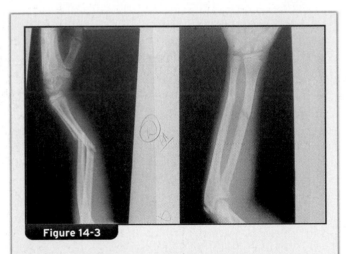

Figure 14-3

X-rays of a victim's forearm showing the fracture before and after setting.

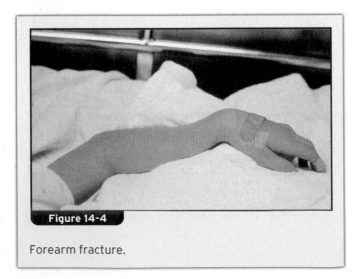

Figure 14-4

Forearm fracture.

Caring for Fractures

1. Perform an initial check for life-threatening conditions. A fracture, even an open fracture, seldom presents an immediate threat to life. Treatment should be deferred until after you have handled any life-threatening conditions such as opening an airway or controlling massive bleeding. A tourniquet is practically never necessary to treat an open fracture, even when an extremity has been mangled beyond all possibility of salvage or a limb has been amputated. Only when all life-threatening conditions have been dealt with is it appropriate to identify and stabilize fractures. Determine what happened and the location of the injury.
2. Gently remove clothing covering the injured area. Cut clothing at the seams if necessary.
3. Examine the area by looking and feeling for D-O-T-S.
   - Look at the injury site. Swelling and black-and-blue marks, which indicate escape of blood into the tissues, may come from the bone end or associated muscular and blood vessel damage. Shortening or severe deformity (*angulation*) between the joints or deformity around the joints, shortening of the extremity, and rotation of the extremity when compared with the opposite extremity indicate a bone injury. Lacerations or even small puncture wounds near the site of a bone fracture are considered open fractures.
   - Feel the injured area. If a fracture is not obvious, gently press, touch, or feel along the length of the bone for deformities, tenderness, and swelling **Figure 14-5**.

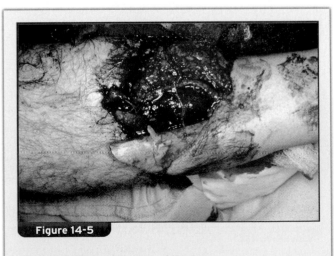

Figure 14-5

Open tibia, fibula fracture of the leg.

4. Check blood flow and nerves. Use the mnemonic CSM (circulation, sensation, movement) as a way of remembering what to do **Skill Drill 14-1** :
   - *Circulation.* For an arm injury, feel for the radial pulse (located on the thumb side of the wrist); use the posterior tibial pulse (located between the inside ankle bone and the Achilles tendon) for a leg injury. A pulseless arm or leg is a significant emergency that requires immediate surgical care. If there is no pulse, gently realign the extremity to try to restore the blood flow. Some experts recommend the capillary refill test. (Press on a fingernail or toenail, then release it. If circulation is normal, the nail bed should return to its normal color within 2 seconds.) Performing the capillary refill test in the dark or the cold may limit its accuracy (**Step ❶**).
   - *Sensation.* This is the most useful early sign. Lightly touch or squeeze one of the victim's toes or fingers and ask the victim what he or she feels (**Step ❷**). Loss of sensation is an early sign of nerve damage.
   - *Movement.* Inability to move develops later. Check for nerve damage by asking the victim to wiggle his or her toes or fingers. If the toes or fingers are injured, do not have the victim attempt to move them (**Step ❸**). A quick nerve and circulatory check is extremely important. The most serious complication of a fracture is inadequate blood flow in an extremity. The major blood vessels of an extremity tend to run close to the bones, which means that any time a bone is broken, the adjacent blood vessels are at risk of being torn by bone fragments or pinched off between the ends of the broken bone. The tissues of the arms and legs cannot survive for more than 3 hours without a continuing blood supply. If you note any disruption in the nerve or circulatory supply, seek immediate medical attention. Major nerve pathways also travel close to bone and may be torn or pinched off between the ends of the broken bone.
5. Stabilize the injured part to prevent movement.
   - If emergency medical services (EMS) will arrive soon, stabilize the injured part with your hands until they arrive.
   - If the EMS will be delayed or if you are taking the victim to medical care, stabilize the injured part with a splint.
6. If the injury is an open fracture, do not push on any protruding bones. Cover the wound and ex-posed bones with a dressing. Place rolls of gauze around the bone and bandage the injury without applying pressure on the bone.
7. Apply an ice pack, if possible, to help reduce swelling and pain.
8. Seek medical care. Call 9-1-1 for any open fractures or large bone fractures (such as the femur) or when transporting the victim would be difficult or would aggravate the injury.

Joint Injuries

A joint is where two or more bones come together.

▶ Dislocations

A *dislocation* occurs when a joint comes apart and stays apart with the bone ends no longer in contact. The shoulders, elbows, fingers, hips, kneecaps (patellas), and ankles are the joints most frequently affected.

Recognizing Dislocations

Dislocations cause signs and symptoms similar to those of fractures: deformity, severe pain, swelling, and inability of the victim to move the injured joint. The main sign of a dislocation is deformity. Its appearance will be different from that of an uninjured joint **Figure 14-6** .

Care for Dislocations

1. Check the CSM. If the end of the dislocated bone is pressing on nerves or blood vessels, numbness or paralysis may exist below the dislocation. Always check the pulses. If there is no pulse in the injured extremity, transport the victim to a medical facility immediately.

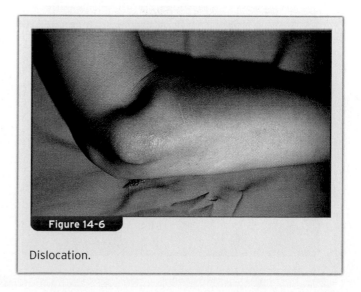

Figure 14-6

Dislocation.

14-1 **Checking CSM in an Extremity**

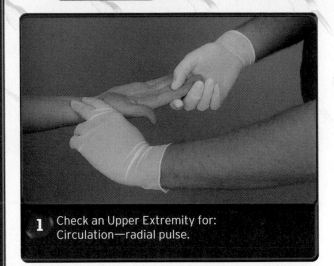

1 Check an Upper Extremity for:
Circulation—radial pulse.

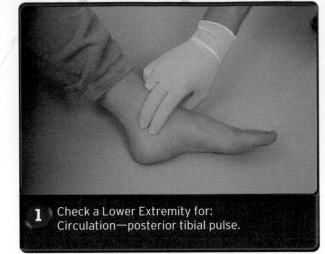

1 Check a Lower Extremity for:
Circulation—posterior tibial pulse.

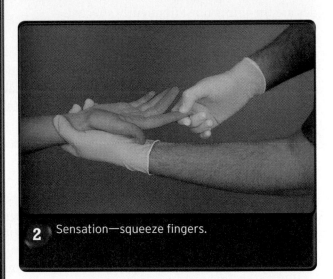

2 Sensation—squeeze fingers.

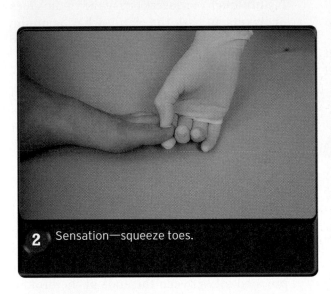

2 Sensation—squeeze toes.

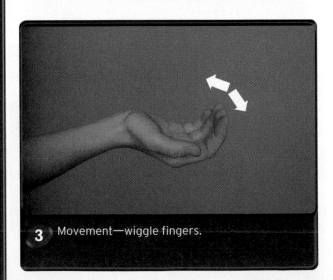

3 Movement—wiggle fingers.

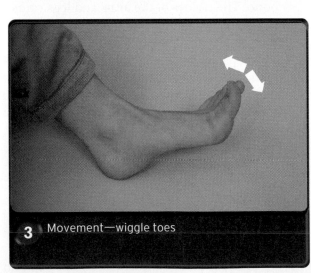

3 Movement—wiggle toes

2. Use the RICE procedures.
3. Use a splint to stabilize the joint in the position in which it was found.
4. Do not try to reduce the joint (put the displaced parts back into their normal positions) because nerve and blood vessel damage could result. For instances when medical help is more than 1 hour away, experts in wilderness medicine have identified easy and safe ways to treat the following dislocations: kneecap, fingers and toes, and anterior shoulder (see Chapter 24).
5. Seek medical care to reduce the dislocation. Call 9-1-1 for dislocations when transporting the victim would be difficult or would aggravate the injury.

▶ Sprains

A sprain occurs when a joint is twisted or stretched beyond its normal range of motion. Bones are held together at joints by tough bands of tissue called ligaments. When a joint is sprained, the ligaments are either partially or completely torn. There are different degrees of sprains, but it is difficult for a first aider to classify the degree of a sprain. Sprains most often occur in the knee and the ankle, but can occur in any joint.

Ankle sprains most often occur when the foot turns inward and stress is placed on the outside (lateral side) of the ankle. A severe lateral ankle sprain, if not correctly treated, can result in a chronically unstable ankle that is prone to sprains. Any ligament or bone injury on the inner side of the ankle usually represents a serious problem and requires medical care.

Recognizing Sprains

It is often difficult to distinguish between a severe sprain and a fracture because their signs and symptoms are similar.

- Severe pain
- Pain prevents the victim from moving or using the joint.
- Swelling
- Skin around the joint may be discolored because of bleeding from torn blood vessels.

Care for Sprains

1. Follow the RICE procedures. Apply an ice pack for 20 minutes; apply compression with an elastic bandage for 3 to 4 hours; repeat the cycles of an ice pack for 20 minutes and 3 hours of compression. Raise the injured part to reduce the flow of blood to the injury. For more information on the RICE procedure, see page 190.

2. Swelling in a joint can lead to stiffness in a matter of hours. It is important to keep a joint from swelling by using cold promptly; it is equally important to help the swelling recede as quickly as possible with a compression and elevation.

Muscle Injuries

Although muscle injuries pose no real emergency, first aiders have ample opportunities to care for them.

▶ Strains

A *muscle strain,* also known as a *muscle pull,* occurs when a muscle is stretched beyond its normal range of motion and tears the muscle. There are different degrees of strains, but it is difficult for a first aider to classify the degree of a strain. When muscle fibers tear, fluid from nearby tissues leaks out and starts to build up near the injury. The area becomes inflamed, swollen, and tender. Inflammation begins immediately after an injury, but it can take 24 to 72 hours for enough tissue fluid to build up to cause pain and stiffness.

Recognizing Strains

Any of the following signs and symptoms may indicate a muscle strain:

- Sudden, sharp pain in the affected muscle
- Extreme tenderness when the area is touched
- Swelling
- Weakness and inability to use the injured part
- Stiffness and pain when the victim moves the muscle
- After a few days, the skin around the injury may be discolored because of bleeding from torn blood vessels.

Care for Strains

To care for strains, simply follow the RICE procedures.

▶ Cramps

A cramp occurs when a muscle goes into an uncontrolled spasm and contraction. Although scientific literature has yet to confirm the causes of muscle cramps, several factors are associated with them. For example, muscle cramping is associated with certain diseases such as diabetes and atherosclerosis. Muscle cramps are often associated with physical activity. Roughly, muscle cramps can be divided into two categories: *night cramps,* which include any cramp occurring at night or while an individual is at rest, and *heat cramps,* which are related to dehydration and electrolyte imbalance. (The electrolytes potassium and sodium carry an electric charge that helps trigger muscles to contract and relax.)

Recognizing Cramps

- Sudden, severe pain, usually in the legs.
- A knotting of the muscle may be felt and sometimes seen.
- Restricts movement

Care for Cramps

Many treatments for cramps are available. Try one or more of the following:

1. Have the victim gently stretch the affected muscle. Because a muscle cramp is an uncontrolled muscle contraction or spasm, a gradual extension of the muscle may help lengthen the muscle fibers and relieve the cramp.
2. Relax the muscle by pressing and massaging it.
3. Apply an ice pack to help relieve the cramping pain (unless you are in a cold environment).
4. Pinch the upper lip hard (an acupressure technique) to reduce calf-muscle cramping.
5. Drink lightly salted cool water (dissolve ¼ teaspoon salt in a quart of water) or a commercial sports drink.

▶ Contusions

A muscle contusion or bruise results from a blow to the muscle.

Recognizing Contusions

- Swelling
- Pain and tenderness
- After a few days, the skin in the area may become discolored due to bleeding from torn blood vessels.

Care for Contusions

1. To care for muscle contusions, follow the RICE procedures.

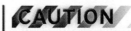

CAUTION

DO NOT give salt tablets to a person with muscle cramps. They can cause stomach irritation, nausea, and vomiting.

▶ Bone Injuries

What to Look For

Fractures (broken bones)
- DOTS (deformity, open wound, tenderness, swelling)
- Inability to use injured part normally
- Grating or grinding sensation felt or heard
- Victim heard or felt bone snap

What to Do

1. Expose and examine the injury site.
2. Bandage any open wound.
3. Splint the injured area.
4. Apply ice or cold pack.
5. Seek medical care: Depending on the severity, call 9-1-1 or transport to medical care.

▶ Joint Injuries

What to Look For

Dislocation or sprain
- Deformity
- Pain
- Swelling
- Inability to use injured part normally

What to Do

Dislocation
1. Expose and examine the injury site.
2. Splint the injured area.
3. Apply ice or cold pack.
4. Seek medical care.

Sprain
1. Use RICE procedures.

▶ Muscle Injuries

What to Look For

Strain
- Sharp pain
- Extreme tenderness when area is touched
- Indentation or bump
- Weaknesss and loss of function of injured area
- Stiffness and pain when victim moves the muscle

Contusion
- Pain and tenderness
- Swelling
- Bruise on injured area

Cramp
- Uncontrolled spasm
- Pain
- Restriction or loss of movement

What to Do

1. Use RICE procedures.

1. Use RICE procedures.

1. Stretch and/or apply direct pressure to the affected muscle.

prep kit

▶ Ready for Review

- Broken bones can be painful and debilitating and can cause lifelong aggravation, disability, and deformity.
- A joint is where two or more bones come together. Joints can be dislocated or sprained.
- Muscles can be strained, bruised, or cramped.

▶ Vital Vocabulary

closed fracture A fracture in which there is no wound in the overlying skin.

cramp A painful spasm, usually of a muscle.

crepitus A grating sound heard and the sensation felt when the fractured ends of a bone rub together.

fracture A break or rupture in a bone.

open fracture A fracture exposed to the exterior; an open wound lies over the fracture.

sprain A trauma to a joint that injures the ligaments.

▶ Assessment in Action

During a softball game, a batter loses her grip while swinging at a pitch. The bat flies through the air and hits a nearby player hard on the arm. Although the skin is not broken, there is tenderness and some swelling.

Directions: Circle Yes if you agree with the statement, circle No if you disagree.

Yes No 1. A splint can help stabilize a broken bone against movement.

Yes No 2. Applying heat reduces bleeding and swelling.

Yes No 3. This is an open fracture.

Yes No 4. If the player can move her arm, she does not need to see a doctor.

Yes No 5. You should look and feel for D-O-T-S.

Answers: **1.** Yes; **2.** No; **3.** No; **4.** No; **5.** Yes

▶ Check Your Knowledge

Directions: Circle Yes if you agree with the statement, circle No if you disagree.

Yes No 1. Apply cold on a suspected sprain.

Yes No 2. The letters RICE stand for rest, ice, compression, and elevation.

Yes No 3. D-O-T-S stands for deformity, open wound, tenderness, and swelling.

Yes No 4. Guarding occurs when motion produces pain.

Yes No 5. Crepitus cannot be heard, but it can be felt by the victim.

Yes No 6. A dislocation is cared for much differently than a fracture.

Yes No 7. Check a suspected fracture by having the victim move the extremity.

Yes No 8. Treat a muscle cramp by stretching the affected muscle.

Yes No 9. CSM stands for cold, swelling, and motion.

Yes No 10. Do not push on a protruding bone.

Answers: **1.** Yes; **2.** Yes; **3.** Yes; **4.** Yes; **5.** No; **6.** No; **7.** No; **8.** Yes; **9.** No; **10.** Yes

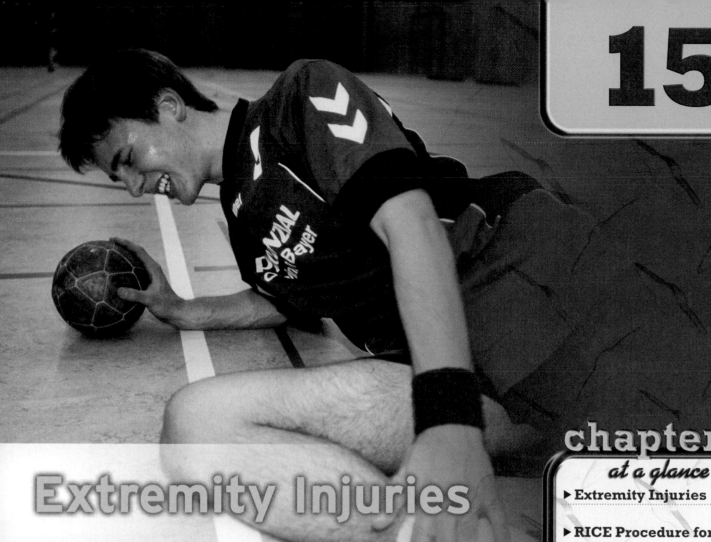

chapter
at a glance
▶ **Extremity Injuries**

▶ **RICE Procedure for Bone, Joint, and Muscle Injuries**

▶ **Shoulder Injuries**

▶ **Elbow Injuries**

▶ **Hand Injuries**

▶ **Finger Injuries**

▶ **Hip-Joint Injuries**

▶ **Thigh Injuries**

▶ **Knee Injuries**

▶ **Lower-Leg Injuries**

Extremity Injuries

Extremity Injuries

Injuries to the extremities are common because people are involved in active lifestyles that include sports and wilderness activities. This chapter focuses on bone, joint, and muscle injuries of the extremities; bleeding, wounds, and other soft-tissue injuries are covered elsewhere. Most of the conditions discussed result from sudden trauma, although some chronic injuries incurred over time, such as tennis elbow, are included.

▶ Assessment

Use these guidelines to assess injuries to the extremities:
- Look for signs and symptoms of fractures and dislocations.
- Examine the extremities, using the mnemonic D-O-T-S (Deformity, Open wound, Tenderness, Swelling). Look at and gently feel the extremity, starting at the distal end (fingers or toes) and working upward.
- Compare one extremity with the other to determine size and shape differences.
- Use the "rule of thirds" for extremity injuries. Imagine each long bone as being divided into thirds. If deformity, tenderness, or swelling is located in the upper or lower third of a long bone, assume that the nearest joint is injured.

- Consider the cause of injury (COI) when evaluating the possibility of a fracture and its location. Forces that cause musculoskeletal injuries are direct forces (for example, a car bumper striking a pedestrian's leg), indirect forces along the long axis of bones (for example, a person falling onto an outstretched hand and fracturing the collar bone), and twisting forces (for example, a person's foot fixed in one spot with the leg suddenly twisting).
- Use the mnemonic CSM as a reminder to check the extremity for Circulation, Sensation, and Movement of fingers or toes.

▶ Types of Injuries

Types of injuries to the extremities range from simple contusions to complex open fractures:

- <u>Contusions</u>, or bruising of the tissue
- <u>Strains</u>, in which muscles are stretched or torn
- <u>Sprains</u>, which involve the tearing or stretching of the joints, causing mild to severe damage to the ligaments and joint capsules
- <u>Tendinitis</u>, which is inflammation of a tendon due to overuse (cord that attaches muscle to bone)
- <u>Dislocations</u>, in which bones are displaced from their normal joint alignment, out of their sockets, or out of their normal positions
- <u>Fractures</u>, which are breaks in bones that may or may not be accompanied by open wounds

Care for Extremity Injuries

1. Use the RICE procedures for injuries described in this chapter (see Skill Drill 15-1, page 193).
2. Apply a splint to stabilize fractures and dislocations.

RICE Procedure for Bone, Joint, and Muscle Injuries

RICE is the acronym for Rest, Ice, Compression, Elevation, the recommended immediate treatment for bone, joint, and muscle injuries. The steps during the first 48 to 72 hours after an injury can do a lot to relieve—even prevent—aches and pains. Treat all extremity bone, joint, and muscle injuries with the RICE procedure. In addition to RICE, fractures and dislocations should be splinted to stabilize the injured area.

▶ R = Rest

Injuries heal faster if rested. *Rest* means the victim does not use or move the injured part. Using any part of the body increases the blood circulation to that area, which can cause more swelling of an injured part. Crutches may be used to rest leg injuries.

▶ I = Ice

An ice pack should be applied to the injured area as soon as possible after the injury for 20 to 30 minutes every 2 or 3 hours during the first 24 to 48 hours. Skin treated with cold passes through four stages: cold, burning, aching, and numbness. When the skin becomes numb, usually in 20 to 30 minutes, remove the ice pack. After removing the ice pack, compress the injured part with an elastic bandage and keep it elevated (the "C" and "E" of RICE).

Cold constricts the blood vessels to and in the injured area, which helps reduce the swelling and inflammation, and it dulls the pain and relieves muscle spasms. Cold should be applied as soon as possible after the injury; healing time often is directly related to the amount of swelling that occurs. Heat has the opposite effect when applied to fresh injuries: It increases circulation to the area and greatly increases the swelling and the pain.

Use either of the following methods to apply cold to an injury:

- Put crushed ice (or cubes) into a double plastic bag, hot water bottle, or wet towel. Secure it in place with an elastic bandage for 20 to 30 minutes. Ice bags can conform to the body's contours.
- Use a chemical "snap pack," a sealed pouch that contains two chemical envelopes. Squeezing the pack mixes the chemicals, producing a chemical reaction that has a cooling effect. Although they do not cool as well as other methods, they are convenient to use when ice is not readily available. They lose their cooling power quickly, however, and can be used only once. Also, they may be impractical because they are expensive.

CAUTION

DO NOT apply an ice pack for more than 20 to 30 minutes at a time. Frostbite or nerve damage can result.

DO NOT apply an ice pack on the back outside part of the knee. Nerve damage can occur.

DO NOT apply cold if the victim has a history of circulatory disease, Raynaud disease (spasms in the arteries of the extremities that reduce circulation), or abnormal sensitivity to cold or if the injured part has been frostbitten previously.

DO NOT stop using an ice pack too soon. A common mistake is the early use of heat, which will result in swelling and pain. Use an ice pack three to four times a day for the first 24 hours, preferably up to 48 hours, before applying any heat. For severe injuries, using ice for up to 72 hours is recommended.

FYI

Heat and Cold: When to Use Which?

Many people use heat devices or ice packs to speed recovery from sports injuries—but when is the right time to use each technique? Cold usually should be applied immediately after an acute injury, such as an ankle sprain. Icing reduces pain, swelling, and muscle spasm immediately after injury, but its use should be discontinued after 2 or 3 days. Heat applications (heat packs, radiant heat, or whirlpool baths) can then be used to reduce muscle spasms and pain. In addition, heat increases blood flow and joint flexibility. Vigorous heat is used to treat chronic injuries, but mild heat can reduce muscle spasm. Heat is also effective for acute back pain, but ice massage is preferred if the back pain persists for 2 weeks or more.

Source: Kaul M P, Herring S A: Superficial heat and cold. *Physician and Sportsmedicine.* 22(12);65.

FYI

Homemade Ice Packs

- Ice bags kept in a freezer freeze solid and cannot be shaped to fit the injured area. One part isopropyl (rubbing) alcohol to three parts water prevents freezing, and the ice bag can be easily molded. Bags can be reused for months.

- An unopened bag of frozen vegetables is inexpensive; keeps its basic shape (unlike ice chips, which melt); molds to the shape of the injured area; is reusable; and is packaged in a fairly puncture-resistant, watertight bag.

- For cold therapy over a fairly large area, soak a face towel in cold water, wring it out, fold it, and place it in a large self-sealing plastic bag. Store the bag in the freezer. To use the cold pack, wrap it in a light cotton towel and apply for 20 minutes, after which it can be refrozen. A washcloth in a smaller bag can be used to treat a smaller area.

- Fill a plastic bag with snow.

- Fill a polystyrene plastic cup with water and freeze it. When you need an ice pack, peel the cup to below ice level; the remaining part of the cup forms a cold-resistant handle. Rub the ice over the injured area (movement is necessary to prevent skin damage). These ice "packs" are inexpensive and convenient and take up little space.

- To make a funnel for filling an ice bag, push out the bottom of a paper cup and fit it into the neck of the ice bag. The ice will slide through the cup and into the bag.

▶ C = Compression

Compressing the injured area squeezes fluid out of the injury site. Compression limits the ability of the skin and of other tissues to expand and reduces internal bleeding. Apply an elastic bandage to the injured area, especially the foot, ankle, knee, thigh, hand, or elbow. Fill the hollow areas with padding such as a sock or washcloth before applying the elastic bandage.

Elastic bandages come in various sizes for different body areas:

- 2-inch width for the wrist, hand, and foot
- 3-inch width for the elbow and arm
- 4-inch width for the ankle, knee, and leg

Start the elastic bandage several inches below the injury and wrap in an upward, overlapping (about one half to three fourths of the bandage's width) spiral, starting with even and somewhat tight pressure, then gradually wrapping more loosely above the injury.

Applying compression may be the most important step in preventing swelling. The victim should wear the elastic bandage continuously for the first 18 to 24 hours (except when cold is applied). At night, have the victim loosen but not remove the elastic bandage.

For an ankle injury, place a horseshoe-shaped pad around the ankle knob and secure it with the elastic bandage. The pad will compress the soft tissues and the bones. Wrap the bandage tightest nearest the toes and loosest above the ankle. It should be tight enough to decrease swelling but not tight enough to inhibit blood flow. For a contusion or a strain, place a pad between the injury and the elastic bandage.

CAUTION

DO NOT apply an elastic bandage too tightly. If applied too tightly, elastic bandages will restrict circulation. Stretch a new elastic bandage to about one third its maximum length for adequate compression. Leave fingers and toes exposed so possible color change can be easily observed. Compare the toes or fingers of the injured extremity with those on the uninjured one. Pale skin, pain, numbness, and tingling are signs that the bandage is too tight. If any of these symptoms appears, immediately remove the elastic bandage. Leave the elastic bandage off until all the symptoms disappear, then rewrap the area less tightly. Always wrap from below the injury and move toward the heart.

▶ E = Elevation

Gravity slows the return of blood to the heart from the lower parts of the body. Once fluids get to the hands or feet, they have nowhere else to go, and those parts of the body swell. Elevating the injured area, in combination with ice and compression, limits circulation to that area, which in turn helps limit internal bleeding and minimize swelling.

It is simple to prop up an injured leg or arm to limit bleeding. Whenever possible, elevate the injured part above the level of the heart for the first 24 hours after an injury. If a fracture is suspected, do not elevate an extremity until it has been stabilized with a splint. Along with the use of RICE procedures, fractures and dislocations should be splinted.

To perform the RICE procedure, follow the steps in **Skill Drill 15-1** :

1. R = Rest. Stop using the injured area.
2. I = Ice. Place an ice pack on the injured area. Use an elastic bandage to hold the ice pack in place for 20 to 30 minutes (**Step ❶**).

3. C = Compression. Remove the ice and apply a compression bandage and leave in place for 3 to 4 hours (**Step ❷**).
4. E = Elevation. Raise the injured area higher than the heart, if possible (**Step ❸**).

Shoulder Injuries

▶ Shoulder Dislocation

Three bones come together at the shoulder: the scapula (shoulder blade), the clavicle (collarbone), and the humerus (upper arm bone). The shoulder is the most freely movable joint in the body. The extreme range of its possible movements makes the shoulder joint highly susceptible to dislocation (separation). A *dislocation* of the shoulder occurs when the bones of the shoulder come apart as a result of a blow or a particular movement. Shoulder dislocation is second in frequency only to finger dislocations.

Recognizing Shoulder Dislocation

- In about 95% of shoulder dislocations, the victim holds the upper arm away from the body, supported by the uninjured arm. This position differentiates a dislocation from a fracture of the humerus, in which the victim holds the arm against the chest.
- The dislocated arm cannot be brought across the chest wall to touch the opposite shoulder (that is, the sling position).
- Extreme pain in the shoulder area.
- In a dislocation, the shoulder looks squared off, rather than rounded.
- An injury to the shoulder resulting in complete loss of function is more apt to be a dislocation than a fracture.
- The victim may describe a history of previous dislocations.
- Numbness or paralysis in the arm from pressure, pinching blood vessels or nerves.

Care for a Shoulder Dislocation

1. Do not try to force, twist, or pull the shoulder back in place because it may cause bone, nerve or blood vessel injury.
2. Place folded or rolled blanket or a pillow between the upper arm and the chest to support the arm.
3. Apply an arm sling and swathe (binder). Use the arm sling which has one end tucked between the arm and body and ties in the back. This keeps pressure off of the area.

skill drill

15-1 The RICE Procedure

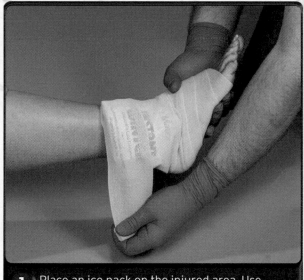

1 Place an ice pack on the injured area. Use an elastic bandage to hold the ice pack in place for 20 to 30 minutes.

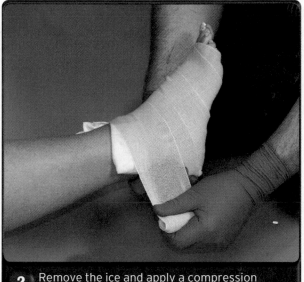

2 Remove the ice and apply a compression bandage and leave in place for 3 to 4 hours.

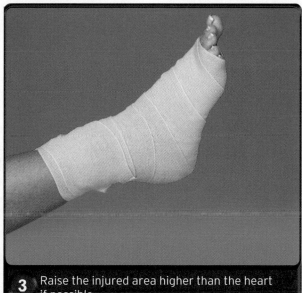

3 Raise the injured area higher than the heart if possible.

4. Apply an ice pack for 20 minutes.
5. Seek immediate medical care.

▶ Clavicle Fracture

Fractures of the clavicle (collarbone) are common and usually are the result of falling with the arm and hand outstretched. The victim falls onto his or her hand, and the force from the fall is transmitted to the shoulder. Most clavicle fractures (80%) occur in the middle third of the bone.

Recognizing a Clavicle Fracture

Usually the fracture is easy to detect because the clavicle lies immediately under the skin and a deformity can be seen.

The victim:
- Fell on an outstretched arm
- Received a direct blow to the clavicle or shoulder

AND if the victim has:
- Severe pain over the injured area
- Been holding the injured arm against the chest with the uninjured arm to stabilize the injury
- Not moved the arm because of the pain
- Swelling
- Visible deformity
- Tenderness
- "Dropped" or drooped shoulder
- Bruising

Care for a Clavicle Fracture

1. Treat for shock.
2. Apply an arm sling and swathe (binder). Use the arm sling which has one end tucked between the arm and body and ties in the back. This keeps pressure off of the area.
3. Apply an ice pack to the area for 20 minutes, three to four times during the next 24 hours.
4. Seek immediate medical care.

▶ Contusions

Direct blows cause contusions, or bruises, about the shoulder. Often called *shoulder pointers*, contusions of this type may cause severe discomfort.

Recognizing Contusions

- Swelling
- Pain at the injury site
- Feeling of firmness when pressure is exerted on the shoulder
- Tenderness
- Discoloration under the skin (black and blue)

Care for Contusions

1. Apply an ice pack to the area for 20 minutes, three to four times during the first 24 hours.
2. Place the arm in a sling and swathe (binder). Use the arm sling which has one end tucked between the arm and body and ties in the back. This keeps pressure off of the area.

▶ Tendinitis

The general cause of tendinitis (inflammation) in the shoulder is continuous overuse or unusual use. Repeated arm movement often results in painful shoulders. Examples of these include many of the throwing sports (such as seen with a baseball pitcher or a football quarterback) and in other sports in which the shoulder is used extensively (such as swimming).

Recognizing Tendinitis

- Constant pain or pain with motion of the shoulder
- Limited motion of the shoulder
- "Crackling" sound when the joint is moved
- Tenderness over the area

Care for Tendinitis

1. Use an ice massage for 10 minutes before and after exercise. Fill a Styrofoam cup with water and freeze. Tear a small amount of foam from the top so ice protrudes. Massage firmly over the injured area in a circle about the size of a baseball.
2. Use a sling and swathe (binder) to rest the shoulder.
3. Use pain medication such as ibuprofen.
4. Seek medical advice if needed.

▶ Humerus Fracture

The shaft of the humerus (upper arm) can be felt throughout its entire length along the inner side of the upper arm.

Recognizing a Humerus Fracture

The victim received a:
- Direct blow to the area
- Twist or fall on the outstretched arm

AND any one or combination of these occurred:
- Severe pain
- Swelling

- Visible deformity. The deformity may be hidden by swelling or by the large muscles surrounding the upper part of the arm.
- Tender if touched
- May be unable to move the arm
- Will hold the arm against the chest for comfort

Care for a Humerus Fracture

1. Treat for shock.
2. Apply an ice pack for 20 minutes.
3. Stabilize the arm by applying one rigid splint on the part of the arm away from the body. Apply an arm sling and swathe (binder).
4. Seek immediate medical care.

Elbow Injuries

▶ Elbow Fractures and Dislocations

All elbow fractures and dislocations should be considered serious and treated with extreme care. Inappropriate care can result in injury to the nearby nerves and blood vessels.

Recognizing Elbow Fractures and Dislocations

- Immediate swelling
- Severe pain
- Possible visible deformity; compare it with the uninjured elbow
- Restricted, painful motion
- Numbness or coldness of the hand and fingers below the elbow

Care for Elbow Fractures and Dislocations

1. Do not move the elbow.
2. Treat for shock.
3. Splint the elbow in the position found in order to prevent nerve and blood vessel damage:
   - If straight, keep the splinted elbow straight.
   - If bent, keep the elbow bent.
4. Apply an ice pack for 20 minutes.
5. Seek immediate medical care.

▶ Tennis Elbow

Tennis elbow results from sharp, quick twists of the wrist (not just from playing tennis). The muscles that bend the wrist back and straighten the fingers all begin in one spot, no bigger than a dime, on the outside bony prominence (protrusion), of the elbow. Tennis elbow, which is an inflammation of the tendons on this outer side of the elbow, can be very painful whenever the wrist and the elbow are used.

Recognizing Tennis Elbow

- Pain increases while using the arm
- Causes gradual grip weakness
- The injured elbow fatigues quicker than normal
- Very tender on outer protusion of elbow

Care for Tennis Elbow

1. Apply heat before an activity; the victim might wear a brace or rubber sleeve on the sore elbow.
2. Apply an ice pack for 20 minutes after completion of the activity.
3. Seek medical advice for appropriate rehabilitation program.

▶ Golfer's Elbow

Repetitive motion produces pain. This injury is the equivalent of the more common tennis elbow but with pain on the inside of the elbow. It is tendinitis affecting the tendons attached to the bony protrusion, on the inside of the elbow.

Recognizing Golfer's Elbow

- Pain increases while using the arm.
- Causes gradual grip weakness
- The injured elbow fatigues quicker than normal.

Care for Golfer's Elbow

1. Apply heat before an activity; the victim might wear a brace or rubber sleeve on the tender elbow.
2. Apply an ice pack for 20 minutes after completion of an activity.
3. Seek medical advice for appropriate rehabilitation program.

▶ Radius and Ulna Fractures

There are two large bones (radius and ulna) in the forearm, and either or both bones may be broken. When only one bone is broken, the other acts as a splint and there may be little or no deformity. However, a marked deformity may be present in a fracture near the wrist. When both bones are broken, the arm usually appears deformed.

Recognizing Radius and Ulna Fracture

The victim has pain in the forearm or wrist from:
- A direct blow
- Falling on an outstretched hand

AND has

- A visible deformity
- Severe pain radiating up and down from the injury site
- An inability to move the wrist or it is painful while moving the wrist

OR

- The wrist is painful on the thumb side and pain continues into next day

Care for Radius and Ulna Fracture

1. Treat for shock.
2. Apply an ice pack to the area for 20 minutes.
3. Apply two rigid splints on both sides of the arm from the tip of the elbow to the fingers. Place the arm in a sling and swathe (binder) with the hand in a thumb-up position.
4. Seek medical care.

▶ Wrist Fracture

The wrist usually is broken when the victim falls with the arm and hand outstretched.

Recognizing a Wrist Fracture

- Injury to the wrist associated with a snapping or popping sensation within the wrist
- Pain in the wrist that is aggravated by movement
- Tenderness
- Swelling
- Unable or unwilling to move the wrist
- Lumplike deformity on the back of the wrist

Care for a Wrist Fracture

1. Use the RICE procedures.
2. Stabilize the wrist with a splint.
3. Seek medical care.

Hand Injuries

▶ Crushed Hand

The hand may be fractured by a direct blow or by a crushing injury.

Recognizing a Crushed Hand

- Pain
- Swelling
- Loss of motion
- Open wounds
- Broken bones

Care for a Crushed Hand

1. Control the bleeding.
2. Apply an ice pack for 20 minutes.
3. Seek medical care.

Finger Injuries

The three bones that make up each finger are the most commonly broken bones in the body. Many of the tendons attached to the finger bones can tear with or without a fracture, and the three joints—the *distal interphalangeal*, the *proximal interphalangeal*, and the *metacarpal phalangeal*—can also be injured. A so-called finger sprain may be a complicated fracture or dislocation.

▶ Finger Fracture

Contrary to popular belief, broken bones—especially the fingers—can move when they are broken.

Recognizing Finger Fractures

The finger or thumb has:

- A visible deformity; finger has a twisted look
- Immediate pain and hurts with or without movement
- Numbness
- Swelling
- Pinpointed tenderness that usually indicates a fracture

Test for a finger fracture:

- If possible, straighten the fingers and place them on a hard surface.
- Tap the tip of the injured finger toward the hand. Pain lower down in the finger or into the hand can indicate a fracture.

Care for Finger Fractures

1. Do not try to realign the finger.
2. Gently apply an ice pack.
3. Splint the finger by either:
   - "Buddy" taping the fractured finger to another for support. For a thumb, tape it with three to four figure-eight patterns around the joint

   OR

   - Keeping the hand and fingers in the position of function (cupping shape as though holding a baseball) with extra padding in the palm. Secure the hand, fingers, and arm to a rigid splint.
4. Seek medical care.

▶ Finger Dislocation

Finger dislocations are common. The same causes of fractured fingers can also cause a dislocated finger.

Recognizing Finger Dislocation

The finger or thumb has:
- A visible deformity
- Immediate pain
- Swelling
- Shortening of the finger
- May be unable to bend the finger in the injured area; motion is impossible

Care for Finger Dislocation

1. Do not try to realign the dislocation.
2. Apply an ice pack.
3. If possible, splint the finger by either:
   - "Buddy" taping the finger for support. For a thumb, tape it with three to four figure-eight patterns around the joint

OR

   - Keeping the hand and fingers in the position of function (cupping shape as though holding a baseball) with extra padding in the palm. Secure the hand, fingers, and arm to a rigid splint.
4. Seek medical care.

▶ Sprained Finger

The upper joints of the fingers have a ligament on each side of the joint.

Recognizing a Sprained Finger

The finger or thumb has been:
- "Jammed" or compressed
- Stepped on
- Forced or twisted sideways

AND the victim:
- Has pain and swelling over a joint (especially tenderness on both sides of a joint)
- Is unable to make a fist
- Has a weakness while curling the injured finger alone
- Experiences a weakness or pain when gripping

Care for a Sprained Finger

1. Apply an ice pack for 20 minutes.
2. Reevaluate after the ice-pack application and seek medical care if pain and weakness exist.

3. Tape fingers with "buddy" taping for support. Tape thumb with three to four figure-eight patterns around joint.

▶ Nail Avulsion

A victim may have had a blow to the nail, the nail may have been torn away by a piece of machinery, or a long toenail may have caught on a loop of carpet or other fixed object. An injury in which a nail is partly or completely torn loose is known as a *nail avulsion*.

Recognizing Nail Avulsion

- The nail may be completely detached or partially held in place by the skin.

Care for a Nail Avulsion

1. Secure the damaged nail in place with an adhesive bandage.
2. If part or all of the nail has been completely torn away, apply antibiotic ointment. Secure a partly torn loose nail with an adhesive bandage. Do not trim away the loose nail. Consult a physician for further advice.

▶ Splinters

Sharp splinters (usually wooden) can be impaled into the skin or under a fingernail or toenail.

Recognizing Splinters

- There is a small puncture wound. The sliver may be seen or in other cases, not seen nor can it be felt.

Care for Splinters

1. If embedded in the skin, use tweezers to remove it. In some cases, you may need to tease it out with sterile needle until the end can be grasped with tweezers or fingers. Clean the wound with soap and water.
2. If the splinter is impaled under a fingernail or toenail and breaks off flush, cut a V-shaped notch in the nail to gain access to the splinter. Remove the embedded splinter by grasping its end with tweezers.

▶ Blood Under a Nail

Blood collects under a fingernail when underlying tissues are bruised (e.g., finger struck by a hammer or caught between a door and its frame).

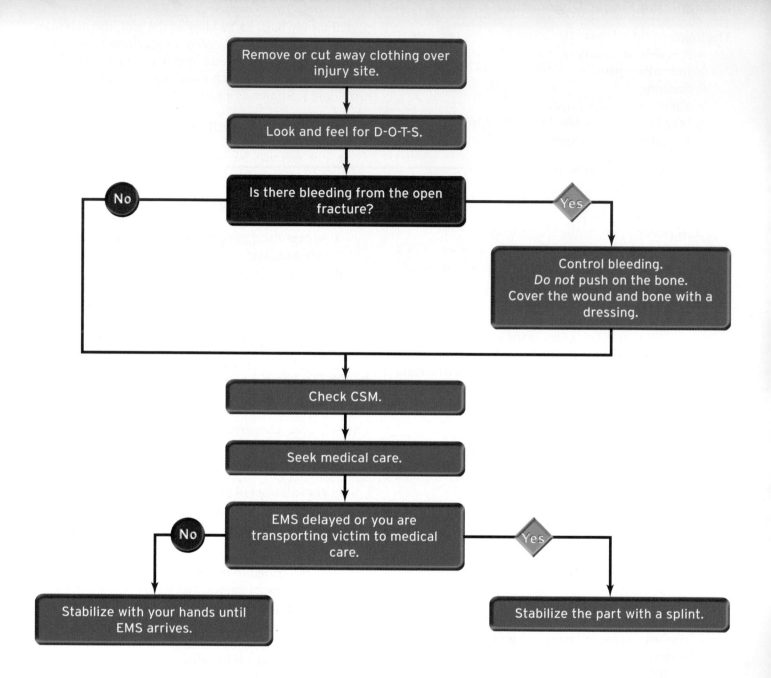

Recognizing Blood Under a Nail

- Excruciating pain exists because of the pressure of the blood pushing against the nail.
- Pain does not disappear until the collection of blood is drained.

Care for Blood Under a Nail

1. Immerse the finger in ice water or apply an ice pack with the hand elevated to reduce pain and swelling.
2. Relieve the pressure under the injured nail by using one of the following methods **Figure 15-1** :
   - Straighten the end of a metal (noncoated) paper clip or use the blunt (eye) end of a sewing needle. Hold the paper clip or needle with pliers, and use a match or cigarette lighter to heat it until the metal is red hot. Press the glowing end of the paper clip or needle against the nail

FYI

Blood Clot Under a Fingernail

Blood clots are common problems. Relieving the pressure of blood under the nails in 45 victims was successfully done using a heated object (first aiders could use a heated paperclip). All victims reported relief of pain after this procedure. No complications of infection or major nail deformities occurred. This method is preferred over removing the nail.

Source: Seaberg D C, Angelos W J, Paris P M: Treatment of subungual hematomas with nail trephination: a prospective study. *Am J Emerg Med* 9:209-210.

so it melts through. Little pressure is needed. The nail has no nerves, so this is a painless procedure **Figure 15-2** .

- By using a rotary action, carefully drill through the nail with the sharp point of a knife. This method is less threatening than the previous method of using heat.

3. Apply a dressing to absorb the draining blood and to protect the injured nail.

▶ Ring Strangulation

Ring strangulation can be a serious problem if it cuts off the blood supply long enough. Permanent damage may result within 4 or 5 hours.

Recognizing Ring Strangulation

- The ring has become tight on the finger after an injury or after some other cause of swelling, such as a local reaction to a bee sting.

Care for Ring Strangulation

Try one or more of the following methods to remove a ring:

- Lubricate the finger with soap and water, grease, oil, butter, petroleum jelly, or some other slippery substance, and then try to remove the ring.
- Immerse the finger in cold water or apply an ice pack for several minutes to reduce the swelling.
- Liberally spray window or glass cleaner onto the finger, and then try to slide the ring off.

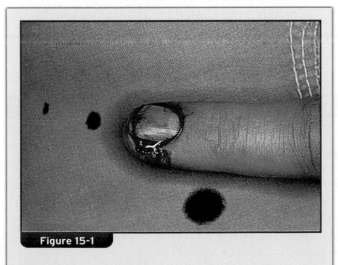

Figure 15-1

Relieve pain by releasing the blood under a nail.

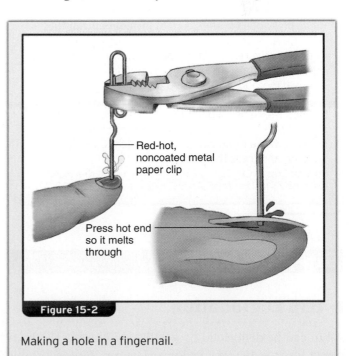

Red-hot, noncoated metal paper clip

Press hot end so it melts through

Figure 15-2

Making a hole in a fingernail.

- Massage the finger from the tip toward the hand to move the swelling; lubricate the finger again and try removing the ring.
- Smoothly wind thread around the finger, starting about an inch from the ring edge and going toward the ring, keeping each round of thread touching the next. Wind smoothly and tightly right up to the edge of the ring. This action will push the swelling toward the hand. Slip the end of the thread under the ring with a matchstick or toothpick, then slowly unwind the thread on the hand side of the ring. You should be able to gently twist the ring over the thread and off the finger.
- Lubricate the finger well, then pass a rubber band under the ring. Hold both ends of the rubber band and, while maintaining tension on the rubber band toward the end of the finger, pull the rubber band around and around the finger.
- Cut the narrowest part of the ring with a ring saw, jeweler's saw, ring cutter, or fine hacksaw blade. Be sure to protect the exposed portions of the finger.
- Inflate an ordinary balloon (preferably a slender, tube-shaped one) about three-fourths full. Tie the end. Insert the victim's swollen finger into the end of the balloon until the balloon evenly surrounds the entire finger. In about 15 minutes, the air pressure in the balloon should return the finger to its normal size and the ring can be removed.

FYI

Ring Removal From an Extremely Swollen Finger

Rings on swollen fingers are not uncommon, but they must be removed or serious problems can result. Generally, the removal method is simply to cut the ring off the finger or to use one of several nondestructive removal methods using string or a rubber band. A new yet simple method that eliminates the swelling and permits the removal of a ring involves wrapping the entire finger starting at the nail and wrapping toward the ring with a tight, elastic band, which reduces the swelling and frees the ring.

Source: Cresap CR: Removal of a hardened steel ring from an extremely swollen finger. *Am J Emerg Med* 13(3):318-320.

Hip-Joint Injuries

▶ Hip Dislocation

A hip can be dislocated by a fall, a blow to the thigh, or direct force to the foot or knee. The hip joint is a stable ball-and-socket joint that requires great force to dislocate. Often a hip is dislocated when the knee strikes the dashboard during a motor vehicle crash. It is difficult to differentiate a hip dislocation from a hip fracture.

Recognizing Hip Dislocation

- Severe pain at the injury site
- Swelling at the injury site
- Hip is flexed and the knee bent and rotated inward toward the opposite hip
- Injury usually quite visible

Care for Hip Dislocation

1. Treat for shock.
2. Stabilize the injury.
3. Check for an ankle pulse (posterior tibial).
4. Seek medical care. This injury is best transported by the EMS.

▶ Hip Fracture

A *hip fracture* is a fracture of the upper end of the femur (thighbone), not the pelvis. A fractured hip usually is caused by a fall. Elderly people, especially women, are susceptible to this type of injury because of brittle bones (*osteoporosis*).

Recognizing a Hip Fracture

- Severe pain in the groin area.
- Inability to lift the injured leg.
- Leg may appear shortened and be rotated with the toes pointing abnormally outward.

Care for a Hip Fracture

1. Treat for shock.
2. Stabilize the injured leg against movement.
3. Monitor the ankle pulse (posterior tibial).
4. Seek immediate medical care. This injury is best transported by the EMS.

Thigh Injuries

▶ Femur Fracture

Because the femur (thighbone) is the largest bone in the body, considerable force is required to break it. Femur injuries can occur in any part of the femur, from the hip to just above the knee joint. A fracture of the femur usually is caused by a fall or a direct blow.

Femur fractures often include open wounds and external bleeding may be severe. If the blood vessels are damaged, the victim may lose 1 or 2 quarts of blood into the thigh. There may be loss of blood circulation to the lower part of the extremity or nerve damage, especially with lower-third femur fractures.

Recognizing a Femur Fracture

- Severe pain at the injury site
- Deformity may occur. The leg may appear shorter.
- Swelling comes from severe damage to blood vessels.
- Victim may report having heard or felt a severe pop or snap at the time of injury.

Care for a Femur Fracture

1. Treat for shock.
2. Cover a wound with a sterile dressing.
3. Stabilize the injured leg against movement.
4. Monitor the ankle pulse (posterior tibial).
5. Seek immediate medical care. This injury is best transported by the EMS.

▶ Muscle Contusion

The muscle group on the front of the thigh is the *quadriceps group* and often gets bruised. Depending upon the force of impact and the muscles involved, the contusion may be of varying degrees of severity.

Recognizing Muscle Contusion

The victim received a direct hit producing:
- Swelling
- Pain and tenderness
- Tightness or firmness of site when pressed
- Visible bruise that may appear hours later

FYI

Thigh Muscle Injuries: Strain or Contusion?

Athletes often injure the large quadriceps muscles of their thighs. According to one report, strains (pulling of the muscle, which causes tears) should be treated first with ice, compression, elevation of the limb, nonsteroidal anti-inflammatory drugs, and use of crutches. After several days, the athlete can start gentle stretching and knee extension but should avoid straight-leg raises. For thigh contusions (direct blow, causing bruising), the knee should be immediately flexed and immobilized in that position for 24 hours. Ice should be applied for the first half hour and intermittently thereafter to slow bleeding and prevent swelling.
Source: Kaeding C C, et al: Quadriceps strains and contusions. *Phys Sportsmed* 23(1):59.

FYI

Charley Horse

The term charley horse came about in the 1880s among baseball players. At that time, the outfield grass of some major league ballparks was mowed by horses pulling lawn mowers. At Ebbet's Field in New York, the horse that did this chore—Charley—had a continual limp. When a baseball player was hit in the leg with a ball or received a blow to his leg muscle that caused him to limp, he was said to be walking like Charley. The muscle blow and the contusion that caused the pain and limping were referred to as a *charley horse*. The term remains popular in the United States.

Care for Muscle Contusion

1. Follow the RICE procedures. Apply an ice pack for 20 minutes, three to four times daily for the next 48 hours.
2. Stretch the muscle by bending the knee toward the victim's chest.

▶ Muscle Strain

When a muscle is overstretched, it can result in a tear, called a *strain*. Different degrees of strains occur, but first aiders will be unable to determine their degree.

Recognizing a Muscle Strain

While running or jumping, the victim:
- Feels a pop or pulling sensation

And later has:
- Tenderness
- Stiffness and pain during movement
- Swelling
- A visible bruise appearing days later

Care for a Muscle Strain

1. Follow the RICE procedures. Apply an ice pack for 20 minutes, three to four times daily for the next 48 hours.
2. Stretch the muscle but do not force stretching.

Knee Injuries

Knee injuries, of which there are many types, are among the most serious joint injuries. Their severity is difficult to determine, thus medical care is necessary if the injury is from being hit or twisted and not from overuse. You probably have seen a physician or an athletic trainer performing stress tests on a player's knee on the sidelines at a football game. Controversy exists about the exact meaning and interpretation of many of the ligament stress tests. First aiders should not perform such tests.

▶ Knee Fracture

A fracture of the knee generally occurs as a result of a fall or a direct blow.

Recognizing a Knee Fracture

Fractures about the knee may occur at the end of the femur, at the end of the tibia, or in the *patella* (kneecap). Determining if a fracture exists is difficult. Some fractured knees may look like a dislocation. Other signs include:

- Deformity
- Tenderness
- Swelling

Care for a Knee Fracture

1. If a pulse can be felt in the ankle (posterior tibial) with no deformity, splint the leg with the knee straight.
2. If a pulse can be felt in the ankle with significant deformity, splint the knee in the position found.
3. Seek medical care. However, if a pulse is absent in the ankle, immediately seek medical care.

▶ Knee Dislocation

A knee dislocation is a serious injury. Deformity will be grotesque.

Recognizing a Knee Dislocation

- Excruciating pain
- Deformity
- Pulse may be absent in the ankle (posterior tibial).
- Do not confuse a knee dislocation with a patella dislocation. A knee dislocation is a much more serious injury.

Care for a Knee Dislocation

1. Stabilize the knee in the position found.
2. Seek medical care immediately.

▶ Patella Dislocation

A dislocated patella (kneecap) can be a very painful injury and must be treated immediately. Some people have repeated kneecap dislocations, just as others have a tendency for shoulder dislocations. A dislocated patella most commonly occurs in teenagers and young adults who are engaged in athletic activities.

Recognizing a Patella Dislocation

A blow or twisting causes the kneecap to be moved to the outside of the knee joint and there is:

- Possible swelling
- An inability to bend or straighten the knee
- Pain
- Deformity; compare it with the other kneecap

Care for a Patella Dislocation

1. Follow the RICE procedures.
2. Do not try to relocate a dislocated kneecap (sometimes the kneecap replaces itself).
3. Splint the knee in the position found.
4. Seek medical care.

▶ Knee Sprain

Ligament injuries occur most often in sports. The knee is very prone to ligament injury, ranging from mild sprains to complete tearing. The knee will be swollen and painful and usually cannot be used normally.

Recognizing a Knee Sprain

At the time of injury, the victim has:

- Severe pain
- The feeling of a pop or snap
- A locking sensation

OR the victim:

- May not be able to walk without limping
- May not be able to bend or straighten the knee

Later, there may be:

- Swelling in the knee
- Bruising

Care for a Knee Sprain

1. Follow the RICE procedures
2. Seek medical care

▶ Knee Contusion

Contusions of the knee are caused by a direct blow or by falling on the knee.

Recognizing a Knee Contusion

After a direct blow to the kneecap, the victim has:

- Pain
- Swelling
- Tenderness
- Bruise marks (black-and-blue discoloration)

Care for a Knee Contusion

1. Follow the RICE procedures.

Muscle Injuries

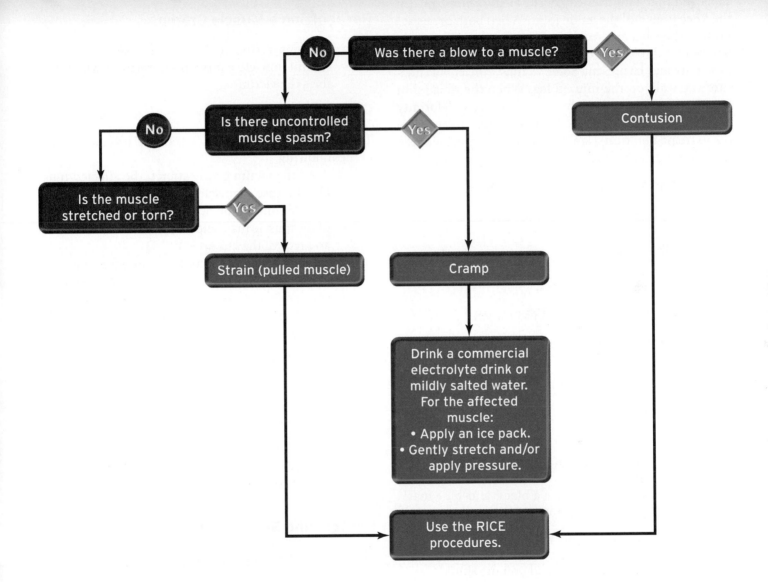

Lower-Leg Injuries

▶ Tibia and Fibula Fractures

Tibia and fibula injuries can occur at any place between the knee joint and the ankle joint. When both bones are broken, there is a marked deformity of the leg. When only one bone is broken, the other acts as a splint, and little deformity may be present. Some victims with a fibula fracture can walk on the injured leg. When the tibia (shin bone) is broken, an open fracture and severe deformity are likely to exist. Injuries to the blood vessels, caused by the extreme deformity, are common with injuries of the tibia and the fibula, and the pain usually is severe.

Recognizing Tibia and Fibula Fractures

A direct blow or twisting forces produce:
- Severe pain
- Swelling
- Visible deformity
- Tenderness when touched

Care for Tibia and Fibula Fractures

1. Stabilize the leg using a splint, either improvised by tying the legs together or a rigid splint (two boards or two SAM splints—one on each side to prevent rotation of the lower leg bones).
2. Apply an ice pack.
3. Seek medical care.

▶ Tibia and Fibula Contusion

Many contusions simply cause a black-and-blue mark and some soreness, then clear up with little attention.

Recognizing a Tibia and Fibula Contusion

- Victim received a hit directly on the shin
- Tender when touched
- Sharp pain

Later has:
- Discoloration (black-and-blue mark)
- Difficulty moving ankle up and down
- Numbness or coldness in toes or foot

Care for a Tibia and Fibula Contusion

1. Expose the injury.
2. Apply the RICE procedures. Use an ice pack for 20 minutes, three to four times daily for first 48 hours.
3. If numbness or tingling exists, seek medical care.

▶ Muscle Cramp

Muscle spasm or cramping usually occurs in the calf and sometimes in the thigh or hamstring. It is a temporary condition of little consequence.

Recognizing a Muscle Cramp

- Happens during or after intense exercise sessions
- Painful, muscle contraction or spasm which disables the victim

Care for Muscle Cramps

There are many treatments for cramps. Try one or more of the following:

1. Have the victim gently stretch the affected muscle. Because a muscle cramp is an uncontrolled muscle contraction or spasm, a gradual extension of the muscle may help lengthen the muscle fibers and relieve the cramp.
2. Relax the muscle by applying pressure to it.
3. Apply ice to the cramped muscle to make it relax (unless you are in a cold environment).
4. Pinch the upper lip hard (an acupressure technique) to reduce calf-muscle cramping.
5. Drink lightly salted, cool water (dissolve ¼ teaspoon salt in a quart of water) or a commercial sports drink.

▶ Shin Splints

Shin splints is a term that describes pain in the front of the lower leg, also called the shin. Shin splints are caused by repetitive stress in the leg such as running and extensive walking.

Recognizing Shin Splints

The shin aches during activity, but:
- The ache subsides significantly after activity stops
- The ache is a result of an increase in the workout routine (eg, running longer, running on hills, etc.)
- Usually a chronic problem that gets worse

Care for Shin Splints

1. Apply an ice pack before an activity. Heat can be applied later, when the victim is well on the way to recovery.
2. Apply pressure with a 3-inch elastic bandage over the sorest point (start below the sore area and spiral wrap up and around the leg).
3. Apply an ice pack for 20 minutes after the activity.

4. Curtail activity until the shin is pain free.

5. Pain medications that are anti-inflammatory drugs may be taken: Use aspirin (adults only) or ibuprofen.

▶ Ankle and Foot Injuries

The ankle and the foot frequently are injured, mainly by twisting, which stretches or tears the supporting ligaments. Incorrect treatment can have consequences that include lifelong disability. In some cases, the damage requires surgical correction. Most ankle injuries are sprains; about 85% of sprains involve the outside (lateral) ligaments and are caused by the ankle having turned or twisted inward **Figure 15-3**.

Recognizing Foot and Ankle Injuries

It is difficult to tell the difference between a severely sprained ankle and a fractured ankle. A useful two-part test can help determine whether an X-ray of the ankle or midfoot is needed:

1. Press along the bones. Pain and tenderness over the back edge or the tip of either of the ankle knob bones (malleolus bones) or the midfoot's outside bone (fifth metatarsal) or inside bone (navicular) may indicate a broken bone.

2. Ask the victim, "Have you tried standing on it?" Putting some weight on the foot may hurt a little, but if the victim is able to do that and take four or more steps, most likely the ankle or foot is sprained. If it is broken, the victim will not want

to put any weight on it and will not be able to take more than four steps.

3. A few additional signs and symptoms may help determine whether an injured ankle or foot is sprained or fractured. These indicators are not hard-and-fast rules but useful guidelines to help you treat foot and ankle injuries.

    - If the victim hops on the good foot and the injured ankle cannot tolerate the jarring, suspect a fracture.
    - Foot injuries usually lead to substantial swelling. It has been observed that ankle sprains tend to swell on only one side of the foot (usually the lateral or outer side), whereas swelling on both sides of the foot usually accompanies fractures.

Care for Foot and Ankle Injuries

Controversy exists about whether to remove a shoe from an injured foot. Those who favor leaving the shoe on believe it acts as a splint and helps retard swelling. However, taking the shoe off allows for a better examination, better checking of the CSM, and better care. A shoe that is left on often does not cover and, thus, cannot compress the injured area that is swelling. If a shoe acts as a compression device, it could also reduce blood circulation in the foot as the swelling increases. In addition, footwear left in place will thwart efforts to apply an ice pack and an elastic bandage. Use the RICE procedures to limit swelling.

Aftercare of an Ankle Injury

1. First 24 to 48 hours: Use the RICE treatment.

2. Within 3 to 7 days: Use a contrast bath if swelling persists. Submerge the ankle for 1 minute in cold water (45° F to 60° F) and then for 4 minutes in warm water (100° F to 105° F). Continue to alternate cold and warm submersions for 15 minutes. Gently move the foot up and down for mobility. This should be done once or twice a day for 1 to 2 weeks.

3. Once the initial swelling has decreased, discontinue immobilization and start range-of-motion exercises, even if the injured ankle cannot bear weight. Joint motion decreases swelling and stiffness and prevents fluid accumulation.

4. Begin with gentle exercises such as bending the ankle up and down 15 times, two or three times a day. Also, try sitting with the legs straight out in

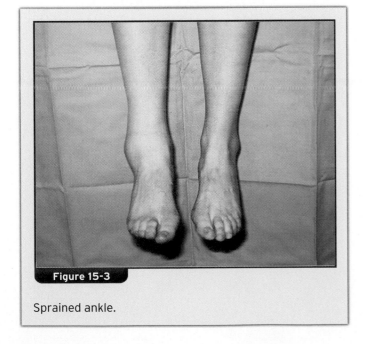

Figure 15-3

Sprained ankle.

Sprains, Strains, Contusions, Dislocations

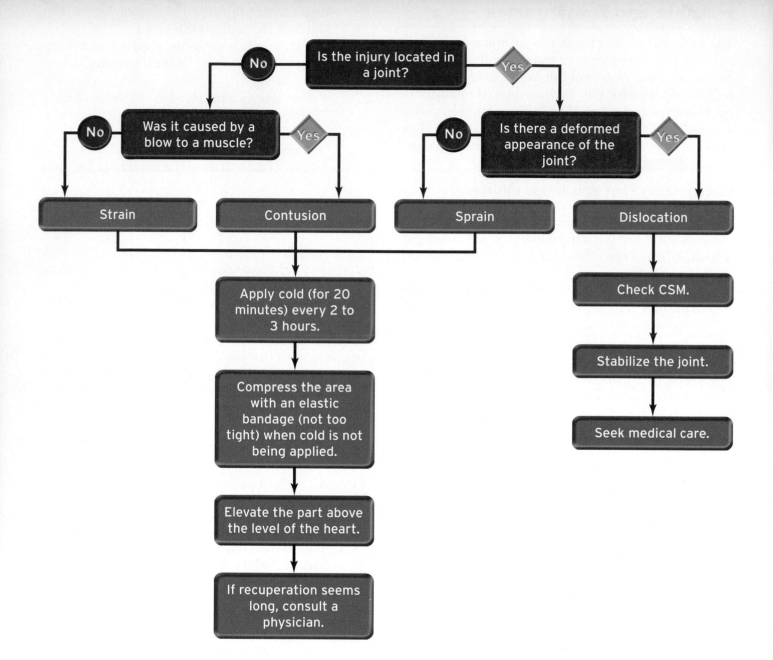

Ankle Injuries

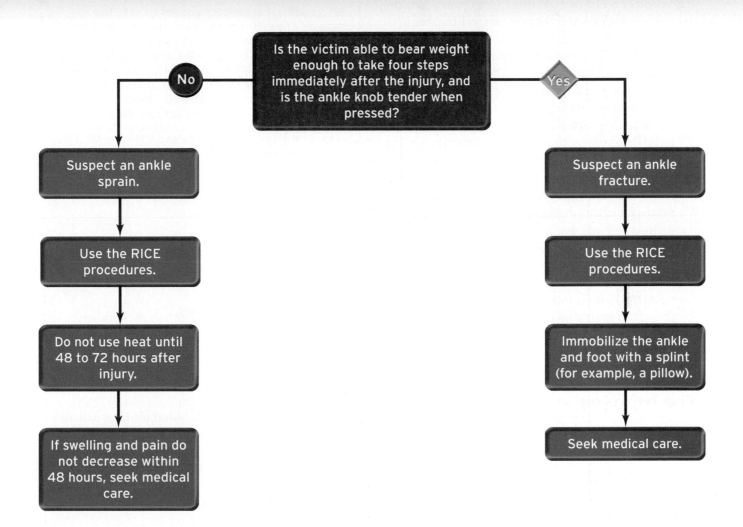

Is the victim able to bear weight enough to take four steps immediately after the injury, and is the ankle knob tender when pressed?

No

Suspect an ankle sprain.

Use the RICE procedures.

Do not use heat until 48 to 72 hours after injury.

If swelling and pain do not decrease within 48 hours, seek medical care.

Yes

Suspect an ankle fracture.

Use the RICE procedures.

Immobilize the ankle and foot with a splint (for example, a pillow).

Seek medical care.

front. Place a towel around the ball of the foot and, sitting upright, hold the ends of the towel. Stretch the foot back toward you and hold for 10 seconds. Then point the toes away and hold for 10 seconds. Stop if pain is felt.

5. Within 7 to 14 days: If there is no pain when the ankle is rotated and there is no swelling, begin to stretch and strengthen the calf and the ankle. Stretch the calf muscles by leaning against a wall with one foot forward. Keep the back leg straight, heel down. Bend the front knee and lean into the wall. Hold for 10 seconds, and then stretch with the other leg forward. This stretch can be done 5 to 10 times on each side, two or three times a day.

6. Avoiding reinjury: Once the ankle has healed—typically within 4 to 6 weeks—consider taping it (after the first injury) or bracing it (more appropriate for chronic sprains). Bracing alternatives include lace-up, gel-filled, and air-stirrup devices. Also, firm high-top shoes may give added support. Continue to stretch and strengthen the ankle and calf muscles with exercises.

7. NSAIDs: Nonsteroidal anti-inflammatory drugs (NSAIDs) greatly help to reduce pain and swelling. Examples of NSAIDs are ibuprofen, naproxen, and aspirin. Analgesics such as acetaminophen relieve only pain, not swelling.

▶ Toe Injuries

The toes can be injured in various ways. The toes can be stepped on or the foot may be kicked against a hard ob-

> ### FYI
>
> **Ankle and Foot Injuries: Is Something Broken?**
> Two symptoms were 93% accurate in predicting a broken ankle bone: (1) inability to bear weight and take four steps immediately after the injury; and (2) tenderness at the back edge or tip of either malleolus bone (the projections on each side of the ankle). Similar symptoms predicted whether a foot bone was broken: (1) pain in the midfoot or tenderness at the base of the fifth metatarsal bone at the outer edge of the foot or at the navicular bone at the inner edge, plus (2) inability to take four steps.
> *Sources:* Stiell I G, Greenberg G H, McKnight R D, et al: Decision rules for the use of radiography in acute ankle injuries: refinement and prospective validation; *JAMA* 269:1127-1132.

ject, resulting in torn-off nails, hematoma formation under the nails, dislocations, or fractures.

Recognizing Toe Injuries

- Pain and swelling
- Deformity may be present

Care for Toe Injuries

For nail avulsions, splinters, blood under a nail, dislocations, and fractures refer to the appropriate sections under finger injuries.

▶ Ready for Review

- Injuries to the extremities are common.
- There are many types of injuries to the extremities, ranging from simple contusions to complex open fractures.
- RICE is the acronym for Rest, Ice, Compression, and Elevation.
- Shoulder injuries include:
  - Shoulder dislocation
  - Clavicle fracture
  - Contusions
  - Tendinitis
- Elbow injuries include:
  - Elbow fractures and dislocations
  - Tennis elbow
  - Golfer's elbow
- Hand injuries include:
  - Crushed hand
- Finger injuries include:
  - Finger fracture
  - Finger dislocation
  - Sprained finger
  - Nail avulsion
  - Splinters
  - Blood under a nail
  - Ring strangulation
- Hip-joint injuries include:
  - Hip dislocation
  - Hip fracture
- Thigh injuries include:
  - Femur fracture
  - Muscle contusion
  - Muscle strain
- Knee injuries include:
  - Knee fracture
  - Knee dislocation
  - Patella dislocation
  - Knee sprain
  - Knee contusion
- Lower-leg injuries include:
  - Tibia and fibula fractures
  - Tibia and fibula contusion
  - Muscle cramp
  - Shin splints
  - Ankle and foot injuries
  - Toe injuries

▶ Vital Vocabulary

Contusions A bruise; an injury that causes a hemorrhage in or beneath the skin but does not break the skin.

Dislocations Bones are displaced from their normal joint alignment, out of their sockets, or out of their normal positions.

Fractures A break or crack in the bone.

Sprains A trauma to the joint that injures the ligaments.

Strains An injury to a muscle caused by a violent contraction or an excessive, forcible stretching.

Tendinitis Inflammation of a tendon due to overuse.

▶ Assessment in Action

You and your sister are playing a friendly game of basketball on a warm summer day. As you dodge around her and attempt a three-point shot, you hear a thud and your sister cry out in pain. She is on the ground with her right ankle twisted underneath her and she is holding out her left arm.

Directions: Circle Yes if you agree with the statement, circle No if you disagree.

Yes No **1.** Due to the way she fell, you suspect that she could have a radius or ulna fracture.

Yes No **2.** You do not have to seek medical care for this injury.

Yes No **3.** You should not apply ice to her arm.

Yes No **4.** You ask your sister if she can bear weight on her ankle. She is able to take five steps toward you. Her ankle is probably sprained.

Yes No **5.** A sprained ankle will benefit from RICE treatment.

Answers: **1.** Yes; **2.** No; **3.** No; **4.** Yes; **5.** Yes

prep kit

▶ Check Your Knowledge

Directions: Circle Yes if you agree with the statement, circle No if you disagree.

Yes   No   **1.** Injuries heal faster if rested.

Yes   No   **2.** Compression increases internal bleeding, helping the injury to heal faster.

Yes   No   **3.** Tennis elbow results from sharp, quick twists of the wrist.

Yes   No   **4.** The three bones in the fingers are very strong and do not break easily.

Yes   No   **5.** The hip joint is easily dislocated.

Yes   No   **6.** Considerable force is required to break the femur.

Yes   No   **7.** A strain is actually a tear in the muscle.

Yes   No   **8.** Knee injuries are not serious.

Yes   No   **9.** Shin splints are a pain that runs down the back of the leg.

Yes   No   **10.** It is difficult to tell the difference between a severely sprained ankle and a fractured ankle.

Answers: **1.** Yes; **2.** No; **3.** Yes; **4.** No; **5.** No; **6.** Yes; **7.** Yes; **8.** No; **9.** No; **10.** Yes

Splinting Extremities

Splinting Extremities

Injured extremities should be stabilized by splinting the extremity in the position it was found. To stabilize means to minimize further injury by holding a body part to prevent movement. All fractures should be stabilized before a victim is moved. The reasons for splinting to stabilize an injured area are to:

- reduce pain.
- prevent damage to muscles, nerves, and blood vessels.
- prevent a closed fracture from becoming an open fracture.
- reduce bleeding and swelling.

All fractures are complicated to some degree by damage to the soft tissue and structures surrounding the bone. The major cause of tissue damage at a fracture site is movement by the end of the broken bone. The end of a broken bone is sharp, and it is important to prevent a fractured bone from moving into soft tissues.

▶ Types of Splints

A splint is any device used to stabilize a fracture or a dislocation. Such a device can be improvised (for example, a folded newspaper), or it can be one of several commercially available splints (for example, SAM splint). Lack of a commercial splint should never prevent you from properly stabilizing an injured extremity. Splinting sometimes requires improvisation.

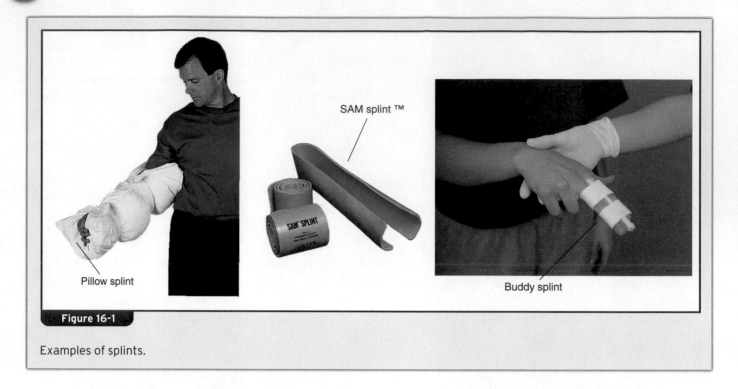

SAM splint ™

Pillow splint

Buddy splint

Figure 16-1

Examples of splints.

A rigid splint is an inflexible device attached to an extremity to maintain stability. It can be a padded board, a piece of heavy cardboard, or a SAM splint molded to fit the extremity. Whatever its construction, a rigid splint must be long enough so that it can be secured well above and below the fracture site. A soft splint, such as a pillow, is useful mainly for stabilizing fractures of the lower leg or the forearm **Figure 16-1**.

A self-splint, or anatomic splint, is almost always available because it uses the body itself as the splint. A self-splint is one in which the injured extremity is tied to an uninjured part (for example, an injured finger to the adjacent finger, the legs together, or an injured arm to the chest).

▶ Splinting Guidelines

All fractures and dislocations should be stabilized before the victim is moved. When in doubt, apply a splint. In order to apply a splint:

1. Cover any open wounds with a sterile dressing before applying a splint.
2. Check the CSM in the extremity. If pulses are absent and medical help is hours away, gently line up a fracture or a dislocation to restore blood flow. Support the limb and move gently to line up the parts. Joints may be left in a position of comfort. Line up the limb above and below the joint, do not force anything into position. Any movement of a fracture is expected to cause pain; you should

be aware of this and warn the victim. You do not have to align the limb perfectly, just align it enough to allow the return of circulation.

3. Determine what to splint by using the rule of thirds. Imagine each long bone as being divided into thirds. If the injury is located in the upper or lower third of a bone, assume that the nearest joint is injured. Therefore, the splint should extend to stabilize the bones above and below the unstable joint. For example, for a fracture of the upper third of the tibia (shinbone), the splint must extend above the knee to include the upper leg, as well as the lower leg, because the knee is unstable. For a fracture of the middle third of a bone, stabilize the joints above and below the fracture (for example, the wrist and elbow for a fractured radius or ulna; the shoulder and elbow for a fractured humerus; the knee and ankle for a fractured tibia or fibula). In addition to splinting an upper extremity fracture, place the injured arm in an arm sling and a swathe (binder).
4. If two first aiders are present, one should support the injury site and minimize movement of the extremity until splinting is completed.
5. When possible, place splint materials on both sides of the injured part, especially when two bones are involved, such as the radius and ulna in the lower arm or the tibia and fibula in the lower leg. This sandwich splint prevents the injured extremity from rotating and keeps the two bones from touching.

With rigid splints, use extra padding in natural body hollows and around any deformities.

6. Apply splints firmly but not so tightly that blood flow into an extremity is affected. Check the CSM before and periodically after the splint is applied. If the pulse disappears, loosen the splint enough so you can feel the pulse. Leave the fingers or toes exposed so the CSM can be checked easily.

7. Use RICE (rest, ice, compression, and elevation) on the injured part. When practical, elevate the injured extremity after it is stabilized to promote drainage and reduce swelling. Do not, however, apply ice packs if a pulse is absent.

If the victim has a possible spinal injury and an extremity injury, the spinal injury takes precedence. Splinting the spine is always a problem. Tell the victim not to move. Then stabilize the spine with rolled blankets or similar objects placed on each side of the neck and torso. In most cases, it is best to wait until emergency medical services (EMS) personnel arrive with proper equipment to handle spinal injuries.

Most fractures do not require rapid transportation. An exception is an arm or a leg without a pulse, which means there is insufficient blood flow to the injured extremity. In that case, immediate medical care is necessary.

Seek medical care for the following injuries or situations:

- Any open fracture
- Any dislocation (injury that causes joint deformity)
- Any joint injury with moderate to severe swelling
- Any injury in which there is deformity, tenderness, or swelling over the bone
- If the victim is unable to walk or bear weight after a lower extremity injury
- If a snap, crackle, or pop was heard at the time of injury
- If the injured area, especially a joint, becomes hot, tender, swollen, or painful
- If you are unsure whether a bone was broken
- If the injury does not improve rapidly, especially over the first few days

CAUTION

DO NOT straighten dislocations or fractures of the spine, elbow, wrist, hip, or knee because of the proximity of major nerves and arteries. Instead, if the CSM assessment findings are normal, splint joint injuries in the position in which you find them.

DO NOT apply traction on open fractures. Instead, cover the wound with a sterile dressing and apply a splint.

▶ Slings

An open triangular bandage can be used as a <u>sling</u>. A folded triangular bandage known as a cravat can be used as a <u>swathe</u> (binder) in conjunction with a sling. A cravat may also be applied using the same procedures as an open triangular sling but placed around the wrist when long splints on an upper arm or forearm may be in the way. To apply an arm sling to the upper arm, forearm, or hand/wrist injuries, follow the steps in **Skill Drill 16-1** :

1. Hold the victim's arm slightly away from the chest, with the wrist and hand slightly higher (about 4 inches) than the tip of the elbow. Place a triangular bandage between the forearm and chest with the point of the triangular bandage toward the elbow and stretch the bandage well beyond the elbow. Pull the upper end of the bandage over the uninjured shoulder (**Step 1**).

2. Bring the lower end of the bandage over the forearm (**Step 2**).

3. Bring the end of the bandage around the neck to the uninjured side and tie to the other end at the hollow above the clavicle on the uninjured side. If possible, secure the point of the bandage at the elbow with a safety pin or twist it into a pigtail which can be tied into a knot or tucked inside the sling (**Step 3**).

4. Place a swathe (binder) around the upper arm and body. The center of the swathe (binder) should be placed over the arm. The hand should be in thumb-up position within the sling and slightly above the level of the elbow (about 4 inches). Place padding underneath both knots for comfort. Adjust the sling to support the hand and wrist, only the fingers should be exposed (**Step 4**).

To apply a sling for clavicle or shoulder injuries, follow the steps in **Skill Drill 16-2** :

1. Hold arm slightly away from the chest, with the wrist and hand slightly higher (about 4 inches) than the tip of the elbow. Place a triangular bandage between the forearm and chest with its point toward the elbow and stretching well beyond it. Pull the upper end over the shoulder on the uninjured side. Bring the other end of the bandage over the forearm and tuck it under the armpit (between the arm and body) on the injured side (**Step 1**).

2. Continue bringing the lower end of the bandage around the victim's back where it is tied to the upper end of the bandage (**Step 2**).

3. Place a swathe (binder) around the chest and forearm rather than the upper arm (**Step 3**).

skill drill

16-1   Arm Sling for Arm Injury

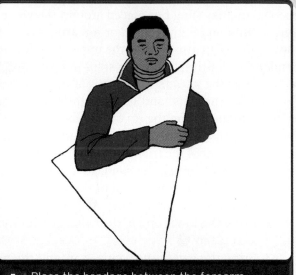

1 Place the bandage between the forearm and chest with the point of the bandage toward the elbow and stretch beyond the elbow. Pull the upper end of the bandage over the uninjured shoulder.

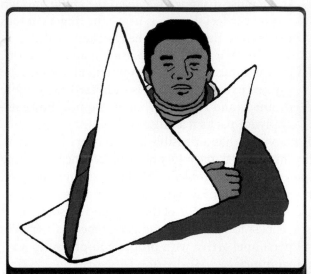

2 Bring the lower end of the bandage over the forearm.

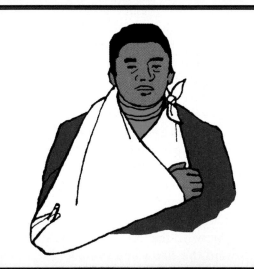

3 Bring the end of the bandage around the neck to the uninjured side and tie to the other end at the hollow above the clavicle on the uninjured side.

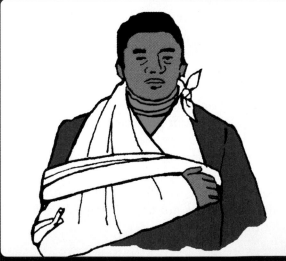

4 Place a swathe around the upper arm and body. The center of the swathe should be placed over the arm. The hand should be in thumb-up position within the sling and slightly above the level of the elbow.

skill drill

16-2 Sling for Clavicle or Shoulder Injury

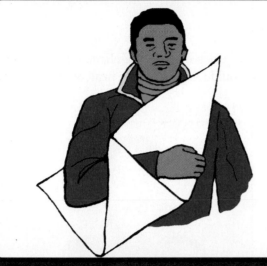

1 Place bandage between the forearm and chest with its point toward the elbow and stretching beyond it. Pull the upper end over the shoulder on the uninjured side. Bring the other end of the bandage over the forearm and tuck it under the armpit on the injured side.

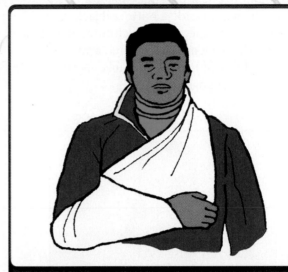

2 Continue bringing the lower end of the bandage around the victim's back where it is tied to the upper end of the bandage.

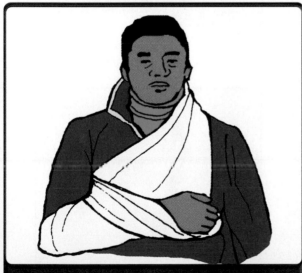

3 Place a swathe around the chest and forearm rather than the upper arm.

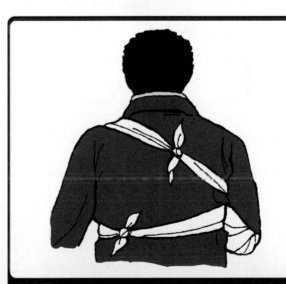

4 The center of the swathe should be placed over the forearm. The hand should be in a thumb-up position within the sling and slightly above the level of the elbow.

4. The center of the swathe (binder) should be placed over the forearm. The hand should be in a thumb-up position within the sling and slightly above the level of the elbow (about 4 inches) (**Step ④**).

If bandages or other resources are unavailable, you may need to improvise a sling (**Figure 16-2**).

- Place the hand inside a buttoned jacket.
- Use a belt, necktie, or other clothing item looped around the neck and the injured arm.
- Pin the sleeve of the shirt or jacket to the clothing in the desired position.

- Turn up the lower edge of the victim's jacket or shirt over the injured arm and pin it to the upper part of the jacket or shirt.

▶ Splinting Specific Areas

Shoulder

Shoulder injuries involve the clavicle (collarbone), the scapula (shoulder blade), or the head of the humerus (up-

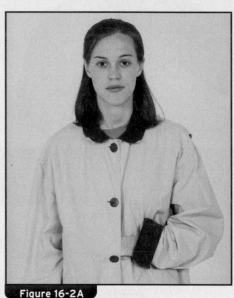
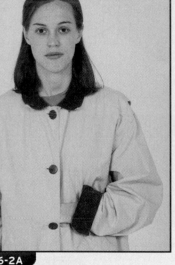
Figure 16-2A

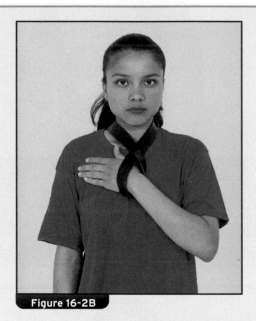
Figure 16-2B

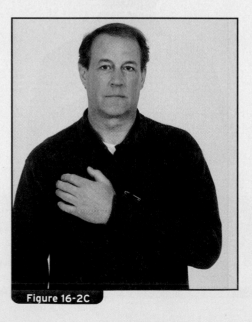
Figure 16-2C

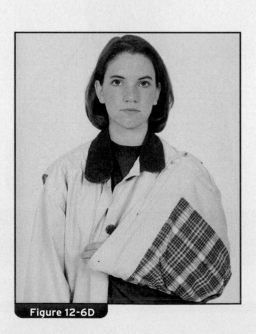
Figure 12-6D

Improvised slings. **A.** A buttoned jacket. **B.** A belt, necktie, or other clothing item looped around the neck and the injured arm. **C.** Sleeve of the jacket or shirt pinned to the clothing. **D.** Lower edge of the victim's jacket or shirt pinned up over the injured arm.

per arm). To stabilize the shoulder and upper arm against movement with a shoulder sling, follow these steps:

1. Support the injured arm slightly away from the chest, with the wrist and hand higher than the elbow.
2. Place an open triangular bandage between the forearm and the chest, with the point stretching well beyond the elbow.
3. Pull the upper end of the bandage over the shoulder on the uninjured side.
4. Bring the lower end of the bandage over the forearm, under the armpit on the injured side, and around the victim's back.
5. Tie the upper and lower ends of the triangular bandage.
6. Check the pulse and fingernail color for signs of circulation loss.
7. The hand should be in a thumb-up position in the sling and slightly above the level of the elbow **Figure 16-3** .

To further stabilize the arm, fold another triangular bandage to make a 3- to 4-inch-wide swathe. Tie one or two swathes (binders) around the upper arm and chest of the victim. This stabilizes the clavicle (collarbone) and most shoulder injuries, as well as upper humerus (upper arm) fractures.

Most shoulder dislocations (about 95%) are anterior, meaning that the top of the humerus pops out in front of the shoulder joint. The victim will hold the arm in a fixed position away from the chest wall. In these cases, the most comfortable splinting method is to place a pillow or rolled blanket between the involved arm and the chest. This fills the space created; you can then use cravats or a roller bandage to secure the arm against the chest. If the injury occurs in a remote setting (hours from medical care), use one of the methods described in Chapter 24 to reduce an anterior shoulder dislocation.

Humerus (Upper Arm)

Fractures of the humerus (upper arm) should be stabilized with a rigid splint. Extend the splint along the outside of the humerus. Then apply a sling and a swathe over the rigid splint, using the chest wall as an additional splint **Skill Drill 16-3** .

1. Gently place injured arm across the chest. If available, tie a rigid splint to the outside of the arm. (**Step ❶**). If a rigid splint is not available, go to Step 2.
2. Place the arm in a sling (**Step ❷**).
3. Secure the arm to the chest with a swathe (folded triangular bandage) (**Step ❸**).

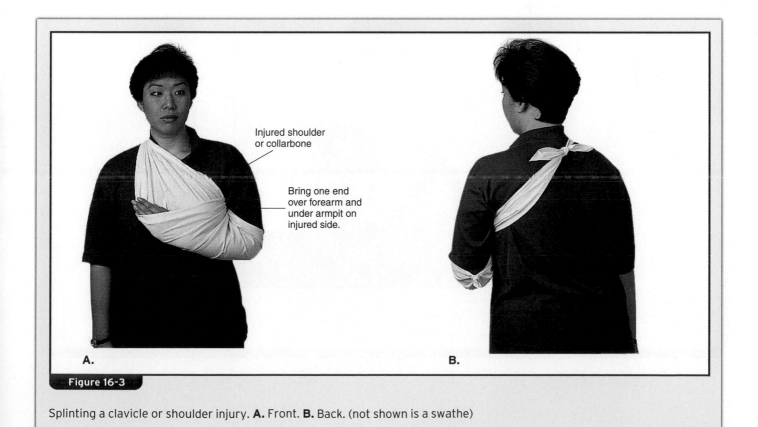

Injured shoulder or collarbone

Bring one end over forearm and under armpit on injured side.

A.   **B.**

Figure 16-3

Splinting a clavicle or shoulder injury. **A.** Front. **B.** Back. (not shown is a swathe)

skill drill

16-3   Splinting—Upper Arm (Humerus)

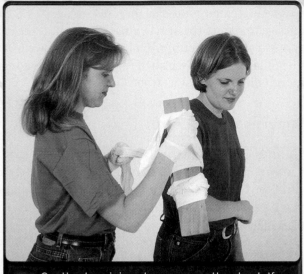

1 Gently place injured arm across the chest. If available, tie a rigid splint to the outside of the arm. If a rigid splint is not available, go to step 2.

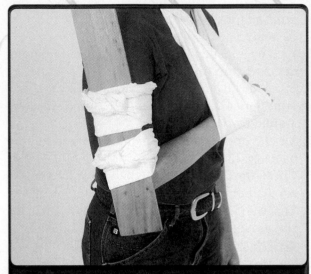

2 Place the arm in a sling.

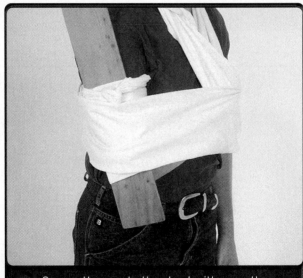

3 Secure the arm to the chest with a swathe (folded triangular bandage).

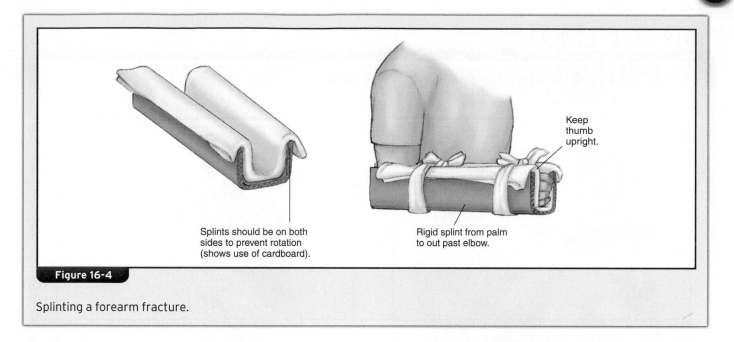

Splints should be on both sides to prevent rotation (shows use of cardboard).

Keep thumb upright.

Rigid splint from palm to out past elbow.

Figure 16-4

Splinting a forearm fracture.

Elbow

An elbow must be stabilized in the position it is found—if bent, splint it bent; if straight, splint it straight (Skill Drill 16-4 and Skill Drill 16-5). If the injured elbow is straight, place a rigid splint along the inside of the arm from hand to armpit. Secure the splint with a roller bandage or several cravat bandages. For a bent elbow, apply a rigid splint diagonally, so that it extends from the humerus (near the armpit) to the wrist, to prevent motion of the elbow. Depending on how bent the elbow is, you can also use a sling and a swathe (binder) for a bent elbow.

To splint an elbow in the bent position, follow the steps in **Skill Drill 16-4** :

1. If the injured elbow is bent, place a rigid splint from the upper arm to the wrist (**Step ❶**).
2. Tie a rigid splint onto the arm with cravat bandages (**Step ❷**).
3. Place the arm in a sling and check CSM (**Step ❸**).

To splint an elbow in the straight position, follow the steps in **Skill Drill 16-5** :

1. If the injured elbow is straight, place a rigid splint along the inside of the arm from the hand to the armpit (**Step ❶**).
2. Secure with a roller bandage or several cravat bandages (**Step ❷**).
3. Check CSM (**Step ❸**).

Forearm

To stabilize a forearm fracture, use one rigid splint extending from the palm of the hand out past the elbow and a second one on the opposite side of the arm. Placing

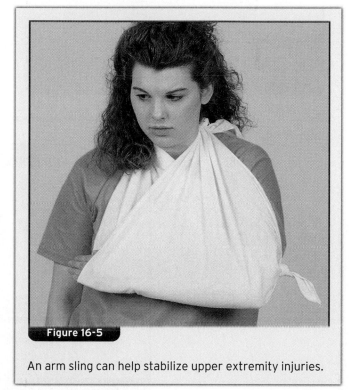

Figure 16-5

An arm sling can help stabilize upper extremity injuries.

splints on both sides of the injured part (sandwich splint) keeps the forearm from twisting or rotating **Figure 16-4** .

Keep the victim's thumb in an upright position so that the two bones in the forearm (the radius and the ulna) do not touch each other (Skill Drill 16-6). Secure the splint with a roller bandage or several cravats. A pillow or a rolled, folded blanket also can be secured to the arm. Put the arm in a sling and secure it with a swathe (binder) around the body **Figure 16-5** .

skill drill

16-4   **Splinting Elbow in Bent Position**

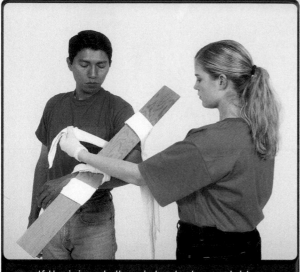

1 If the injured elbow is bent, place a rigid splint from the upper arm to the wrist.

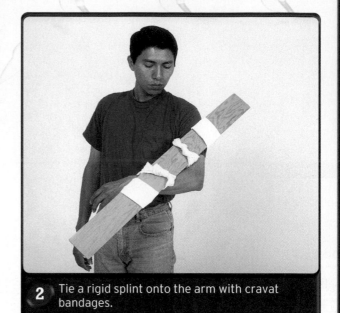

2 Tie a rigid splint onto the arm with cravat bandages.

3 Place the arm in a sling.

skill drill

16-5   Splinting Elbow in Straight Position

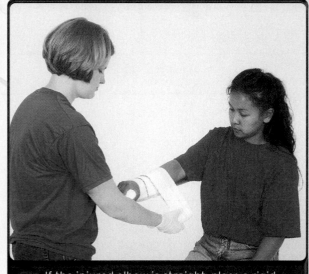

1 If the injured elbow is straight, place a rigid splint along the inside of the arm from the hand to the armpit.

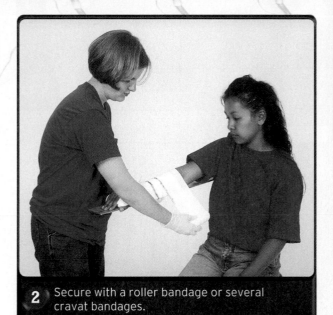

2 Secure with a roller bandage or several cravat bandages.

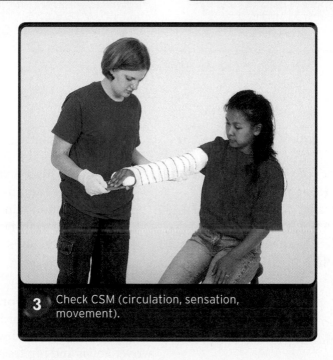

3 Check CSM (circulation, sensation, movement).

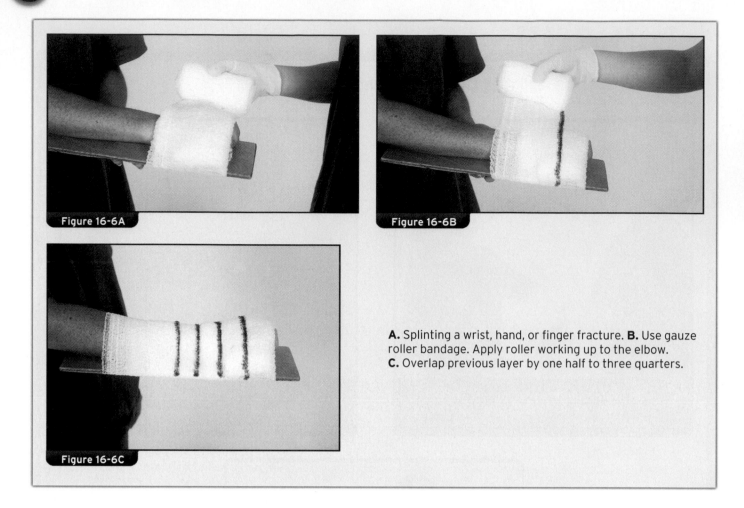

Figure 16-6A

Figure 16-6B

Figure 16-6C

A. Splinting a wrist, hand, or finger fracture. **B.** Use gauze roller bandage. Apply roller working up to the elbow. **C.** Overlap previous layer by one half to three quarters.

To splint the forearm, follow the steps in **Skill Drill 16-6**:

1. Place splints on both sides of a forearm to prevent rotation of the forearm (**Step ❶**).
2. Secure with a cravat or roller bandage (**Step ❷**).
3. Place the arm in a sling. A binder or swathe around the body is recommended. Keep the thumb in the upright position (**Step ❸**).

Wrist, Hand, and Fingers

To stabilize the wrist, hand, and fingers, use one of the following three methods:

- Place the injured hand in the position of function (hand looks like it is holding a baseball) by placing a rolled pair of socks or a roller bandage in the palm. Then attach a rigid splint that extends past the tips of the fingers along the forearm **Figure 16-6**.

- Place the hand in the position of function, mold a pillow around the hand and forearm, and tie the pillow in place with cravats or a roller bandage. Then place the arm in a sling and a swathe (binder), with the thumb in an upright position.
- Splint fingers by taping them together (buddy taping), with gauze separating the fingers.

Pelvis and Hip

If you suspect a pelvis or hip fracture, stabilize the victim as you found him or her. Treat the victim for shock, do not lift the legs, and wait for the EMS ambulance to arrive. Pelvis and hip fractures require a long backboard (spine board).

Femur (Thigh)

A fractured femur is best splinted with a traction splint, which requires special training to use. Traction splints are seldom available except on ambulances.

skill drill

16-6   Splinting—Forearm (Radius/Ulna)

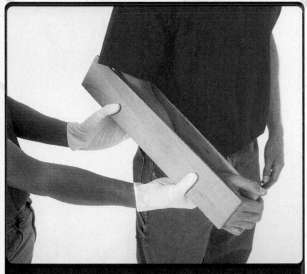

1 Place splints on both sides of a forearm to prevent rotation of the forearm.

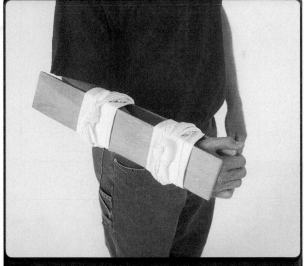

2 Secure with a cravat or roller bandage.

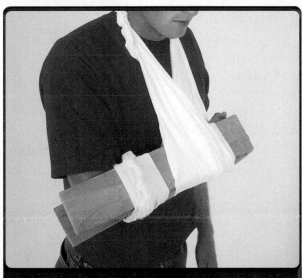

3 Place the arm in a sling. A binder or swathe around the body is recommended. Keep the thumb in the upright position.

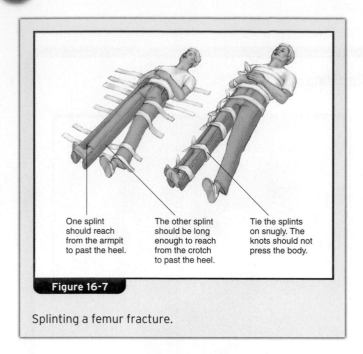

Figure 16-7

One splint should reach from the armpit to past the heel.

The other splint should be long enough to reach from the crotch to past the heel.

Tie the splints on snugly. The knots should not press the body.

Splinting a femur fracture.

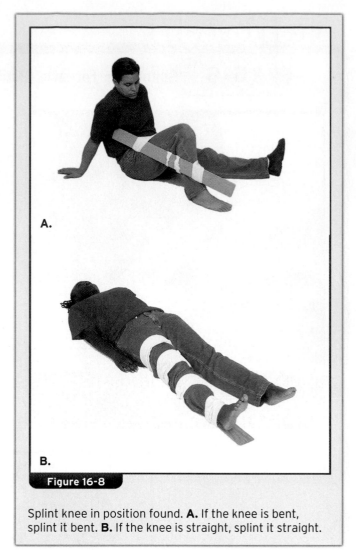

A.

B.

Figure 16-8

Splint knee in position found. **A.** If the knee is bent, splint it bent. **B.** If the knee is straight, splint it straight.

First aiders can use one of two methods to splint a fractured femur:

- Place a folded blanket or pillows between the victim's legs for padding, then tie the injured leg to the uninjured leg with several cravats or bandages.
- Place one board long enough to extend from the groin to the foot between the victim's legs. Place another board, long enough to extend from the armpit to the foot, along the victim's side. The boards must be well padded along their entire lengths. Tie the boards to the leg and body securely. This will stabilize the hip and the knee against movement **Figure 16-7**.

Knee

Always stabilize an injured knee in the position that you find it. If the knee is straight, splint it straight; if it is bent, splint it bent **Figure 16-8**.

For a straight knee, there are three options: (1) tie one long, padded board that extends from the hip to the ankle underneath the leg; (2) tie two boards along the sides of the leg, one between the victim's legs that extends from the groin to the foot and the other on the outer side that extends from the hip to the foot; or (3) tie the injured leg to the uninjured one.

For a bent knee, tie a long board extending from just below the hip to just above the ankle to prevent motion of the knee. Or, place a pillow or a rolled blanket beneath the knee and tie the injured leg to the uninjured leg.

To splint a knee in the straight position, follow the steps in **Skill Drill 16-7**:

1. Carefully lift the injured leg and place a rigid splint (long board) under the leg that extends from the buttocks to beyond the foot (**Step ❶**).
2. Place cravat bandages under the rigid splint and place soft padding under the knee and ankle (**Step ❷**).
3. Tie the cravat bandages. Do not tie the knots over the injured area (**Step ❸**).

To splint a knee in the bent position, follow the steps in **Skill Drill 16-8**:

1. Place a rigid splint (long board) against the injured leg. Do not place the splint against the knee (**Step ❶**).
2. Tie a cravat bandage around the splint and lower leg (**Step ❷**).
3. Tie a cravat bandage around the splint and thigh (**Step ❸**).
4. Tie knots over the splint, not over the leg (**Step ❹**).

skill drill

16-7 Splint a Knee in the Straight Position

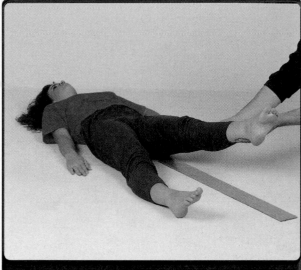

1 Lift the injured leg and place a rigid splint (long board) under the leg. The splint should extend from the buttocks to beyond the foot.

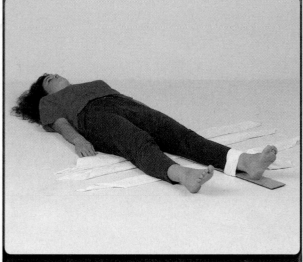

2 Place cravat bandages under the rigid splint and place soft padding under the knee and ankle.

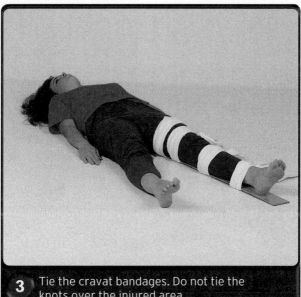

3 Tie the cravat bandages. Do not tie the knots over the injured area.

skill drill

16-8   Splint a Knee in the Bent Position

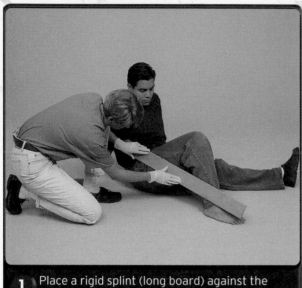

1 Place a rigid splint (long board) against the injured leg. Do not place the splint against the knee.

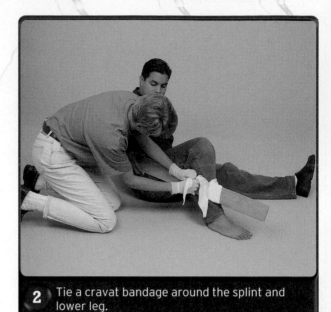

2 Tie a cravat bandage around the splint and lower leg.

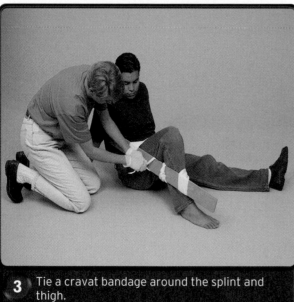

3 Tie a cravat bandage around the splint and thigh.

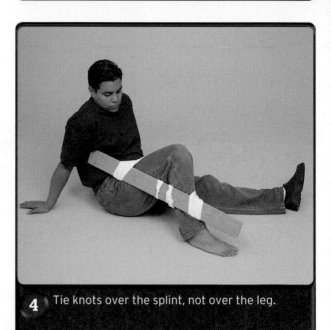

4 Tie knots over the splint, not over the leg.

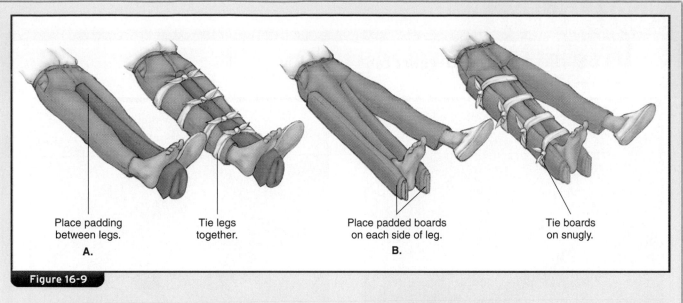

Place padding between legs. **A.**

Tie legs together.

Place padded boards on each side of leg. **B.**

Tie boards on snugly.

Figure 16-9

Two methods of splinting tibia and fibula fractures: **A.** Self-splint (left) **B.** Two boards (right).

Lower Leg

Stabilize the lower leg with two boards that extend from the upper thigh to the bottom of the foot. Or, place a folded blanket or pillow between the victim's legs for padding, and then tie the injured leg to the uninjured leg with several swathes, cravats, or bandages **Figure 16-9**.

To splint the lower leg using the self-splint method, follow the steps in **Skill Drill 16-9**:

1. Place padding (such as a folded blanket) between the legs. Push the cravat bandages under the leg with a thin board (**Step ❶**).
2. Tie the legs together (**Step ❷**).
3. Tie knots between the legs, over the padding (folded blanket) (**Step ❸**).

To splint the leg using rigid splints, follow the steps in **Skill Drill 16-10**:

1. Place one rigid splint (board) on the outside (lateral) and another inside (medial). Push the cravat bandages under the leg and splints with a thin board (**Step ❶**).
2. Tie both splints and leg together with cravat bandages (**Step ❷**).
3. Tie knots on top of the splint (board) (**Step ❸**).

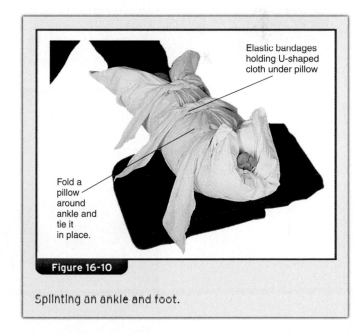

Elastic bandages holding U-shaped cloth under pillow

Fold a pillow around ankle and tie it in place.

Figure 16-10

Splinting an ankle and foot.

Ankle and Foot

Treat ankle and foot injuries with the RICE procedures. To further stabilize an ankle, wrap a pillow or folded blanket around the ankle and foot and tie with cravats **Figure 16-10**.

skill drill

16-9   Splinting—Lower Leg

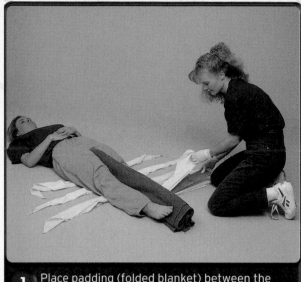

1 Place padding (folded blanket) between the legs. Push the cravat bandages under the leg with a thin board.

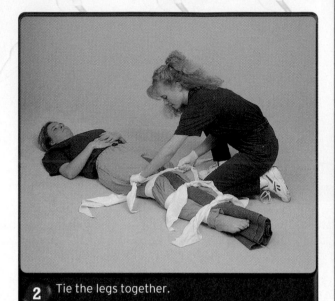

2 Tie the legs together.

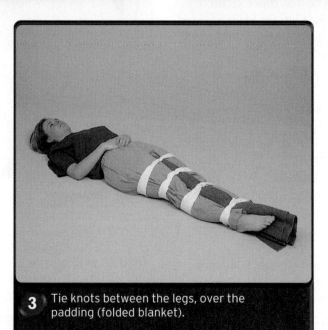

3 Tie knots between the legs, over the padding (folded blanket).

skill drill

16-10   Splinting—Leg

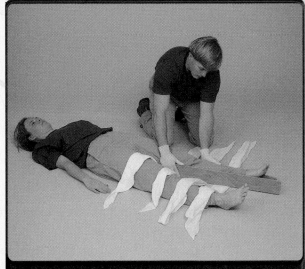

1 Place one rigid splint (board) on the outside (lateral) and another inside (medial). Push the cravat bandages under the leg with a thin board.

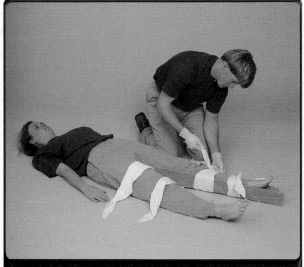

2 Tie both splints and leg together with cravat bandages.

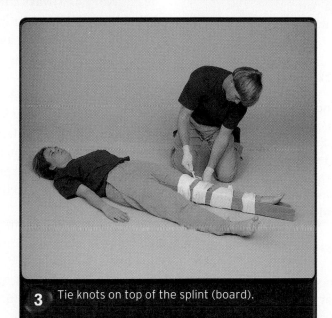

3 Tie knots on top of the splint (board).

prep kit

▶ Ready for Review

- Until medical care is available, stabilize the injury by splinting the extremity in the position found.
- A splint is any device used to stabilize a fracture or dislocation.
- When in doubt, apply a splint.
- A sling is any bandage or material that helps support the weight of an injured area.

▶ Vital Vocabulary

<u>sling</u> A triangular bandage applied around the neck to support an injured upper extremity; any material long enough to suspend an upper extremity by passing the material around the neck; used to support and protect an injury of the arm, shoulder, or clavicle.

<u>splint</u> Any support used to immobilize a fracture or to restrict movement of a part.

<u>swathe</u> A cravat tied around the body to decrease movement of a part.

▶ Assessment in Action

You are out with your best friend at a dog park walking her Irish wolfhound. Your friend is animated and engrossed in your conversation. Suddenly, a rabbit leaps out of the hedges and the dog lurches forward, pulling your friend and causing her to trip and let go of the leash. You call to the dog, which becomes obedient again, and then you notice that your friend has a deformity of her forefinger.

Directions: Circle Yes if you agree with the statement, circle No if you disagree.

Yes   No   1. You should immediately stabilize the finger until medical care is available.

Yes   No   2. You should splint the finger to prevent a possible closed fracture from becoming an open fracture.

Yes   No   3. Splinting increases blood flow to the fracture, thus speeding up the healing process.

Yes   No   4. If you do not have a commercial splint, you should never improvise one.

Yes   No   5. You can wrap two fingers together with adhesive tape.

Answers: 1. Yes; 2. Yes; 3. No; 4. No; 5. Yes

▶ Check Your Knowledge

Directions: Circle Yes if you agree with the statement, circle No if you disagree.

Yes   No   1. All fractures are complicated to some degree by damage to the soft tissue and structures surrounding the bone.

Yes   No   2. A rigid splint should never be used on an extremity.

Yes   No   3. All fractures and dislocations should be stabilized before the victim is moved.

Yes   No   4. Always check the CSM in the extremity.

Yes   No   5. Shoulder injuries can involve the clavicle, scapula, and the tibia.

Yes   No   6. An elbow must be stabilized in the position it is found.

Yes   No   7. Always straighten an injured knee before splinting it.

Yes   No   8. First aiders should always use traction splints on leg fractures.

Yes   No   9. Buddy taping is when you tape two fingers together with gauze separating the fingers.

Yes   No   10. You can make a temporary sling by pinning a shirt or coat sleeve to the front of the coat or shirt.

Answers: 1. Yes; 2. No; 3. Yes; 4. Yes; 5. No; 6. Yes; 7. No; 8. No; 9. Yes; 10. Yes

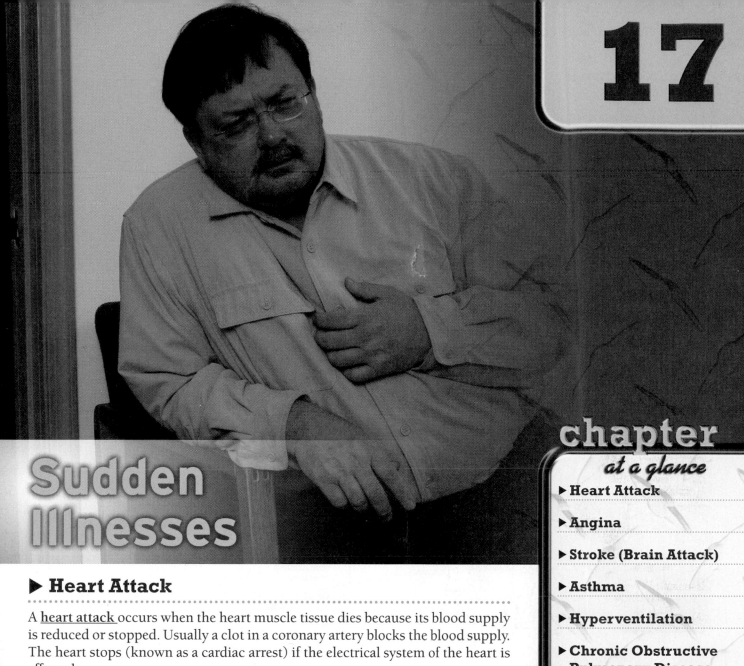

Sudden Illnesses

▶ Heart Attack

A <u>heart attack</u> occurs when the heart muscle tissue dies because its blood supply is reduced or stopped. Usually a clot in a coronary artery blocks the blood supply. The heart stops (known as a cardiac arrest) if the electrical system of the heart is affected.

Recognizing a Heart Attack

Whether a heart attack is occurring is difficult to determine. Because medical care at the onset of a heart attack is vital to survival and the quality of recovery, if you suspect a heart attack for any reason, seek medical attention *at once.* **Figure 17-1** shows a heart with a clot in an artery.

The possible signs and symptoms of a heart attack include:
- Pressure, squeezing, or pain in the center of the chest that lasts more than a few minutes or that goes away and comes back; some victims have no chest pain
- Pain spreading to the shoulders, neck, or arms
- Dizziness, sweating, nausea
- Shortness of breath

Not all of these warning signs occur in every heart attack. Many victims deny that they might be experiencing something as serious as a heart attack. Do not

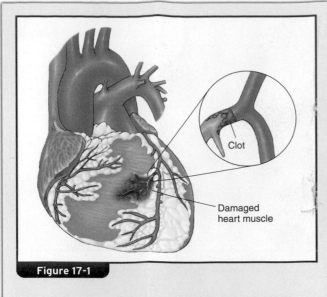

Figure 17-1

A heart attack occurs when a clot prevents blood flow to a part of the heart.

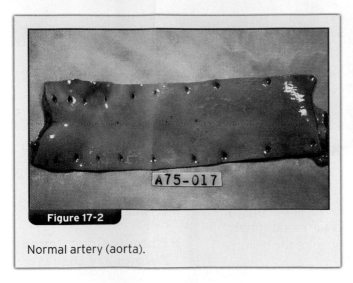

Figure 17-2

Normal artery (aorta).

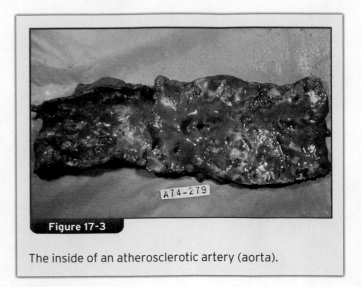

Figure 17-3

The inside of an atherosclerotic artery (aorta).

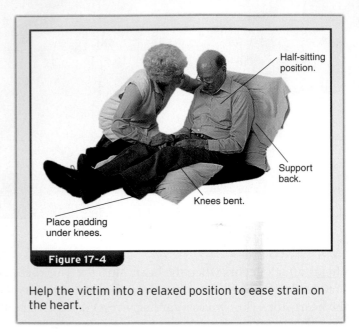

Figure 17-4

Help the victim into a relaxed position to ease strain on the heart.

take "no" for an answer. Delay can seriously increase the risk of major damage. Insist on taking prompt action.

Victims with heart attack symptoms who are brought to a hospital by ambulance receive clot-dissolving drugs (thrombolytics) sooner than those arriving by other means **Figure 17-2** and **Figure 17-3**. Reducing the time from the onset of a heart attack to the administration of thrombolytic drugs is beneficial and decreases the amount of heart damage.

Care for Heart Attack Victims

Treat a suspected heart attack in the following manner:

1. Call 9-1-1 or go to the nearest hospital emergency department that offers 24-hour emergency cardiac care. Medications to dissolve a clot are available but must be given early.

2. Monitor breathing. Give cardiopulmonary resuscitation (CPR) if necessary and if you are properly trained.

3. Help the victim to the most comfortable resting position, usually sitting **Figure 17-4**. Loosen clothing around the neck and midriff. Be calm and reassuring.

4. If the victim is alert, able to swallow, and not allergic to aspirin, give one adult aspirin or two to four chewable children's aspirin.

5. Find out whether the victim is using nitroglycerin. Nitroglycerin tablets, spray, or ointment can relieve chest pain from angina but not from a heart attack. Nitroglycerin dilates the coronary arteries, which increases blood flow to the heart muscle. It also lowers blood pressure and dilates the

veins, thus decreasing the work of the heart and the heart muscle's need for oxygen. *Caution:* Because nitroglycerin lowers blood pressure, the victim should sit or lie down once it is taken. Nitroglycerin usually may be repeated for a total of three doses in 10 minutes if the first dose does not relieve the pain. Keep in mind, though, that the victim might have already taken some nitroglycerin. Also, nitroglycerin is prescribed in different strengths—three tablets of one strength might be a mild dose, whereas three tablets of another strength might be a very high dose.

6. If the victim is unresponsive, check breathing and start CPR if needed.

▶ Angina

Chest pain called <u>angina pectoris</u> can result from coronary heart disease just as a heart attack does (Table 17-1). Angina occurs when the heart muscle does not get as much blood as it needs, which leads to a lack of oxygen.

Angina is brought on by physical exertion, exposure to cold, or emotional stress. It seldom lasts longer than 10 minutes and almost always is relieved by nitroglycerin. In contrast, chest pain from a heart attack is as likely to happen at rest as during activity; the pain lasts longer than 10 minutes and is not relieved by nitroglycerin. Nitroglycerin is the drug used most often to dilate the coronary arteries and increase the blood supply to the heart. It is often prescribed by physicians for patients with angina.

Recognizing Angina

It can be difficult to differentiate a heart attack from angina even for physicians. Typical signs of angina include:

- Chest pain described as crushing, squeezing, or like somebody standing on the victim's chest.
- Pain can spread to the jaw, the arms (frequently the left arm), and mid-back.
- Pain usually lasts from 3 to 10 minutes, but rarely longer than 15 minutes.
- Can be associated with shortness of breath, nausea, or sweating.
- Victim feels anxious.

Care for People With Angina

Use the following guidelines in caring for a victim suffering from angina.

1. If a victim has his or her own nitroglycerin, assist the victim in using it appropriately. Refer to the Caution under the Care for Heart Attack section.

FYI

No Chest Pain in One Third of Heart Attacks

A study of hundreds of thousands of heart attack victims found that as many as one third had no chest pain and that they were less likely to seek help and twice as likely to die.

The study found that women, people of color, people older than 75 years, and people with previous heart failure, stroke, or diabetes were most likely to have painless heart attacks. Although doctors have long known about painless heart attacks, many said they did not realize the number was so high.

Patients with chest pain were more than twice as likely to be diagnosed at admission and to receive clot-busting drugs or undergo angioplasty to open clogged arteries.

Source: Canto JG, Shlipak MG, Rogers WJ, et al: Prevalence, clinical characteristics, and mortality among patients with myocardial infarction presenting without chest pain. *JAMA* 283:3223-3229.

FYI

Dangerous Morning Hours

Many studies in the past decade have demonstrated diurnal variation in the onset of acute cardiovascular disorders (such as heart attack, cardiac death). The results consistently show an increased incidence of acute cardiac events in the morning hours (6:00 AM to noon) and a low incidence at night. Some data suggest another late afternoon or evening peak of incidence.

Source: Peckova M, et al: Circadian variation in the occurrence of cardiac arrests. *Circulation* 98(1):31-39.

FYI

Monday Morning Heart Attacks

Studies show that heart attacks occur most frequently in the morning and during the winter months. In one study, 5,596 heart attacks and sudden cardiac deaths were recorded in Augsburg, Germany, from 1958 through 1990. The increased risk of heart attack was highest among people employed outside the home, especially in blue collar jobs, and the incidence of heart attack peaked on Mondays. Sundays had the lowest heart attack rate for all workers. There was no significant daily variation in heart attacks among nonworking people.

Source: Willich SN, Lowel H, Lewis M, Hormann A, Amtz HR, Keil U: Weekly variation of acute myocardial infarction: increased Monday risk in the working population. *Circulation* 90(7):87.

FYI

Risk Factors for Heart Disease

Several factors contribute to an increased risk of heart attack and stroke. The more risk factors present, the greater the possibility that a person will develop heart disease.

Risk Factors You Cannot Change

- *Heredity:* Tendencies appear in family lines.
- *Sex:* Men have a greater risk, although heart attack is still the leading cause of death among women.
- *Age:* Most heart attack victims are 65 years or older.

Risk Factors You Can Change

- *Cigarette smoking:* Smokers have more than twice the risk of heart attack as nonsmokers.
- *High blood pressure:* This condition adds to the heart's workload.
- *High blood cholesterol level:* Too much cholesterol in the blood can cause a buildup on the walls of the arteries.

Other Risk Factors You Can Change or Control

- *Diabetes:* This condition affects the blood's cholesterol and triglyceride levels.
- *Obesity:* Being overweight influences blood pressure and blood cholesterol, can result in diabetes, and can place added strain on the heart.
- *Physical inactivity:* Inactive people have twice the risk of heart attack as active people.
- *Stress:* All people feel stress but react in different ways. Excessive, long-term stress can lead to physical problems in some people.

FYI

Why Don't They Call?

A study of heart attack victims who waited for more than 20 minutes before getting help were asked why they delayed. Their answers included the following:

- They thought the symptoms would go away.
- The symptoms were not severe enough.
- They thought it was a different illness.
- They were worried about medical costs.
- They were afraid of hospitals.
- They feared being embarrassed.
- They wanted to wait for a better time.
- They did not want to find out what was wrong.

The average time that elapsed between symptom onset and hospital arrival was 2 hours; 28% waited at least 1 hour, 33% waited 1 to 3 hours, 15% waited 3 to 6 hours, and 23% waited more than 6 hours. The researchers noted that the main reason for delay seemed to be uncertainty in interpreting heart attack symptoms. Most victims reported they were not sure their symptoms were severe enough to merit action as drastic as calling 9-1-1.

The same study concluded that one way to shorten out-of-hospital delay is to encourage victims with heart-related symptoms to use EMS rather than slower transportation methods.

Source: Meischke H, Eisenberg MS, Schaeffer SM, Larsen MP: Reasons patients with chest pain delay or do not call 911. A*nn Emerg Med* 25(2):193–197.

Table 17-1   Chest Pain

Cause of pain	Characteristics	Care
Muscle or rib pain from exercise or injury	Reproduced by movement Tender spot when pressed	Rest Aspirin or ibuprofen
Respiratory infection (pneumonia, bronchitis, pleuritis)	Cough Fever Sore throat Production of sputum	Antibiotics
Indigestion	Belching Heartburn Nausea Sour taste	Antacids
Angina pectoris	Lasts less than 10 minutes (but pain is similar to that of a heart attack)	Rest Victim's nitroglycerin
Heart attack (myocardial infarction)	Lasts more than 10 minutes Pressure, squeezing, or pain near center of the chest Pain spreads to shoulders, neck, or arms Lightheadedness, fainting, sweating, nausea, shortness of breath	Call EMS Check Breathing Resting position Victim's nitroglycerin

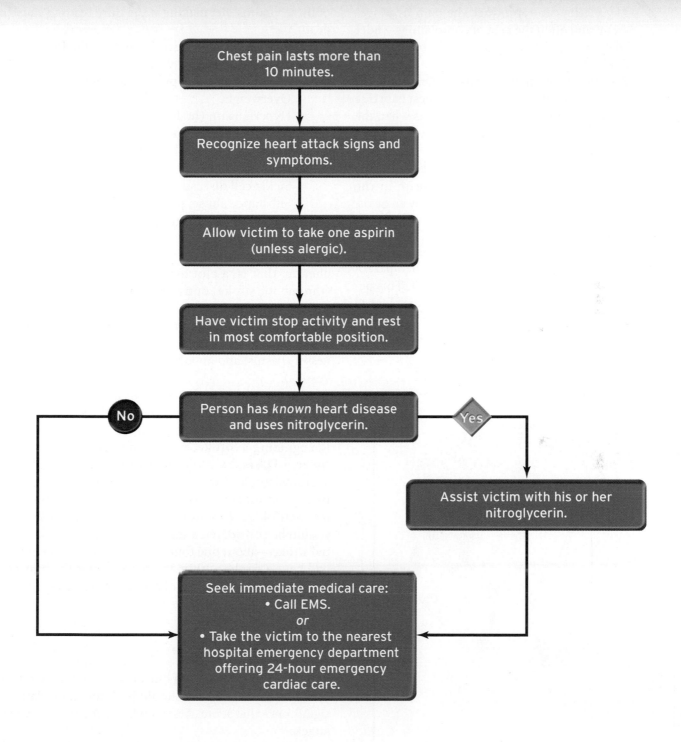

2. If the pain does not quickly subside (5–10 minutes), suspect a heart attack and care for the victim accordingly. Many causes of chest pain have nothing to do with the heart, including:

- Muscle or rib pain due to exercise or injury: The victim can reproduce the pain by movement, and often the area of complaint is tender when pressed. Rest and aspirin or ibuprofen relieves the pain.
- Respiratory infections such as pneumonia, bronchitis, pleuritis, or lung injury: Chest pain due to these conditions usually worsens when the victim coughs or breathes deeply. Fever and colored sputum might be present.
- Indigestion, usually accompanied by belching, heartburn, nausea, and a sour taste in the mouth: This type of pain is relieved by antacids.

▶ Stroke (Brain Attack)

A <u>stroke</u>, also called a brain attack, occurs when part of the blood flow to the brain is suddenly cut off. This occurs when arteries in the brain rupture or become blocked so part of the brain does not receive the blood flow it needs **Figure 17-5**. Deprived of oxygen-rich blood, nerve cells in the affected area of the brain cannot function and die within minutes. Because dead brain cells are not replaced, the devastating effects of strokes often are permanent. Each year, approximately 700,000 Americans suffer a new or recurrent stroke, and approximately one fourth of these victims die, making it the third leading cause of death.

The risk factors for a stroke include the following:

- Age (older than 50 years)
- Use of birth control pills and age older than 30 years
- Overweight
- Hypertension (high blood pressure)
- High blood cholesterol levels
- Diabetes
- Heart disease
- Sickle cell disease
- Substance abuse, particularly crack cocaine
- Family history of strokes or transient ischemic attacks (TIAs)

The most common type of stroke (about 80%) is ischemic, that is, a clot forms in an artery in the brain (thrombotic stroke) or travels from the heart to the brain and plugs the artery (embolic stroke). In about 20% of cases, a blood vessel ruptures (hemorrhagic stroke). Other causes include tumors pressing on blood vessels, blood vessel spasms, and aneurysms (ballooning out of blood vessels).

Transient ischemic attacks are closely associated with strokes. Because TIAs have many of the same signs and symptoms, they often are confused with strokes (see Recognizing a Stroke, next). The main difference between a TIA and a stroke is that the symptoms of a TIA are transient, lasting from several minutes (75% last less than 5 minutes) to several hours, with a return to normal neurologic function. TIAs are ministrokes. A TIA should be considered a serious warning sign of a potential stroke—about one third of all people who have a TIA will have a stroke within 2 to 5 years after the first TIA. Any signs and symptoms of a TIA should be reported to a physician.

Recognizing a Stroke

The next time you think about stroke, think brain attack. The symptoms of stroke should have the same alarming significance that acute chest pain has in identifying a heart attack:

- Weakness, numbness, or paralysis of the face, an arm, or a leg on one side of the body **Figure 17-6**
- Blurred or decreased vision, especially in one eye
- Problems speaking or understanding
- Dizziness or loss of balance

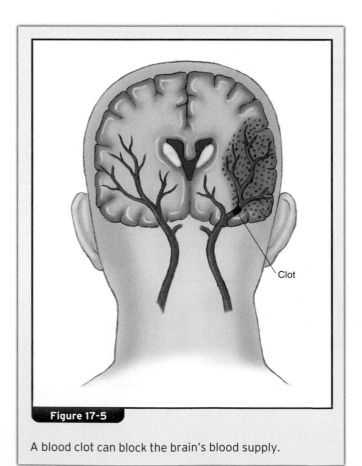

Clot

Figure 17-5

A blood clot can block the brain's blood supply.

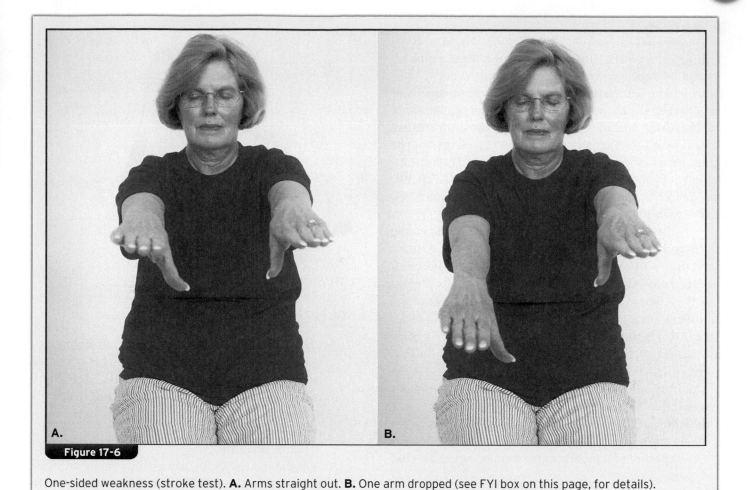

Figure 17-6

One-sided weakness (stroke test). **A.** Arms straight out. **B.** One arm dropped (see FYI box on this page, for details).

- Sudden, severe, and unexplained headache
- Deviation of the eyes from PEARL (pupils equal and reactive to light), which might mean the brain is being affected by lack of oxygen

FYI

Los Angeles Stroke Screen

Los Angeles paramedics use a proven method for quickly identifying stroke victims, and so can first aiders. When you suspect a stroke, apply these three simple tests for one-side paralysis:

1. Arm strength (both arms): the victim closes his eyes and holds both arms out with palms down, and slowly counts to five. If one arm does not move and the other drifts down, suspect a stroke.
2. Facial smile: the victim smiles or shows teeth. If one side of the face does not move as well as the other side, suspect a stroke.
3. Hand grip (both hands): the victim grips one of your fingers in each of his hands at the same time. If grip strength is not equal, suspect a stroke.

Care for a Stroke Victim

First aid for a stroke victim is limited to supportive care:

1. Call 9-1-1. Minimize brain damage by getting the victim to medical care.
2. If the victim is unresponsive, open the airway and check breathing. If there is no breathing, give CPR.
3. If the victim is responsive, lay the victim down with the head and shoulders slightly elevated.
4. Place a victim who is unresponsive but breathing in the recovery position to keep the airway open and to permit secretions and vomit to drain from the mouth.

CAUTION

DO NOT give a stroke victim anything to drink or eat. The throat can be paralyzed, which restricts swallowing.

▶ Asthma

Asthma is a chronic, inflammatory lung disease characterized by repeated breathing problems. People with asthma have acute episodes (some call them attacks or flares) when the air passages in their lungs get narrower, and breathing becomes more difficult. The problems are caused by an oversensitivity of the air passages in the lungs, which overreact to certain triggers and become inflamed and clogged. Asthma affects an estimated 10 million people in the United States and accounts for 6,000 deaths each year.

The condition is most common in children and young adults and tends to improve or resolve with age. Asthma is the number one prehospital emergency in children. It can occur in infants who are as young as a few weeks; about one half of all children with asthma experience the condition during their first 2 years of life. Adult-onset asthma tends to be chronic. Viral infections are a common cause of the onset of acute asthma in children younger than 6 months.

Asthma has three components: airway obstruction, airway inflammation, and overly sensitive airways. Some of the known triggers of asthma include the following:

- Respiratory tract infection
- Exposure to temperature extremes, especially cold air
- Strong odors, perfumes, talcum powder, deodorizers, and paint
- Occupational exposures: dust, fumes, and smoke
- Certain drugs: aspirin, nonsteroidal anti-inflammatory drugs, yellow dye No. 5, and beta blockers
- Exercise
- Emotional stress
- Allergens: pollen, mold, dust mites, animal dander, and tobacco smoke
- Air pollution: ozone and sulfur dioxide

Recognizing Asthma

Asthma varies a great deal from one person to another. Symptoms can range from mild to moderate to severe and can be life threatening. The episodes can come occasionally or often. Between episodes the person has no breathing difficulties. The signs of an asthma attack include the following:

- Coughing
- Cyanosis (bluish skin)
- Inability to speak in complete sentences without pausing for breath
- Nostrils flaring with each breath
- Difficulty breathing, including wheezing

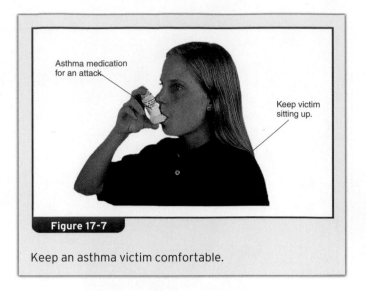

Asthma medication for an attack

Keep victim sitting up.

Figure 17-7

Keep an asthma victim comfortable.

Care for People With Asthma

1. Place the victim in a comfortable, upright position and leaning slightly forward. This is known as the tripod position. Generally the victim will indicate what position is most tolerable; usually sitting up is best because that position makes it easier to breathe.
2. Monitor breathing.
3. Ask the victim about any asthma medication he or she is using 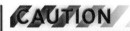. Most people with asthma have some form of asthma medication, usually administered through physician-prescribed, handheld inhalers.
4. If the victim does not respond well to his or her inhaled medication or is having an extreme asthma attack that does not subside (known as status asthmaticus), seek medical care immediately.

Asthma is common and is treated fairly easily. Although asthma is a complex condition that can warrant use of several different medications, the preferred method of initial care for children and adults is use of their inhaled bronchodilators.

> ⚠ **CAUTION**
>
> DO NOT wait too long to seek medical help for the victim of a severe asthma attack.

▶ Hyperventilation

Fast, deep breathing, called hyperventilation, is common during emotional stress. The victim might be hysterical or quite calm. Other factors that can cause rapid breathing include untreated diabetes, severe shock, certain poisons, and brain swelling due to injury or high altitude.

Recognizing Hyperventilation

Signs of hyperventilation include the following:
- Dizziness or lightheadedness
- Numbness
- Tingling of the hands and feet
- Shortness of breath
- Breathing rate faster than 40 breaths per minute

FYI

Breathing Into a Paper Bag

If you are advised to breathe into a paper bag—a popular remedy for anxiety-related hyperventilation (fast breathing)—do not do it. Tests on healthy people show that bag rebreathing rarely restores blood gas balance but often causes dangerous stress to the heart and respiratory system, especially in people with a chronic respiratory disease.

Source: Callaham M: Hypoxic hazards of traditional paper bag rebreathing in hyperventilating patients. *Ann Emerg Med* 18(6):622-628.

Care for Hyperventilation Victims

If you encounter someone who is hyperventilating, two steps can help him or her.
1. Calm and reassure the victim.
2. Encourage the person to breathe slowly, using the abdominal muscles: inhale through the nose, hold the full inhalation for several seconds, then exhale slowly.

▶ Chronic Obstructive Pulmonary Disease

Chronic obstructive pulmonary disease (COPD) is a broad term applied to emphysema, chronic bronchitis, and related lung diseases. The incidence of COPD is very high in North America, and the most common causative factor is cigarette smoking.

Chronic obstructive pulmonary disease describes a disease that makes it hard for a person to breathe because the normal flow of air into and out of the person's lungs is partially obstructed.

Because COPD takes many years to develop before a person notices difficulty breathing, COPD is usually considered a disease of older adults and is most commonly diagnosed in people older than 60 years.

Chronic bronchitis is caused by chronic infection, which can be brought on by irritations such as tobacco smoke. The bronchi become thick, unable to stretch, and partially blocked. Early symptoms include a cigarette cough or a cough due to a cold. Later, more severe symptoms include difficult breathing, increased sputum, and severe coughing.

Emphysema often occurs with chronic bronchitis. The alveoli of the lungs are partially destroyed, and the lungs have lost their elasticity, making it difficult for the victim to exhale. Common symptoms include coughing, wheezing, and shortness of breath. Breathing is extremely difficult for people with emphysema.

Recognizing Chronic Obstructive Pulmonary Disease

The signs and symptoms of COPD are similar to those of asthma. Most victims will wheeze; coughing and shortness of breath might be more prominent in COPD than in asthma. Many people with COPD depend on a constant low level of artificially supplied oxygen to maintain breathing.

Care for People With Chronic Obstructive Pulmonary Disease

Use the following guidelines when caring for someone with COPD:
1. Persons with COPD usually will have their own physician-prescribed medications. Assist the victim to take any prescribed medications.
2. Place the victim in the sitting position that provides the greatest comfort.
3. Encourage the victim to cough up any secretions.
4. Encourage the victim to drink fluids.
5. For acute breathing distress, obtain immediate medical assistance. The victim might need oxygen, which is available from the EMS and at hospital emergency departments.

▶ Fainting

A sudden, brief loss of responsiveness not associated with a head injury is known as <u>syncope</u> (simple fainting) or <u>psychogenic shock</u>.

Simple fainting is common and benign and can have physical or emotional causes. Fainting can happen suddenly when blood flow to the brain is interrupted. The nervous system dilates blood vessels to three to four times their normal size and allows blood to pool in the legs and lower body.

Fainting

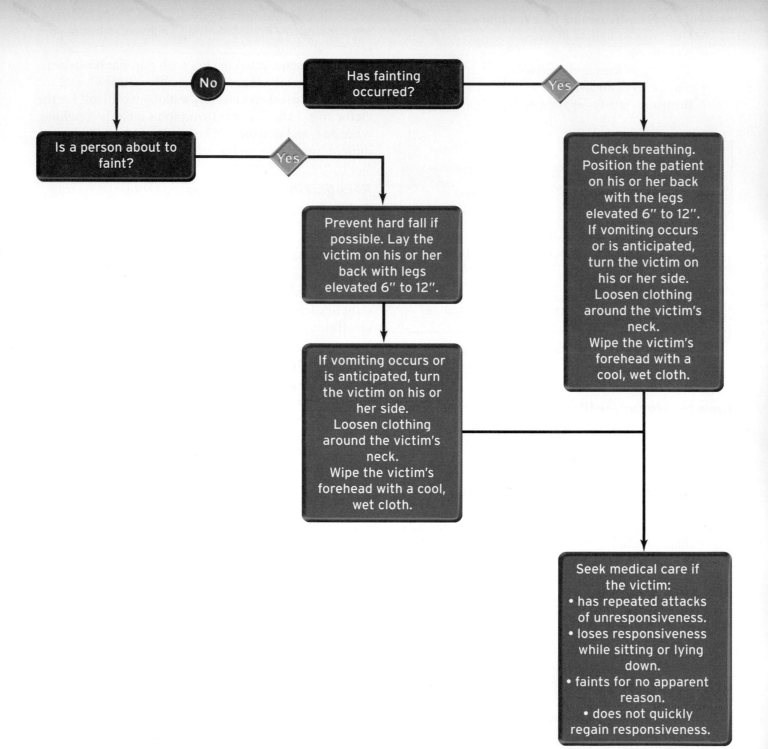

Has fainting occurred?

No → **Is a person about to faint?**

Yes → Check breathing. Position the patient on his or her back with the legs elevated 6" to 12". If vomiting occurs or is anticipated, turn the victim on his or her side. Loosen clothing around the victim's neck. Wipe the victim's forehead with a cool, wet cloth.

Is a person about to faint? — **Yes** → Prevent hard fall if possible. Lay the victim on his or her back with legs elevated 6" to 12".

Prevent hard fall if possible. Lay the victim on his or her back with legs elevated 6" to 12". → If vomiting occurs or is anticipated, turn the victim on his or her side. Loosen clothing around the victim's neck. Wipe the victim's forehead with a cool, wet cloth.

Seek medical care if the victim:
- has repeated attacks of unresponsiveness.
- loses responsiveness while sitting or lying down.
- faints for no apparent reason.
- does not quickly regain responsiveness.

Syncope, or simple fainting, can be precipitated by unpleasant emotional stimuli such as the sight of blood or strong fear. It usually occurs when the victim is in the upright position.

Most fainting episodes are associated with decreased blood flow causing deficient oxygen or glucose in the brain. The decreased blood flow can be caused by low blood sugar (**hypoglycemia**), a slow heart rate (vagal reaction, in which the vagus nerve, which slows the heart rate, is overstimulated by fright, anxiety, drugs, or fatigue), heart-rhythm disturbances, dehydration, heat exhaustion, anemia (low blood clot), or bleeding.

Sitting or standing for a long time without moving, especially in a hot environment, can cause blood to pool in dilated vessels, which results in a loss of effective circulating blood volume, causing the blood pressure to drop. As the blood flow to the brain decreases, the person loses consciousness and collapses.

Recognizing Fainting

A person who is about to faint usually will have one or more of the following signs and symptoms:
- Dizziness
- Weakness
- Seeing spots
- Visual blurring
- Nausea
- Pale skin
- Sweating

Care for Fainting Victims

If a person appears about to faint:
1. Prevent the person from falling.
2. Help the person lie down and raise the person's legs 6 to 12 inches. This position increases venous blood flow back to the heart, which in turn pumps more blood to the brain.
3. Loosen tight clothing at the neck and waist.
4. Stay with the victim until he or she recovers.

If fainting has happened:
1. Monitor breathing.
2. Loosen tight clothing and belts.
3. If the victim fell, check for injuries.
4. Raise the victim's legs 6 to 12 inches.
5. After recovery, have the victim sit for a while, and when he or she is able to swallow, give cool, sweetened liquids to drink and help the victim to slowly regain an upright posture.
6. Fresh air and a cold, wet cloth for the face usually aid recovery.

Most fainting episodes are not serious, and the victim recovers quickly. Seek medical care, however, if the victim:

- has had repeated attacks of unresponsiveness
- does not quickly regain responsiveness
- loses responsiveness while sitting or lying down
- faints for no apparent reason

> **CAUTION**
>
> DO NOT splash or pour water on the victim's face.
> DO NOT use smelling salts or ammonia inhalants.
> DO NOT slap the victim's face in an attempt to revive him or her.
> DO NOT give the victim anything to drink until he or she has fully recovered and can swallow.

▶ Seizures

A **seizure** results from an abnormal stimulation of the brain's cells causing uncontrollable muscle movements. Several medical conditions increase the instability or irritability of the brain and can lead to seizures, including the following:
- Epilepsy
- Heatstroke
- Poisoning
- Electric shock
- Hypoglycemia
- High fever in children
- Brain injury, tumor, or stroke
- Alcohol withdrawal, drug abuse, or overdose

Most people with seizures have idiopathic epilepsy; that is, the cause of the seizures is not known. Because seizure types are so different, they require different first aid actions, and some require no action at all. There are four types of seizures.

- Generalized tonic-clonic seizures (grand mal seizures) are characterized by loss of consciousness, muscle contraction, and sometimes tongue biting, loss of bladder control, and mental confusion. The generalized tonic-clonic seizure is often frightening to witness. The seizure usually is followed by a period of coma or drowsiness.
- Focal motor seizures usually cause one part of the body—such as one side of the face or an arm—to twitch.
- Complex partial seizures are characterized by an altered personality state and are often preceded by dizziness or a peculiar metallic taste in the mouth. In some people, these seizures can cause sudden, unexplained attacks of rage; in others, they are manifested by automatic (involuntary) types of behavior.

- Absence seizures usually occur in children and are rarely an emergency. They are characterized by a brief loss of consciousness. The child suddenly stares off into space for a few seconds and then returns immediately to consciousness.

Because of the nature of the electrical discharge in the brain, generalized tonic-clonic seizures usually follow a typical sequence. Many victims experience an aura, a strange sensation lasting a few seconds. The aura can consist of auditory or visual hallucinations, a peculiar taste in the mouth, or a painful sensation in the abdomen. The victim then loses consciousness and has contractions of the muscles of the extremities, trunk, and head. The attack usually lasts 2 to 5 minutes. It might be followed by deep sleep, headache, and muscle soreness.

The following information is important to obtain from the seizure victim, the family, or bystanders:

- Does the victim have a history of seizures? Does the victim take medication for seizures? Has the victim been taking the medication according to instructions?
- What did the seizure look like? How long did the seizure last? Was the seizure preceded by an aura?
- Does the victim have a recent or remote history of head injury? Trauma can irritate parts of the brain, causing seizures. More than half the victims of acute head injuries will experience a seizure within 1 year following the injury.
- Does the victim abuse alcohol or drugs? Seizures often occur during withdrawal from alcohol and barbiturates.
- Has the victim recently had a fever, headache, or stiff neck? These signs and symptoms could indicate meningitis (an infection of the nervous system).
- Does the victim have a history of diabetes, heart disease, or stroke?

Epilepsy is not a mental illness, and it is not a sign of low intelligence. It also is not contagious. Between seizures, a person with epilepsy can function as normally as a person who does not have epilepsy.

Recognizing Seizures

Regardless of the type of seizure, it is important to recognize when a seizure is occurring or whether one has occurred. Refer to Table 17-2 for detailed information on the different types of seizures and how they present. Gather as much information as you can from family members and bystanders in order to verify that a seizure occurred and to obtain a description of how it developed.

Care for People Who Have Seizures

The Epilepsy Foundation lists the following first aid procedures for seizures:

1. Cushion the victim's head; remove items that could cause injury if the person bumped into them.
2. Loosen any tight clothing, especially around the neck.
3. Roll the victim onto his or her side.
4. Look for a medical tag (bracelet or necklace).
5. As the seizure ends, offer your help. Most seizures in people with epilepsy are not medical emergencies. They end after a minute or two without harm and usually do not require medical attention.
6. Call 9-1-1 if any of the following exists or occurs:
   - A seizure occurs in someone who is not known to have epilepsy (that is, there is no epilepsy or seizure disorder identification). It could be a sign of serious illness.
   - A seizure lasts more than 5 minutes.
   - The victim is slow to recover, has a second seizure, or has difficulty breathing afterward.
   - The victim is pregnant or has another medical condition.
   - There are any signs of injury or illness.

Status epilepticus is defined as two or more seizures without an intervening period of consciousness. Status epilepticus is an emergency situation and requires immediate medical attention. Repeated, uncontrolled seizures can lead to aspiration, brain damage, fractures, and severe dehydration. In adults, the most common cause of status epilepticus is failure to take prescribed medicines for epilepsy.

CAUTION

DO NOT give the victim anything to eat or drink.

DO NOT restrain the victim.

DO NOT put anything between the victim's teeth during the seizure.

DO NOT splash or pour any liquid on the victim's face.

DO NOT move the victim to another place (unless it is the only way to protect the victim from injury).

▶ Diabetic Emergencies

Diabetes is a condition in which insulin, a hormone produced by the pancreas that helps the body use the energy in food, is lacking or ineffective. Insulin is needed to take sugar from the blood and carry it into the cells to be used.

Table 17-2 Seizures: Recognition and First Aid

Seizure type	What it looks like	What it is not	What to do	What not to do
Generalized tonic-clonic seizure (formerly called grand mal)	Sudden cry, fall, rigidity, followed by muscle jerks, shallow breathing or temporarily suspended breathing, bluish skin, possible loss of bladder or bowel control; usually lasts a couple of minutes. Normal breathing then starts again. There could be some confusion and/or fatigue, followed by return to full consciousness.	• Heart attack • Stroke	Look for medical tag. Protect from nearby hazards. Loosen tie or shirt collar. Protect head from injury. Turn on side to keep airway clear. Reassure when consciousness returns. If single seizure lasted less than 5 minutes, ask if hospital evaluation is wanted. If multiple seizures, or if one seizure lasts longer than 5 minutes, call an ambulance. If the person is pregnant, injured, or diabetic, call for aid at once.	Do not put any hard implement in the mouth. Do not try to hold the tongue. It cannot be swallowed. Do not try to give liquids during or just after seizure. Do not use rescue breathing unless breathing is absent after muscle jerks subside or unless water has been inhaled. Do not restrain.
Absence seizure (formerly called petit mal)	A blank stare, lasting only a few seconds; most common in children. Can be accompanied by rapid blinking or some chewing movements. Child is unaware of what's going on during the seizure but quickly returns to full awareness once it has stopped.	• Daydreaming • Lack of attention • Deliberate ignoring of adult instructions	No first aid necessary, but if this is the first observation of the seizure(s), seek medical evaluation.	
Simple partial seizure	Jerking might begin in one area of the body, arm, leg, or face. Cannot be stopped, but patient stays awake and aware. Jerking can proceed from one area of the body to another and sometimes spreads to become a generalized tonic-clonic seizure. Partial sensory seizures might not be obvious to an onlooker. Patient experiences a distorted environment. Patient might see or hear things that are not there, and might feel unexplained fear, sadness, anger, or joy. Might have nausea, experience odd smells, and have a generally funny feeling in the stomach.	• Acting out, bizarre behavior • Hysteria • Mental illness • Psychosomatic illness • Parapsychological or mystical experience	No first aid necessary unless seizure becomes generalized tonic-clonic, then give first aid as indicated for generalized tonic-clonic seizures. No action needed other than reassurance and emotional support. Medical evaluation should be recommended.	

(continued)

Table 17-2   Continued

Seizure type	What it looks like	What it is not	What to do	What not to do
Complex partial seizure (formerly called psychomotor or temporal lobe seizure)	Usually starts with blank stare, followed by chewing, followed by random activity. Person appears unaware of surroundings, might seem dazed and mumble. Unresponsive. Actions clumsy, not directed. Might pick at clothing, pick up objects, try to take clothes off. Might run, appear to be afraid. Same set of actions usually occur with each seizure. Lasts a few minutes, but postseizure confusion can last substantially longer. No memory of what happened during seizure period.	• Drunkenness • Drug intoxication • Mental illness • Disorderly conduct	Speak calmly and reassuringly to patient and others. Guide gently away from obvious hazards. Stay until person is completely aware of environment. Offer to help get person home.	Do not grab or hold the person unless sudden danger (such as a cliff edge or an approaching car) threatens. Do not shout. Do not expect verbal instructions to be obeyed.
Atonic seizure (formerly called a drop attack)	Person suddenly collapses. After 10 seconds to a minute, person recovers, regains consciousness, and can stand and walk again.	• Clumsiness • Normal childhood stage • In a child, lack of good walking skills • In an adult, drunkenness, acute illness	No first aid needed (unless fall results in injury), but a child should be given a thorough medical evaluation.	
Myoclonic seizure	Sudden brief, massive muscle jerks that can involve the whole body or parts of body. Can cause person to drop things or fall off a chair.	• Clumsiness • Poor coordination	No first aid needed, but patient should be given a thorough medical evaluation.	
Infantile spasms	Clusters of quick, sudden movements that start between 3 months and 2 years. If child is sitting up, head will fall forward, and arms will flex forward. If lying down, knees will be drawn up, with arms and head flexed forward as if the child is reaching for support.	• Normal movements • Colic	No first aid needed, but a doctor should be consulted.	

Source: Epilepsy Foundation. Reprinted with permission.

Seizures

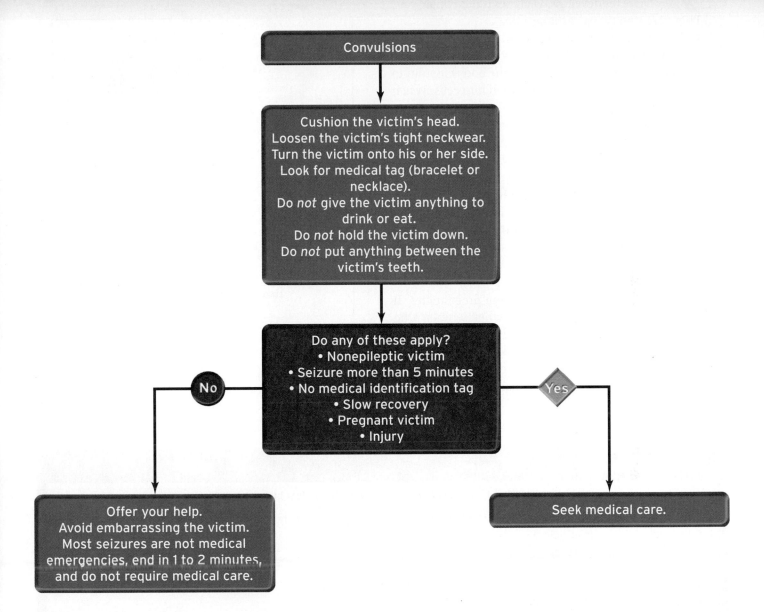

Convulsions

Cushion the victim's head.
Loosen the victim's tight neckwear.
Turn the victim onto his or her side.
Look for medical tag (bracelet or necklace).
Do *not* give the victim anything to drink or eat.
Do *not* hold the victim down.
Do *not* put anything between the victim's teeth.

Do any of these apply?
• Nonepileptic victim
• Seizure more than 5 minutes
• No medical identification tag
• Slow recovery
• Pregnant victim
• Injury

No

Yes

Offer your help.
Avoid embarrassing the victim.
Most seizures are not medical emergencies, end in 1 to 2 minutes, and do not require medical care.

Seek medical care.

When excess sugar remains in the blood, the body cells must rely on fat as fuel. Blood sugar (glucose) is a major body fuel, and when it cannot be used, it builds up in the blood, overflows into the urine, and passes out of the body unused—the body loses an important source of fuel **Table 17-3**. Diabetes develops. Diabetes is not contagious.

There are two types of diabetes:

- Type 1 (formerly called juvenile-onset or insulin-dependent diabetes): People with type 1 diabetes require external (not made by the body) insulin to allow sugar to pass from the blood into cells. When deprived of external insulin, the person becomes quite ill and will die without treatment.
- Type 2 (formerly called adult-onset or non-insulin-dependent diabetes): People with type 2 diabetes tend to be overweight. They are not dependent on external insulin to allow sugar into cells. However, if their insulin level is low, the lack of sugar in the cells increases sugar production and sugar in the blood to very high levels. Glucose then spills into the urine, drawing fluid with it and resulting in dehydration.

Gestational diabetes occurs in some pregnancies. It usually ends after a baby is born, but when women who had gestational diabetes get older, type 2 diabetes can develop. Gestational diabetes results from the body's resistance to the action of insulin. This resistance is caused by hormones produced during pregnancy. Gestational diabetes is usually treated with diet, but some women need insulin.

The body is continuously balancing sugar and insulin **Figure 17-8**. Too much insulin and not enough sugar leads to low blood sugar and possibly insulin shock.

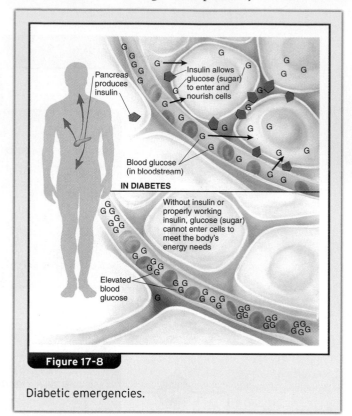

Figure 17-8

Diabetic emergencies.

Table 17-3	**Diabetic Emergencies**	
	Diabetic coma (high blood sugar)	Insulin shock (low blood sugar)
Cause	Not enough insulin; too much sugar	Too much insulin; not enough sugar
Insulin level	Insufficient	Excessive
Onset of symptoms	Gradual	Sudden
Skin	Flushed, dry, warm	Pale, clammy
Breath	Fruity odor	Normal
Thirst	Severe	Normal
Urination	Frequent	Normal
Behavior		Appearance of intoxication: combativeness, bad temper, anger, confusion, disorientation
Other symptoms	Drowsiness, vomiting, heavy breathing, eventual stupor or unconsciousness	Sudden hunger, eventual stupor, or unresponsiveness
First aid	• If in doubt, give sugar. • Give fluids to fight dehydration. • Take victim to hospital.	Give sugar. Seek medical care.

Insulin shock results from severe low blood sugar, causing coma and possibly death. Too much sugar and not enough insulin leads to high blood sugar, and possibly diabetic coma (Figure 17-9). Diabetic coma results from lack of insulin, causing severe high blood sugar and production of chemicals called ketones. Ketones cause a sweet or fruity odor on the breath.

▶ Low Blood Sugar

A low blood sugar level, called hypoglycemia, is sometimes referred to as an insulin reaction. This condition can be caused by too much insulin, too little or delayed food intake, exercise, alcohol, or any combination of these factors.

Recognizing Low Blood Sugar

The American Diabetes Association lists the following signs and symptoms of insulin reaction and hypoglycemia as diabetic emergencies requiring first aid:

- Sudden onset
- Staggering, poor coordination
- Anger, bad temper
- Pale skin
- Confusion, disorientation
- Sudden hunger
- Excessive sweating
- Trembling
- Eventual unresponsiveness

Care for People Who Have Low Blood Sugar

Give sugar using the rule of 15s (later in this section) for an insulin reaction if all three conditions are present:

- The victim is a known diabetic, and
- The victim's mental status is altered, and
- The victim is awake enough to swallow.

Give the victim fast-acting sugars of 10 to 15 grams, such as:

- One tube of glucose gel (Figure 17-10)
- Two to five glucose tablets
- Two large lumps or teaspoons of sugar
- One-half can of regular soda
- 4 oz of orange juice
- 2 tablespoons of raisins
- Five to seven Lifesavers
- Six jelly beans
- 10 gumdrops
- 6 to 8 oz of skim or 1% milk
- Two teaspoons of honey or corn syrup

An injectable medication called glucagon, available by a physician's prescription, raises blood sugar quickly.

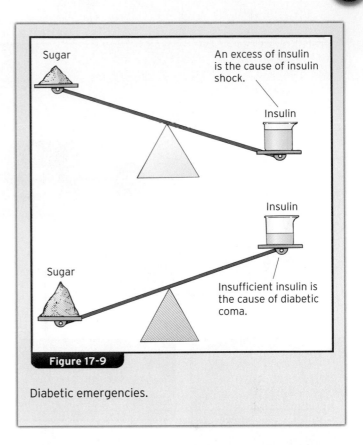

Figure 17-9

Diabetic emergencies.

An excess of insulin is the cause of insulin shock.

Insufficient insulin is the cause of diabetic coma.

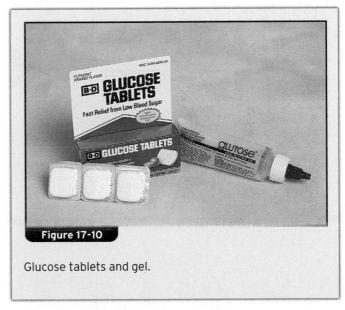

Figure 17-10

Glucose tablets and gel.

A family member or friend should learn when and how to inject glucagon in an emergency.

"Rule of 15s" for Insulin Reaction (Hypoglycemia)

1. Give the victim 15 grams of carbohydrate (sugar).
2. Wait 15 minutes.
3. If there is no improvement, give the victim 15 more grams of carbohydrate.
4. If there is no improvement, seek medical care.

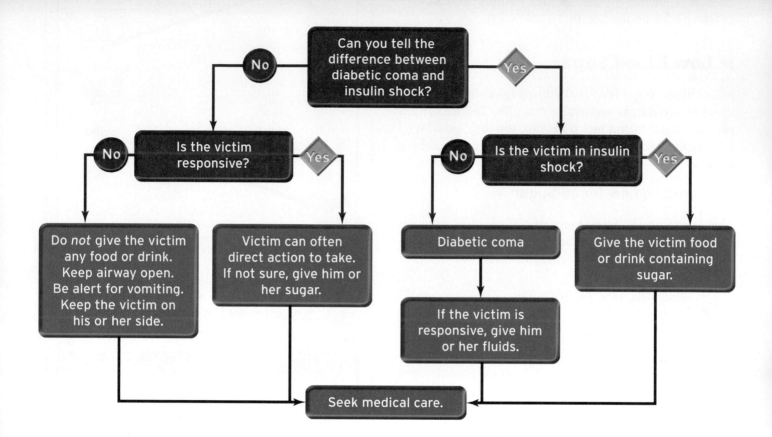

▶ High Blood Sugar

Hyperglycemia, which can lead to diabetic coma, is the opposite of hypoglycemia. Hyperglycemia occurs when the body has too much sugar in the blood. This condition can be caused by insufficient insulin, overeating, inactivity, illness, stress, or a combination of these factors.

Recognizing High Blood Sugar

The American Diabetes Association lists the following signs and symptoms of diabetic coma, hyperglycemia, and acidosis as diabetic emergencies requiring first aid:

- Gradual onset
- Drowsiness
- Extreme thirst
- Very frequent urination
- Flushed skin
- Vomiting
- Fruity breath odor
- Heavy breathing
- Eventual unresponsiveness

Care for People Who Have High Blood Sugar

1. If you are uncertain whether the victim has a high or low blood-sugar level, give the person sugar-containing foods or drinks.
2. If improvement is not seen in 15 minutes, take the victim to the hospital.

▶ Abdominal Complaints

People with gastrointestinal problems usually complain about one or more of the following symptoms:

- Abdominal pain that is aching, cramping, sharp, or dull. It might be constant, or it can come and go. The pain could indicate a mild problem or an acute problem requiring immediate surgery.
- Nausea and vomiting. Vomiting is the ejection of the stomach's contents through the mouth. Nausea is a feeling of the need to vomit.
- Diarrhea or constipation. Diarrhea is the frequent passage of loose, watery stools. Constipation is the opposite of diarrhea; stools are infrequent, hard, and difficult to pass.

Abdominal Pain

The abdomen is the area between the nipple line and the groin. Abdominal organs are hollow or solid. Hollow organs are tubes, such as the stomach and the intestines, through which material passes, conducting food through the body. Solid organs are solid masses of tissue in which much of the chemical work of the body takes place. The liver and spleen, and gallbladder are solid organs. The peritoneum is a thin membrane lining the entire abdominal cavity. Inflammation of the peritoneum is called peritonitis.

There are many possible causes of abdominal pain—some not so serious and some life threatening. They often can be serious enough to require emergency surgery.

Abdominal problems are so difficult to diagnose that even skilled physicians can have trouble pinpointing an exact cause. It is neither feasible nor useful for a first aider to distinguish among the many causes of abdominal pain because first aid usually will be similar regardless of the cause.

Recognizing Abdominal Pain

A first aider should ask himself or the victim the following questions:

- When did the pain start? Where is it located?
- Is the pain constant, or does it come and go? Constant pain can be more serious than a cramping pain. Constant abdominal pain suggests inflammation of an organ; cramping suggests obstruction of a hollow organ.
- Does belching or passing gas relieve the pain? If so, the intestine might be affected.
- Does the victim feel nauseated, or does he or she have a good appetite?
- Is there diarrhea or vomiting?
- Does the victim feel warm (feverish)?
- Does anyone near the victim have similar symptoms?
- For a female, is there any chance of pregnancy? Any pain with pregnancy should be treated as an emergency.
- Is the abdomen rigid to the touch? A rigid abdomen can be a sign of an emergency condition.

Care for People With Abdominal Pain

Care for people with abdominal complaints includes the following:

1. Give the victim only clear fluids (anything you can see through, except alcohol and caffeine). Have the victim slowly sip the fluids.
2. Give the victim an antacid.
3. If practical, place a hot-water bottle against the victim's abdomen or have the victim soak in a warm bath.
4. Recognize the possibility of vomiting and be prepared for it. Keep the victim on the left side to help prevent vomiting.
5. Keep the victim in a comfortable position, usually lying down with knees bent (unless the victim is nauseated).

6. Seek medical care if any of the following applies:
   - Pain is constant for more than 6 hours.
   - The victim is unable to drink fluids.
   - The victim is or might be pregnant.
   - The abdomen is rigid and painful.
   - The abdomen is swollen.
   - More pain occurs after you press your fingers on the victim's abdomen and suddenly release it.
   - There is bloody, blood-stained, or black stool.
   - The victim has a fever.
   - Pain began around the belly button and later moved to the lower right part of the abdomen. This is a sign of appendicitis.

> **CAUTION**
>
> DO NOT give enemas and laxatives, which can worsen the condition or cause complications such as a ruptured bowel.
>
> DO NOT give fluids other than clear fluids as long as the pain continues.
>
> DO NOT give solid foods.
>
> DO NOT give milk products.

▶ Nausea and Vomiting

Nausea (upset stomach) and vomiting (throwing up) often occur with conditions such as mild altitude sickness, motion sickness, brain injury, intestinal viruses, eating or drinking too much, and being emotionally upset. In minor illnesses, nausea and vomiting should clear up in a day. Persistent nausea and vomiting can signal more serious illnesses such as appendicitis, food poisoning, or bowel obstruction. In general, if the condition lasts longer than 1 or 2 days, the victim could become dehydrated (lose too much fluid). Young children and elderly people can be more seriously affected.

Recognizing Nausea and Vomiting

First aiders should determine the answers to the following questions:
- Is there abdominal pain?
- Is there blood or brown, grainy material in the vomit?
- Is there diarrhea? Vomiting and diarrhea together usually indicate a self-limited viral infection.
- Are there signs of dehydration (for example, the victim is dizzy when standing; has dry, cracked lips; is very thirsty)?

- Does anyone else near the victim have similar symptoms?
- Has the victim had a recent head injury?

Care for People With Nausea and Vomiting

Caring for someone with nausea and vomiting includes the following steps:

1. Give the victim small amounts of clear fluids (for example, sports drinks, clear soups, flat soda, apple or cranberry juice), except alcohol and caffeine.
2. If the victim is able to keep fluids down, offer carbohydrates (for example, bread, cereal, pasta) first—they are easier to digest. Avoid milk products and meats for 48 hours.
3. Have the victim rest and avoid exertion until he or she is able to eat solid foods easily.
4. Prevent inhalation of vomit by positioning the victim on his or her side to allow drainage. Inhaled vomit can result in severe pneumonia.
5. Seek medical care if:
   - blood or brown, grainy material appears in the vomit.
   - there is constant abdominal pain.
   - the victim faints when standing.
   - the victim is unable to keep fluids down for more than 24 hours.
   - the victim has severe, projectile vomiting (vomit shoots out in large quantities).
   - the vomiting follows a recent head injury.

> **CAUTION**
>
> DO NOT give solid foods until the victim can take fluids without vomiting and starts to feel hungry.
>
> DO NOT give milk products.

Recognizing Motion Sickness

Signs of motion sickness include:
- nausea.
- paleness of the skin.
- cold sweats.
- vomiting.
- dizziness.
- headache.
- fatigue.

Care for People Who Have Motion Sickness

1. If the victim is prone to motion sickness, he or she should sit near the midsection of a plane, boat, bus, train, or car. People susceptible to motion sickness should not read; should look far ahead to the horizon, not to the sides; and should avoid overeating.
2. Try an antihistamine 1 hour before traveling (follow label directions).

▶ Diarrhea

Diarrhea is the (usually more than four times a day) passage of loose, watery, or unformed stools. Diarrhea can be a symptom of intestinal infection (bacterial, viral, or parasitic), food poisoning, or food sensitivity or allergy, among other ailments. Dehydration can occur if the body loses too much fluid through the stool and the victim cannot drink enough fluid to keep up with the fluid losses from the diarrhea. Elderly and very young people are especially prone to dehydration, which can result in dangerous chemical imbalances. Replacing fluids and electrolytes such as sodium and potassium is of primary importance for any person with diarrhea. Diarrhea flushes bacteria and parasites out of the body. Letting diarrhea run its course is best because then bacteria or parasites are not trapped in the intestines.

Recognizing Diarrhea

First aiders treating persons with diarrhea should determine the answers to the following questions:

- Was the victim recently exposed to untreated, possibly contaminated water or food?
- Is there blood or mucus in the stool? Their presence can signal more serious problems.
- Are there signs of dehydration (for example, the victim is dizzy when standing; has dry, cracked lips; is very thirsty)?
- Does the victim have cramping abdominal pain?
- Does the victim lose bowel control (sometimes)?
- Is the victim feverish (sometimes)?
- Does anyone else near the victim have similar symptoms?

Care for People Who Have Diarrhea

Care for people with diarrhea includes the following steps:

1. Have the victim drink lots of clear fluids (8 to 10 eight-ounce glasses daily). This is the single most important treatment.

2. When the victim can tolerate clear fluids, give mild foods such as soup and gelatin. Later, the BRAT diet—bananas, rice, applesauce, toast—is recommended.
3. Bismuth can help in most cases (follow label directions). Be aware that bismuth can turn the stool and the tongue black. People sensitive to aspirin should not use it. If the person cannot let the diarrhea run its course, over-the-counter medications will calm the bowel, reducing movement of food through the intestines.
4. Seek medical care if:
   - the victim has bloody stools, which might appear black (keep in mind that bismuth preparations can cause black stools).
   - there is no improvement after 24 hours.
   - the victim has a fever.
   - the victim has severe, constant abdominal pain.
   - the victim is severely dehydrated.

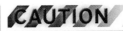

CAUTION

DO NOT give milk products and meats for 48 hours after diarrhea stops.

DO NOT give caffeine, which stimulates the intestine and causes urination, furthering dehydration.

▶ Constipation

Constipation is the passage of hard, dry stools. Most physicians define constipation as two or fewer bowel movements a week, of which 25% require straining. Constipation is rarely more than a passing discomfort in otherwise healthy people. Normal bowel movements can occur three times a day or once every 3 days. Minor changes in diet, fluid intake, activity, or emotional state can cause bowel movement changes. Rectifying any of those changes will also relieve constipation in most cases. Bowel stimulants or laxatives are rarely needed.

Recognizing Constipation

The following are signs of constipation:

- Bloating sensation of abdomen. A very painful or visibly swollen abdomen is a more serious problem than simple constipation.
- Hard, dry stools. Small strings of blood are not unusual if the stool was painful to evacuate.

Care for People With Constipation

Care for those with constipation includes the following:

1. Have the victim eat more fiber (fresh or dried fruits, vegetables, bran). Fiber causes the colon to contract. Over-the-counter fiber products such as Metamucil and Citrucel can be used, but the label directions should be followed.
2. Make sure the victim drinks plenty of fluids (8 to 10 eight-ounce glasses daily). Excessively hard stools often are the result of dehydration.
3. Encourage the victim to remain active. Activity such as walking stimulates colon contractions.
4. If there is no improvement, try one of the following:
   - Milk of magnesia (a mild laxative and stool softener)
   - Caffeine, which stimulates colon contractions

5. Seek medical care if the victim experiences any of the following:
   - Severe abdominal pain
   - Visibly swollen or very painful abdomen
   - Fever
   - Vomiting

CAUTION

DO NOT give laxatives such as Epsom salts to people with severe abdominal pain or vomiting.

DO NOT give alcohol.

DO NOT give binding foods, such as bananas, cheese, and applesauce.

▶ Heart Attack

What to Look For
- Chest pressure, squeezing, or pain
- Pain spreading to shoulders, neck, jaw, or arms
- Dizziness, sweating, nausea
- Shortness of breath

What to Do
1. Help victim take his or her prescribed medication.
2. Call 9-1-1.
3. Help victim into a comfortable position.
4. Give one adult or two to four children's aspirin.
5. Monitor breathing.

▶ Angina

What to Look For
- Chest pain similar to a heart attack
- Pain seldom lasts longer than 10 minutes

What to Do
1. Have victim rest.
2. If victim has his or her own nitroglycerin, help the victim use it.
3. If pain continues beyond 10 minutes, suspect a heart attack and call 9-1-1.

▶ Stroke

What to Look For
- Sudden weakness or numbness of the face, an arm, or a leg on one side of the body
- Blurred or decreased vision
- Problems speaking
- Dizziness or loss of balance
- Sudden, severe headache

What to Do
1. Call 9-1-1.
2. If responsive, help victim into a comfortable position with head and shoulders slightly raised.
3. If unresponsive, move onto his or her side.

▶ Breathing Difficulty

What to Look For
- Abnormally fast or slow breathing
- Abnormally deep or shallow breathing
- Noisy breathing
- Bluish lips
- Need to pause while speaking to catch breath

What to Do

Unknown reason
1. Help victim into a comfortable position.
2. Call 9-1-1.

Asthma attack
1. Help victim into a comfortable position.
2. Help victim use inhaler.
3. Call 9-1-1 if victim does not improve.

Hyperventilating
1. Encourage victim to inhale, hold breath a few seconds, then exhale.
2. Call 9-1-1 if condition does not improve.

254

▶ Fainting

What to Look For

- Sudden, brief unresponsiveness
- Pale skin
- Sweating

What to Do

1. Check breathing.
2. Check for injuries if victim fell.
3. Raise feet 6 to 12 inches.
4. Call 9-1-1 if needed.

▶ Seizures

What to Look For

- Sudden falling
- Unresponsiveness
- Rigid body and arching of back
- Jerky muscle movement

What to Do

1. Prevent injury.
2. Loosen any tight clothing.
3. Roll victim onto his or her side.
4. Call 9-1-1 if needed.

▶ Diabetic Emergencies

What to Look For

Low blood sugar
- Develops very quickly
- Anger, bad temper
- Hunger
- Pale, sweaty skin

High blood sugar
- Develops gradually
- Thirst
- Frequent urination
- Fruity, sweet breath odor
- Warm and dry skin

What to Do

1. If uncertain about high or low sugar level, give sugar.
2. Repeat in 15 minutes if no improvement.
3. Call 9-1-1 if conditions do not improve.

▶ Pregnancy Emergencies

What to Look For

- Vaginal bleeding
- Cramps in lower abdomen
- Swelling of face or fingers
- Severe continuous headache
- Dizziness or fainting
- Blurring of vision or seeing spots
- Uncontrollable vomiting

What to Do

Vaginal bleeding or abdominal pain or injury
1. Keep victim warm.
2. For vaginal bleeding, place sanitary napkin or sterile or clean pad over opening of vagina.
3. Send blood soaked pad and tissues with victim to medical care.
4. Seek medical care.

▶ Ready for Review

- A heart attack occurs when the heart muscle tissue dies because its blood supply is reduced or stopped.
- Angina pectoris can result from coronary heart disease just as a heart attack does.
- A stroke occurs when part of the blood flow to the brain is suddenly cut off.
- Asthma is chronic, inflammatory lung disease characterized by repeated breathing problems. Hyperventilation is fast, deep breathing and is common during emotional stress.
- COPD is a broad term applied to emphysema, chronic bronchitis, and related lung diseases.
- Fainting or psychogenic shock is a sudden brief loss of responsiveness not associated with head injury.
- A seizure results from an abnormal stimulation of the brain's cells causing uncontrollable muscle movements.
- Diabetes is a condition in which insulin is lacking or ineffective.
- Hypoglycemia is very low blood sugar and can be caused by too much insulin, too little or delayed food intake, exercise, alcohol, or a combination of these factors.
- Hyperglycemia occurs when the body has too much sugar in the blood and can be caused by insufficient insulin, overeating, inactivity, illness, stress, or a combination of these factors.
- People with gastrointestinal problems usually complain of pain, nausea, vomiting, diarrhea, or constipation.
- Nausea (upset stomach) and vomiting (throwing up) often occur with conditions such as mild altitude sickness, motion sickness, brain injury, intestinal viruses, eating or drinking too much, and being emotionally upset.
- Diarrhea is the frequent passage of loose, watery, or unformed stools and can be a symptom of intestinal infection, food poisoning, food allergy, or other ailments.
- Constipation is the passage of hard, dry stools and is rarely more than a passing discomfort in otherwise healthy people.

▶ Vital Vocabulary

angina pectoris A spasmodic pain in the chest, characterized by a sensation of severe constriction or pressure on the anterior chest; associated with insufficient blood supply to the heart, aggravated by exercise or tension, and relieved by rest or medication.

asthma A condition marked by recurrent attacks of breathing difficulty, often with wheezing, due to spasmodic constriction of the air passages, often as a response to allergens or to mucous plugs in the bronchioles.

diabetes A general term referring to disorders characterized by excessive urine excretion, excessive thirst, and excessive hunger.

heart attack Lay term for a condition resulting from blockage of a coronary artery and subsequent death of part of the heart muscle; an acute myocardial infarction; sometimes called simply a coronary.

hyperglycemia An abnormally increased concentration of sugar in the blood.

hypoglycemia An abnormally diminished concentration of sugar in the blood.

psychogenic shock A fainting spell resulting from transient decrease in blood flow to the brain.

seizure A sudden attack or recurrence of a disease; a convulsion; an attack of epilepsy.

status epilepticus The occurrence of two of more seizures without a period of complete consciousness between them.

stroke A brain injury due to blockage of blood flow causing permanent damage.

syncope Fainting; a brief period of unresponsiveness.

▶ Assessment in Action

A 50-year-old coworker is experiencing chest pain and nausea. He says that it started about an hour ago and has not let up. He believes it might just be indigestion. He describes the pain as "something pressing on my chest."

Directions: Circle Yes if you agree with the statement, circle No if you disagree.

Yes No 1. Have him lie down for 30 minutes to see if the pain subsides.

Yes No 2. Check to see if his pupils are unequal.

Yes No 3. His signs could indicate a heart attack.

Yes No 4. Help the victim take an aspirin, and call 9-1-1.

Yes No 5. Heart attack victims often resist the idea that they need medical care.

Answers: 1. No; 2. No; 3. Yes; 4. Yes; 5. Yes

prep kit

▶ Check Your Knowledge

Directions: Circle Yes if you agree with the statement, circle No if you disagree.

Yes　No　**1.** Heart attack victims can experience chest pain.

Yes　No　**2.** You can help the victim of chest pain take his or her nitroglycerin.

Yes　No　**3.** A responsive stroke victim should lie down with his or her head slightly raised.

Yes　No　**4.** Asthma victims may have a prescribed inhaler.

Yes　No　**5.** A victim who is breathing fast (hyperventilation) should be encouraged to breathe slowly by holding inhaled air for several seconds and then exhaling slowly.

Yes　No　**6.** Raise the feet of a person who has fainted 6 to 12 inches.

Yes　No　**7.** Some seizure victims display a rigid arching of the back.

Yes　No　**8.** A person having seizures always requires medical attention.

Yes　No　**9.** If in doubt about the type of diabetic emergency a victim is experiencing, give sugar to a responsive victim who can swallow.

Yes　No　**10.** Nitroglycerin can relieve chest pain associated with angina.

Answers: **1.** Yes; **2.** Yes; **3.** Yes; **4.** Yes; **5.** Yes; **6.** Yes; **7.** Yes; **8.** No; **9.** Yes; **10.** Yes

Poisoning

Poison

A <u>poison</u> (also known as a toxin) is any substance that impairs health or causes death by its chemical action when it enters the body or comes in contact with the skin.

▶ Types of Poisons

Poisons are classified by how they enter the body:
- Ingested (swallowed)—through the mouth
- Inhaled (breathed)—through the lungs
- Absorbed (contact)—through the skin
- Injected—through needlelike device (for example, snake's fangs)

▶ Ingested (Swallowed) Poisons

<u>Ingested poisoning</u> occurs when the victim swallows a toxic substance. Fortunately, most poisons have little toxic effect or are ingested in such small amounts that severe poisoning rarely occurs. However, the potential for severe or fatal poisoning is always present. About 80% of all poisonings happen by ingesting a toxic substance.

Swallowing nonfood substances is so common among children that it is unusual for a child to reach the age of 5 years without ingesting a nonfood substance at least once. Although many nonfood substances such as dirt and paper are not

chapter
at a glance

▶ **Poison**

▶ **Alcohol Emergencies**

▶ **Drug Emergencies**

▶ **Carbon Monoxide Poisoning**

▶ **Plant-Induced Dermatitis: Poison Ivy, Poison Oak, and Poison Sumac**

harmful, others present definite health threats. Some have the potential to block the airway. Others are poisonous. Hundreds of thousands of poisonings occur in the United States each year, but only a small percentage progress to severe or life-threatening conditions. Over 50% of all poison cases occur in children younger than six years of age.

Analgesics (pain medications) account for the largest category of poisoning exposures. Basically, any substance that is accessible to a child is a potential poison. Analgesic products that contain acetaminophen, for example, are involved in poisoning incidents more often than other analgesics, not because acetaminophen is more toxic but because products that contain acetaminophen outsell products that contain other analgesics **Figure 18-1**.

It is important not to confuse poisoning frequency with poisoning severity. Plants and mushrooms, for example, account for about 3.1% (about 75,000 cases) of the total poisoning exposures reported each year. However, plant and mushroom ingestion result in only 0.02% of serious poisonings and 1 death each year. Therefore, most exposures to plants are minor, with harmless effects. On the other hand, gun-blueing products (agents containing selenious acid that are used to maintain the blue color of gun barrels) were involved in 100 poisoning episodes and resulted in 4 deaths (death rate of 4%). So despite fewer exposure episodes, the potential for harm is much greater. Fortunately, most poison ingestions involve products with minor toxic effects or amounts so small that severe poisoning rarely occurs **Table 18-1**.

Recognizing Ingested Poisoning

The following are signs of ingested poisoning.
- Abdominal pain and cramping
- Nausea or vomiting
- Diarrhea
- Burns, odor, or stains around and in the mouth
- Drowsiness or unconsciousness
- Poison container nearby

Care for Ingested Poisoning Victims

Follow these steps to care for someone who has ingested poison:
1. Determine critical information:
   - Age and size of the victim
   - What was swallowed (container label; save vomit for analysis)
   - How much was swallowed (for example, a taste, half a bottle, a dozen tablets)
   - When it was swallowed
2. If a corrosive or caustic (that is, acid or alkali) substance was swallowed, immediately dilute it by

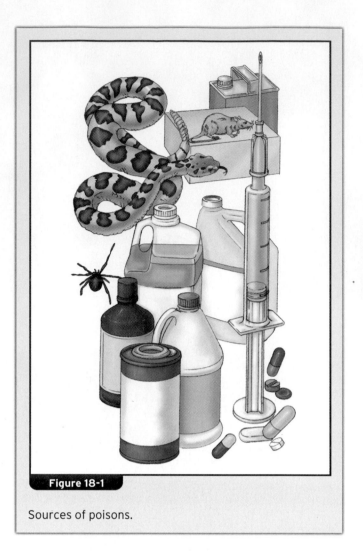

Figure 18-1

Sources of poisons.

having the victim take frequent sips of cold water or milk (up to at least one or two 8-ounce glasses). Cold water or milk tend to absorb heat better than room-temperature or warmer liquids. Heat may be given off as these substances are diluted.
3. For a responsive victim, immediately call the **poison control center**, using the national toll-free number, 1-800-222-1222. The number automatically connects the caller to the local poison control center, 24 hours a day, 7 days a week. Some poisons do not cause harm until hours later, whereas others cause damage immediately. More than 75% of poisonings can be treated by following instructions received by telephone from a poison center. The center staff also will advise you whether medical care is needed. Poison control centers routinely follow up calls to check for additional symptoms or unexpected effects.
4. For an unresponsive victim, call 9-1-1 and check the victim's breathing and treat accordingly.

Table 18-1   Substances Most Frequently Involved in Human Exposures

Substance	Annual number	Percentage of total exposures*
Analgesics	279,955	11.5
Cleaning substances	229,040	9.4
Cosmetics and personal care products	224,792	9.2
Sedatives/hypnotics/antipsychotics	129,885	5.3
Foreign bodies	122,011	5.0
Topicals	113,489	4.7
Cough and cold preparations	108,814	4.5
Antidepressants	103,155	4.2
Insecticides/pesticides (includes rodenticides)	102,754	4.2
Bites/envenomations	97,263	4.0
Plants	74,811	3.1
Alcohols	74,268	3.0
Cardiovascular drugs	74,145	3.0
Antihistamines	72,762	3.0
Food products, food poisoning	69,915	2.9
Antimicrobials	64,768	2.7
Vitamins	62,562	2.6
Hydrocarbons	54,766	2.2
Hormones and hormone antagonists	48,359	2.0

*Despite a high frequency of involvement, these substances are not necessarily the most toxic, but rather can be the most readily accessible. Percentages are based on the total number of human exposures rather than the total number of substances.
Source: American Association of Poison Control Centers.

5. Place the victim on his or her side (recovery position) **Figure 18-2** . For ingested poisoning, the left-side position is best because it positions the end of the stomach where it enters the small intestine (pylorus) straight up. Gravity will delay (by as much as 2 hours) the advance of the poison into the small intestine, where absorption into the victim's circulatory system is faster. The side position also helps prevent aspiration (inhalation) into the lungs if vomiting begins. Do not induce vomiting.

6. Give **activated charcoal** **Figure 18-3** if advised to do so by staff at a poison center. It is the single most effective agent in prehospital settings for most swallowed poisons. Activated charcoal acts like a sponge to bind and keep the poison in the digestive system, preventing its absorption by the blood. Doses of activated charcoal every 2 to 6 hours have been shown to increase the elimination of certain drugs faster than does a single dose. Activated charcoal is a black, tasteless, odorless, insoluble, inert powder that is the product of organic vegetable matter, usually wood pulp, burned at high temperatures, and then exposed to steam and strong acids. A network of tiny pores on each particle increases the surface area enormously, which enables activated charcoal to bind many commonly ingested toxic materials. Although activated charcoal can appear similar to burnt-toast

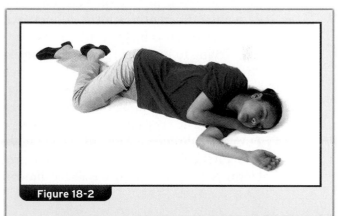

Figure 18-2

The left-side position delays the advance of the poison into the small intestine.

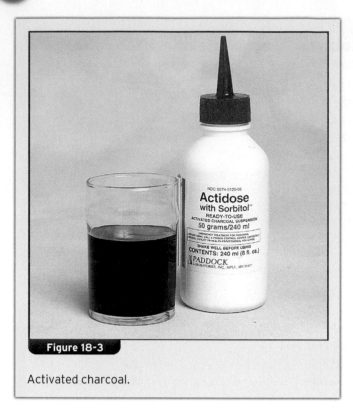

Figure 18-3

Activated charcoal.

several brand names. Although activated charcoal is an inexpensive, safe, and effective means for decreasing the absorption of poison, pharmacies do not routinely stock it. It can be obtained from emergency equipment suppliers over the Internet.

7. Save poison containers, plants, and the victim's vomitus to help medical personnel identify the poison.

scrapings and charcoal briquettes, these items cannot be used for treating poisoning nor can capsules of it be sold as digestive aids. Activated charcoal does not absorb all drugs well. Acids and alkalis (for example, bleach, ammonia), potassium, iron, alcohol, methanol, kerosene, and cyanide require different treatment. A drawback of activated charcoal is its grittiness and its appearance. Trying to improve the taste or consistency by adding chocolate syrup, sherbet, ice cream, milk, or other flavoring agents only decreases the charcoal's binding capacity. Place the charcoal mixture in an opaque container and have the victim sip it through a straw to make it more palatable. First aiders should give only the premixed form. Activated charcoal is available through

CAUTION

DO NOT induce vomiting. Reasons for not using syrup of ipecac include:

- Waiting for vomiting to begin can take 20 to 30 minutes, during which time some poison can pass into the small intestine.
- Additional treatment will be delayed until vomiting stops.
- The victim could inhale the vomitus.
- Vomiting caused by syrup of ipecac removes 30-50% of the poison from the stomach but leaves 50-70%.

CAUTION

DO NOT give water or milk to dilute poisons other than caustic or corrosive substances (acids and alkalis) unless told to do so by staff at a poison center. Fluids can dissolve a dry poison such as tablets or capsules more rapidly and fill up the stomach, forcing the stomach contents (the poison) into the small intestine, where it will be absorbed faster.

CAUTION

DO NOT gag or tickle the back of the victim's throat with a finger or a spoon handle. That method is usually ineffective in causing vomiting, and any vomiting produced is not very forceful.

DO NOT give dish soap, raw eggs, or mustard powder. They are not effective.

DO NOT use syrup of ipecac.

Swallowed Poison

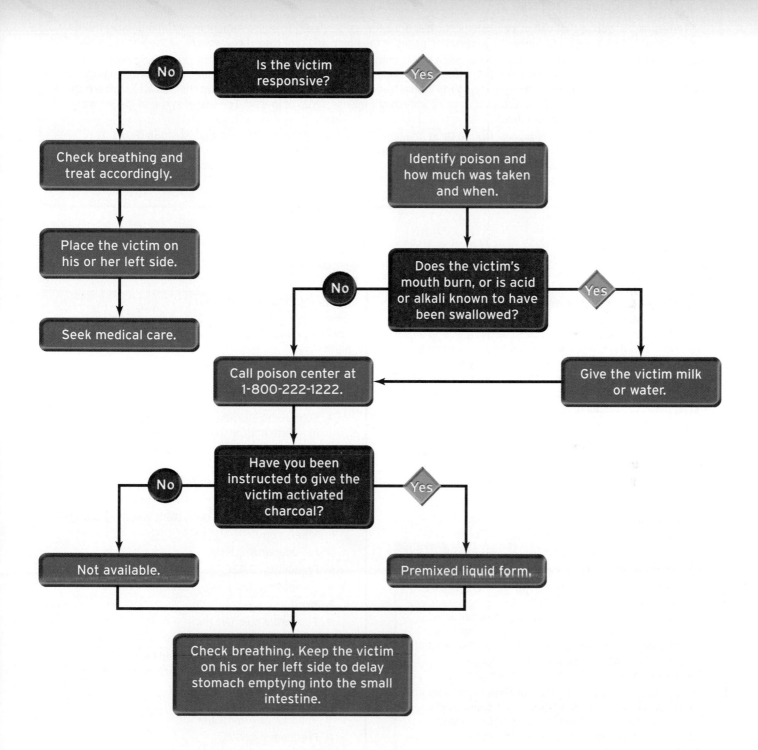

Is the victim responsive?

No → Check breathing and treat accordingly. → Place the victim on his or her left side. → Seek medical care.

Yes → Identify poison and how much was taken and when.

→ Does the victim's mouth burn, or is acid or alkali known to have been swallowed?

Yes → Give the victim milk or water.

No → Call poison center at 1-800-222-1222.

→ Have you been instructed to give the victim activated charcoal?

No → Not available.

Yes → Premixed liquid form.

→ Check breathing. Keep the victim on his or her left side to delay stomach emptying into the small intestine.

FYI

Syrup of Ipecac No Longer Recommended

Since 1965, syrup of ipecac had been recommended by poison centers and physicians for most swallowed poisons. When taken by mouth, it can induce vomiting. In November 2003, the American Academy of Pediatrics (AAP) announced its new guideline on syrup of ipecac. The AAP determined that syrup of ipecac no longer has a place in the home management of poisoning cases. Noting that use of syrup of ipecac had not been associated with improvement in victim outcome, the AAP recommended that parents no longer keep syrup of ipecac in the home and that they throw away any they have on hand.

The AAP says "there has never been any evidence that vomiting helps children who eat or drink something poisonous. Also, most emergency rooms have stopped using syrup of ipecac in favor of activated charcoal—which binds to poisons in the stomach and prevents them from entering the bloodstream." They continue by saying that there is also concern that people with eating disorders such as anorexia or bulimia might misuse syrup of ipecac. The use of syrup of ipecac was based on intuition rather than science.

In addition, in June 2003, the Nonprescription Drug Advisory Panel of the Food and Drug Administration (FDA) recommended that syrup of ipecac be removed from over-the-counter status.

Sources: Bond GR: Home syrup of ipecac use does not reduce emergency department use or improve outcome. *Pediatrics* 112:1061-1064. American Academy of Pediatrics Committee on Injury, Violence, and Poison Prevention. Poison treatment in the home. *Pediatrics* 112(5):1182-1185.

FYI

Activated Charcoal in the Home

Activated charcoal is recognized as the treatment of choice for many ingested poisonings. Activated charcoal use in the home has been limited by concerns that parents would not administer it properly and that children would refuse to take it. Researchers concluded that activated charcoal can be given successfully by the lay public in the home.

Source: Spiller HA, Rodgers GC Jr. Evaluation of administration of activated charcoal in the home. *Pediatrics* 108(6):E100.

CAUTION

DO NOT follow the first aid procedures or recommendations on a container label without first getting confirmation from a medical source. Many labels are incorrect or out of date.

DO NOT try to neutralize a poison. Giving weak acids, such as lemon juice or vinegar, is not safe, contrary to the advice given on many drain cleaner and lye product labels. Chemical neutralization releases large quantities of heat that can burn sensitive tissues.

DO NOT think that a specific antidote exists for most poisons. An antidote is a substance that counteracts a poison's effects. Few poisons have specific antidotes that will effectively block their toxic effects.

DO NOT think that there is a universal antidote. No product is effective in treating most or all poisons.

FYI

Commonly Ingested Plants

According to the American Association of Poison Control Centers, the five most commonly ingested plants are:

1. Peace lily
   - *Spathiphyllum* species
   - Frequency: 2,972
   - Symptoms: Burning in mouth and throat, swelling of mouth and/or tongue, nausea, vomiting, diarrhea
2. Holly
   - *Ilex* species
   - Frequency: 2,597
   - Symptoms: Nausea, persistent vomiting, diarrhea
3. Philodendron
   - *Philodendron* species
   - Frequency: 2,421
   - Symptoms: Same as peace lily
4. Poinsettia
   - *Euphorbia pulcherrima*
   - Frequency: 2,206
   - Symptoms: Skin irritation and blistering, abdominal pain, nausea and/or vomiting, diarrhea
5. Pokeweed, inkberry
   - *Phytolacca Americana*
   - Frequency: 1,697
   - Symptoms: Burning sensation of lips, mouth, and tongue; digestive upset and cramps

Alcohol Emergencies

▶ Alcohol Intoxication

Alcohol is a depressant, not a stimulant. It affects a person's judgment, vision, reaction time, and coordination. In very large amounts, it can cause death by paralyzing the respiratory center of the brain.

Alcohol is the most commonly used and abused drug in the United States, possibly even the world. It is also one of the most lethal because it is implicated as a cofactor in up to 40% of drownings, over 40% of traffic deaths (Figure 18-4), 67% of homicides, and 33% of suicides. It directly affects more than 12 million people annually (10% of all males and 3% of all females) and causes more than 200,000 deaths. Alcohol abuse is a major national health problem, ranking with heart disease and cancer. Lack of data makes it difficult to assess the actual number of alcohol-related injuries. It is estimated, however, that about 25% of the patients treated in hospital emergency departments were for intoxication alone. Nearly 50% of patients in trauma centers were injured while under the influence of alcohol.

Helping an intoxicated person is often difficult because the person could be belligerent and combative. However, it is important that people who abuse alcohol be helped and not labeled as drunks. Their condition can be quite serious, even life threatening.

Occasionally, a person will have consumed so much alcohol that there are signs of central nervous system depression. In such cases, complete respiratory support might be necessary. Death can result from the excessive consumption of alcohol.

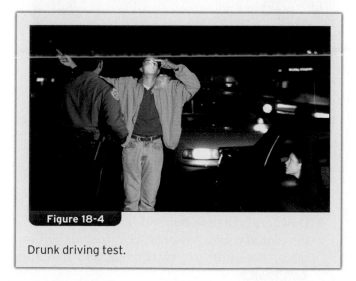

Figure 18-4

Drunk driving test.

The consumption of alcohol is deeply embedded in our society. Because of the widespread use of alcohol, people whose lives are affected directly or indirectly by alcohol abuse should be educated so they can recognize problems and know what to do in an emergency.

Recognizing Intoxication

Although the following signs indicate alcohol intoxication, some might also mean illness or injury other than alcohol abuse, such as diabetes or heat injury:

- The odor of alcohol on a person's breath or clothing
- Unsteady, staggering walking
- Slurred speech and the inability to carry on a conversation
- Nausea and vomiting
- Flushed face

Seizures can result from alcohol ingestion or alcohol withdrawal. Any seizures related to alcohol require medical evaluation. Diabetic coma can mimic alcohol intoxication, as poisoning and neurologic problems.

Care for Intoxicated Individuals

Helping an intoxicated person can be difficult because the person might be belligerent or combative. First aid for an intoxicated person includes these steps:

1. Look for any injuries. Alcohol can mask pain.
2. Monitor breathing and treat accordingly.
3. If the intoxicated person is lying down, place him or her in the recovery (left-side) position to reduce the likelihood of vomiting and aspiration of vomit and to delay the absorption of alcohol into the bloodstream. Be sure to check that the victim is breathing and does not have a spinal injury before you move him or her. The recovery position can be used for responsive and unresponsive persons.
4. Call the poison center for advice or the local emergency number for help. It might be best to let EMS personnel decide whether the police should be alerted.
5. If the victim becomes violent, leave the scene and find a safe place until police arrive.
6. Provide emotional support.
7. Assume that an injured or unresponsive victim has a spinal injury and needs to be stabilized against movement. Because of decreased pain perception, an intoxicated victim cannot be assessed reliably. If you suspect a spinal injury, wait for EMS personnel to arrive. They have the proper equipment and training to stabilize and move a victim.

FYI

Preventing Poisoning

Follow these precautions to reduce the risk of poisoning:

1. Household products and medicines should be kept out of reach and out of sight of children, preferably in a locked cabinet or closet. When an adult who is using household products or taking medicine leaves the room, even briefly, he or she should move the containers to a safe place.

2. Medicines should be stored separately from other household products and kept in their original containers—never in cups or soft-drink bottles.

3 All products should be properly labeled, and the label should be read before use.

4. A light should be turned on when giving or taking medicine.

5. Because children tend to imitate adults, adults should avoid taking medications in their presence.

6. Medicines should be referred to by their correct names. Do not tell children that medicines are candy. They are not candies.

7. Medicine cabinets should be cleaned out periodically. Old medicines should be disposed of by flushing them down the drain, and the container should be rinsed with water and discarded.

8. Use household substances in child-resistant packaging. Prescription medicines should be kept in safety packaging.

To avoid poisonings among elderly persons:

1. Always read the label and follow instructions when taking medicine.

2. Turn on a light at night when taking medicine.

3. Never mix medicines and alcohol, and never take more than the prescribed amount of medicine.

4. Do not borrow a friend's medicine or take old medicines.

5. Inform the physician what other medicines are being taken to avoid the risk of adverse drug interactions.

Source: US Consumer Product Safety Commission.

CAUTION

DO NOT let an intoxicated person sleep on his or her back.

DO NOT leave an intoxicated person alone unless they become violent.

DO NOT try to handle a hostile intoxicated person by yourself. Find a safe place, and then call the police for help.

Figure 18-5

Cocaine.

8. Because many intoxicated people have been exposed to the cold, suspect hypothermia (dangerously low body temperature) and move the person to a warm place whenever possible. Remove wet clothing, and cover the person with warm blankets. Handle a hypothermic victim gently because rough handling could induce a heart attack.

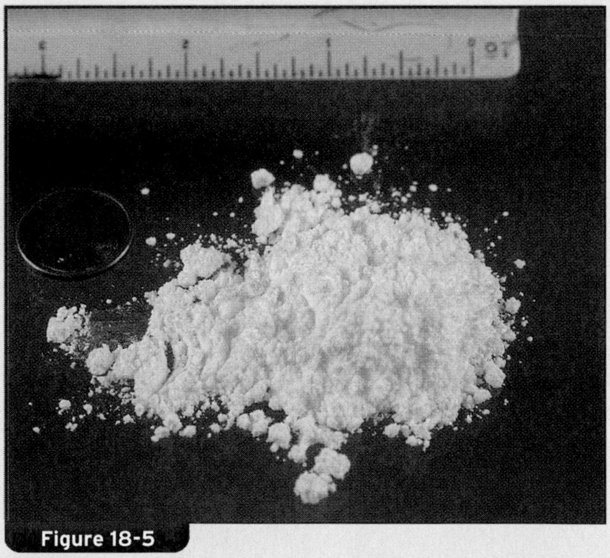

Drug Emergencies

Drugs are classified according to their effects on the user:

- Uppers are stimulants of the central nervous system. They include amphetamines, cocaine, and caffeine **Figure 18-5**.

- Downers (sedative-hypnotic) are depressants of the central nervous system. They include barbiturates, tranquilizers, marijuana, and narcotics **Figure 18-6**.

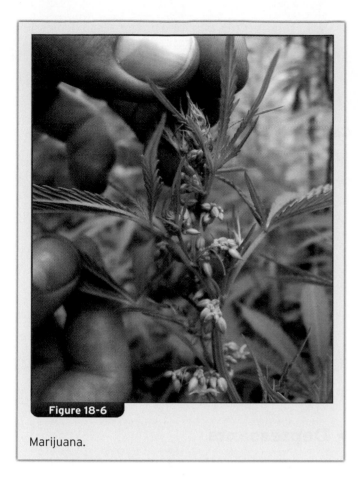

Figure 18-6

Marijuana.

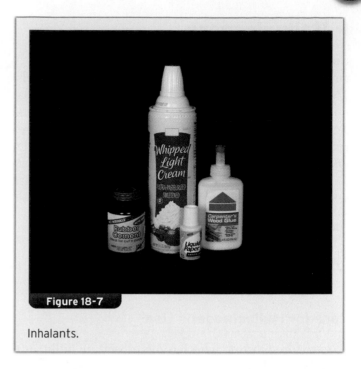

Figure 18-7

Inhalants.

- Hallucinogens alter and often enhance the sensory and emotional information in the brain centers. They include LSD (lysergic acid diethylamide), mescaline, peyote, and PCP (phencyclidine hydrochloride, or angel dust). Marijuana also has some hallucinogenic properties.
- Volatile chemicals usually are inhaled and can cause serious damage to many body organs. They include plastic model glue and cement, paint solvent, gasoline, spray paint, and nail polish remover **Figure 18-7** .

▶ Sympathomimetics

Sympathomimetics are stimulants. A stimulant is any agent that produces an excited state. Amphetamine and methamphetamine (ice) are commonly taken by mouth. They are also injected in many cases. They typically are taken to make the user feel good, improve task performance, suppress appetite, or prevent sleepiness. Sympathomimetic drugs are frequently called uppers.

Cocaine can be taken in a number of different ways—through the nose, by injection, and by smoking. Crack is pure cocaine and is smoked. Smoked crack produces the most potent effect. Cocaine is one of the most addictive substances known.

Recognizing Sympathomimetic Use

Someone using sympathomimetics would exhibit the following characteristics:
- Displays disorganized behavior, hyperactivity, restlessness, and sometimes anxiety or great fear.
- Paranoia (which can put you, the sympathomimetic user, and others in danger) and delusions are common with abuse.

Care for Sympathomimetic Users

To care for someone who has used sympathomimetics, follow these steps:
1. Check breathing.
2. Call the poison center for advice or 9-1-1 for help.
3. Check for injuries.
4. Keep the person on the left side to reduce the likelihood of vomiting and aspiration of vomitus and to delay absorption of drugs.
5. Provide reassurance and emotional support.
6. If the person becomes violent, seek safety until the police arrive. Let law enforcement officers handle dangerous situations.
7. Seek medical care.

▶ Hallucinogens

Hallucinogens produce changes in mood and sensory awareness—a person might hear colors and see sounds. They can cause hallucinations and bizarre behavior that might make users dangerous to themselves and others. Acute cases need medical attention. Users should be protected from hurting themselves. The classic hallucinogen is lysergic acid diethylamide (LSD). Abuse of another hallucinogen, PCP, or angel dust, is dangerous since it causes severe behavioral changes.

Recognizing Hallucinogens Use

The user reports:
- visual hallucinations.
- intensity of both vision and hearing.

Care for Hallucinogens Use

To care for someone who has overdosed on hallucinogens, follow these steps:
1. Check breathing.
2. Call the poison center for advice or 9-1-1 for help.
3. Check for injuries.
4. Keep the person on the left side to reduce the likelihood of vomiting and aspiration of vomit and to delay absorption of drugs.
5. Provide reassurance and emotional support.
6. If the person becomes violent, seek safety until the police arrive. Let law enforcement officers handle dangerous situations.
7. Seek medical care.

▶ Marijuana

The flowering hemp plant called marijuana is abused throughout the world. It has been estimated that as many as 20 million people use marijuana daily in the United States.

Recognizing Marijuana Overdose

Keep the following in mind if you suspect a marijuana overdose.
- Inhaling produces euphoria, relaxation, and drowsiness.
- Short-term memory loss is impaired, as is capacity to do complex thinking and work.

- In some people, euphoria progresses to depression and confusion.
- Altered perception of time is common.
- Anxiety and panic can occur.
- Very high doses produce hallucinations.

Care for Marijuana Overdose Victims

To care for someone who has overdosed on marijuana, do the following:
1. Check breathing.
2. Call the poison center for advice or 9-1-1 for help.
3. Check for injuries.
4. Keep the person on the left side to reduce the likelihood of vomiting and aspiration of vomit and to delay absorption of drugs.
5. Provide reassurance and emotional support.
6. If the person becomes violent, seek safety until the police arrive. Let law enforcement officers handle dangerous situations.
7. Seek medical care.

▶ Depressants

Depressants are often prescribed as a part of legitimate medicine. They are easy to obtain. People sometimes solicit prescriptions from several physicians. This class of drug includes opiates (narcotics) and sedative-hypnotics (barbituates and tranquilizers). Sedative-hypnotics are prescribed as anaesthetics, sedatives, and anti-anxiety treatments.

Recognizing Sedative-Hypnotic Drug Use

Effects of sedative-hypnotic drug overdose are similar to those of alcohol.
- Drowsiness and sleepiness
- Slurred speech
- Slow breathing rate

Opiates

The pain relievers called opiates are named for the opium in poppy seeds, the origin of heroin, codeine, and morphine. On the list of frequently abused drugs, they have been joined by a number of synthetic opiates, with origins in the laboratory—with most of them having legitimate medical uses. With the exception of heroin, which is illegal in the United States, many addicts started using any of the opiates with an appropriate medical prescription.

Recognizing Opiates Overdose

Someone who has overdosed on opiates might exhibit the following signs:

- Reduced breathing rate
- Pinpoint pupils
- Sedated condition and unresponsiveness

Care for Depressant Overdose

To care for someone who has overdosed on a sedative-hypnotic drug, do the following:

1. Check breathing.
2. Call the poison center for advice or 9-1-1 for help.
3. Check for injuries.
4. Keep the person on the left side to reduce the likelihood of vomiting and aspiration of vomit and to delay absorption of drugs.
5. Provide reassurance and emotional support.
6. If the person becomes violent, seek safety until the police arrive. Let law enforcement officers handle dangerous situations.
7. Seek medical care.

▶ Abused Inhalants

Inhaling glue or other solvents (gasoline, lighter fluid, nail polish) produces effects similar to those from ingesting alcohol. Persons who sniff these substances can die of suffocation. In addition, some inhalants can cause death by changing the rhythm of the heartbeat and can cause permanent brain damage.

Recognizing Abused Inhalant

Someone who has abused an inhalant might exhibit the following signs:

- Mild drowsiness to unresponsiveness
- Slurred speech and clumsiness
- Seizures
- Slow breathing rate
- Smell of solvents

Care for Someone Who Has Abused an Inhalant

Someone who has abused an inhalant should be treated thusly:

1. Check breathing.
2. Call the poison center for advice or 9-1-1 for help.
3. Check for injuries.
4. Keep the person on the left side to reduce the likelihood of vomiting and aspiration of vomit and to delay absorption of drugs.
5. Provide reassurance and emotional support.
6. If the person becomes violent, seek safety until the police arrive. Let law enforcement officers handle dangerous situations.
7. Seek medical care.

Carbon Monoxide Poisoning

Carbon monoxide (CO), because of its common presence in our environment, along with its insidious nature, is the leading cause of poisoning death in the United States each year. Carbon monoxide is an odorless, colorless, nonirritating gas produced by the incomplete combustion of carbon-based fuels. According to a report from the Centers for Disease Control and Prevention, each year more than 500 Americans die from unintentional CO poisoning, and more than 2,000 commit suicide by intentionally poisoning themselves. CO poisoning sends 10,000 to the hospital annually.

People who ride long distances in older, poorly maintained cars are at increased risk. Rust is a major factor in damaging an automobile's exhaust system and creating holes in the car's body, through which CO can enter. Many deaths involve people sleeping inside a running car, often after alcohol consumption. Many deaths also involve parking in remote areas.

Persons in a closed room where there is cigarette smoking experience mild increases in the level of CO in their blood. Less familiar and, therefore, more dangerous sources of CO are faulty furnaces, water heaters, and kerosene heaters. Recreational fires, whether open-flame, charcoal, or hibachi grills, also give off CO.

Victims of CO poisoning are often unaware of its presence. The gas is invisible, tasteless, odorless, and nonirritating. It is produced by the incomplete burning of organic material such as gasoline, wood, paper, charcoal, coal, and natural gas.

Carbon monoxide poisons its victims by causing hypoxia, or lack of oxygen, in two ways. First, the hemoglobin in red blood cells is about 200 times more likely to bind to CO than to oxygen if both are present in the blood; thus, even a small amount of CO can greatly reduce the amount of oxygen carried in the bloodstream. Second, CO does not allow the cells to use what little oxygen is delivered. In short, CO deprives the body parts that need oxygen the most—the heart and the brain.

FYI

Carbon Monoxide After Hurricane Katrina

Hurricane Katrina made landfall on August 29, 2005, on the Gulf Coast of the United States, causing loss of life, widespread property damage, and power outages. After hurricanes, some residents use portable generators and other gasoline-powered appliances for electrical power and cleanup. These devices produce carbon monoxide (CO), and improper use can cause CO poisoning. From August 29 through September 24, a total of 51 cases of CO poisoning were reported by hyperbaric oxygen facilities in Alabama, Louisiana, and Mississippi. CO poisoning can be prevented by reducing exposure to CO through appropriate placement and ventilation of gasoline-powered engines.
Source: CDC. *MMWR Morb Mortal Wkly Rep* 54(39):996-998.

FYI

Carbon Monoxide Detectors Can Save Lives

The US Consumer Product Safety Commission recommends that consumers purchase and install CO detectors with labels showing they meet the requirements of the Underwriters Laboratories (UL) voluntary standard (UL 2034). The standard requires detectors to sound an alarm when the CO concentration reaches a potentially hazardous level.

Properly working CO detectors can provide an early warning before the deadly gas builds up to a dangerous level. Exposure to a low concentration during several hours can be as dangerous as exposure to a high carbon monoxide level for a few minutes. The detectors detect both conditions. Each home should have at least one CO detector in the area outside individual bedrooms. CO detectors are as important as smoke detectors to home safety.
Source: US Consumer Product Safety Commission. Carbon monoxide detectors can save lives. October 5, 2004. Available at: *http://www.cpsc.gov/CPSCPUB/PUBS/5010.html.* Accessed November 3, 2005.

Recognizing Carbon Monoxide Poisoning

It is difficult to determine whether a person is a CO poisoning victim. Sometimes, a complaint of having the flu is really a symptom of CO poisoning. Although many symptoms of CO poisoning resemble those of the flu, there are differences. For example, CO poisoning does not cause low-grade fever or generalized aching or involve the lymph nodes.

The signs and symptoms of CO poisoning are as follows:

- Headache
- Ringing in the ears (tinnitus)
- Chest pain (angina)
- Muscle weakness
- Nausea and vomiting
- Dizziness and visual changes (blurred or double vision)
- Unresponsiveness
- Respiratory and cardiac arrest

The traditionally cited sign of CO poisoning is cherry-red skin and lips. This sign is uncommon, however, and occurs only at death; therefore, it is a poor initial indicator of CO poisoning. The following are earmarks of possible CO poisoning:

- The symptoms come and go.
- The symptoms worsen or improve in certain places or at certain times of the day.
- People around the victim have similar symptoms.
- Pets seem ill.

Care for Carbon Monoxide Poisoning Victims

1. Get the victim out of the toxic environment and into fresh air *immediately*.
2. Call 9-1-1, who will send EMS personnel who will be able to give the victim 100% oxygen, improving oxygenation and disassociating the linkage between the CO and the hemoglobin. For a responsive victim, it takes 4 to 5 hours with ordinary air (21% oxygen) or 30 to 40 minutes with

Carbon Monoxide Poisoning Deaths Associated With Camping

Exposure to CO is responsible for more fatal, unintentional poisonings in the United States than any other agent, with the highest incidence occurring during the cold-weather months. Although most of these deaths occur in residences or motor vehicles, two incidents among campers in Georgia illustrate the danger of CO in outdoor settings.

Case 1

A 51-year-old man, his 10-year-old son, a 9-year old boy, and a 7-year-old girl were found dead inside a zipped-up, 10-foot by 14-foot, 2-room tent at their campsite in southeast Georgia (a pet dog also died). A propane gas stove, still burning, was found inside the tent; the stove apparently had been brought inside to provide warmth.

Case 2

A 34-year-old man and his 7-year-old son were found dead inside their zipped-up tent at a group camping site in central Georgia. They were discovered by other campers. A charcoal grill was found inside the tent; the grill apparently had been brought inside to provide warmth after it had been used outside for cooking.

During 1990 to 1994, in the United States, portable fuel-burning camp stoves and lanterns were involved in 10 to 17 CO poisoning deaths each year, and charcoal grills were involved in 15 to 27 deaths each year. During this same time, an annual average of 30 fatal CO poisonings occurred inside tents or campers.

Source: Centers for Disease Control and Prevention. *MMWR Morb Mortal Wkly Rep* 48:705-706.

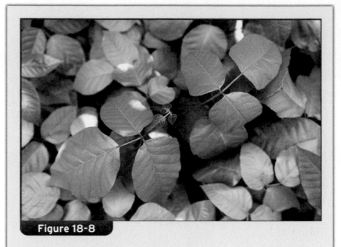

Figure 18-8

Poison ivy, found in all 48 contiguous states in the United States.

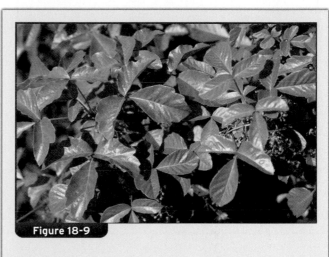

Figure 18-9

Poison oak.

100% oxygen to reverse the effects of CO poisoning.
3. Monitor breathing.
4. Place an unresponsive breathing victim in the recovery position.
5. Seek medical care. All suspected CO victims should obtain a blood test to determine the level of CO.

Plant-Induced Dermatitis: Poison Ivy, Poison Oak, and Poison Sumac

About 85% of the population is sensitive to poison ivy, poison oak, and poison sumac. If a person reaches adulthood without experiencing a reaction, the risk falls from 85% to 50%. With more people venturing into the outdoors, episodes of dermatitis caused by exposure to poison ivy, poison oak, and poison sumac are increasing **Figure 18-8**, **Figure 18-9**, **Figure 18-10**. (Actually, more than 60 plants can cause allergic reactions, but these three are by far the most common offenders.) Of those who do react, 15–25% will have incapacitating swelling and blistering eruptions that require medical care **Figure 18-11**. There is no routine test to determine an individual's degree of sensitivity—a history of dermatitis is the most reliable indicator.

The resin (urushiol) of these plants is a colorless or slightly yellow, light oil. It runs in resin canals just under

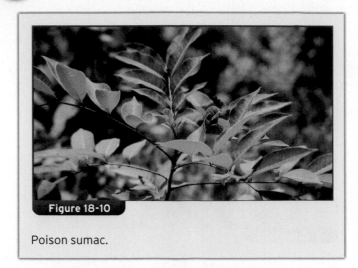

Figure 18-10

Poison sumac.

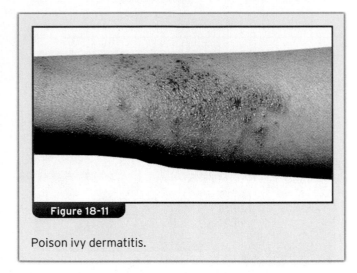

Figure 18-11

Poison ivy dermatitis.

from a campfire in which these leaves are burning often are affected by airborne oil.

Most people cannot identify these irritating plants. Poison ivy and poison oak are low bushes or climbing vines with waxy, broad, green leaves in the summer that change to brown to red in the fall. The leaflets of poison ivy and poison oak grow in groups of three (three leaves radiating from a single attachment point), giving rise to the warning, "leaves of three, let them be." Poison ivy flourishes throughout most of the United States, except in Alaska and Hawaii; poison oak is found on the West and East coasts and some South Central areas of the United States. Poison sumac is found chiefly in damp, swampy areas in the eastern United States. These plants tend not to grow at elevations higher than 5,000 feet or in hot, dry deserts. A helpful method of identifying these plants is the black spot test. When the sap is exposed to the air, it turns brown in a matter of minutes and black by the next day.

Allergic people can come in contact with the urushiol of these plants from their clothes or shoes, pet fur, or the smoke from burning plants. Contrary to popular belief, no one can develop a rash by touching the fluid from the blisters (their own or others') because the fluid in the blister does not contain the oily resin. Any apparent spreading is actually a delayed reaction to contact with the resin.

Recognizing Plant-Induced Dermatitis

Most people do not realize they have come in contact with a poisonous plant until the rash erupts. Reactions can range from mild to severe.

- Mild: itching
- Mild to moderate: itching and redness
- Moderate: itching, redness, and swelling
- Severe: itching, redness, swelling, and blisters

Severity is important, but so is the amount of skin affected. The greater the amount of skin affected, the greater the need for medical care. A day or two is the usual time between contact and the onset of signs and symptoms.

Care for Plant-Induced Dermatitis Victims

To care for someone who has been in contact with poisonous plants:

1. People who know they have been in contact with a poisonous plant should wash the skin with soap and water as soon as possible (within 5 minutes for sensitive people and within 1 hour for moderately sensitive people). Unfortunately, most victims do not know about their contact until several hours or days later, when the itching and rash begin. Use soap and water to cleanse the skin of the

the surface, from the roots through the stems, into the leaves and flowers, and just under the surface of the fruit. It is not present in the nectar. The leaves of the plants are fragile and easily ruptured by high winds or by humans or animals brushing against them. The oil immediately oozes onto the surface.

The light oil generally is not visible on human skin. If present on the sole of a shoe, on the palm of a hand or glove, or on the surface of an animal's fur, it can be spread by direct contact. On some objects, the oil can stay in an active form for months or years. Urushiol can be on the handle of a rake for years and still bond to human skin within five or 10 minutes. Poison ivy leaves have been kept for up to five years with no loss of virulence. Contaminated clothing has caused rashes even after more than one year. Smoke from burning plants can produce severe dermatitis. Firefighters and picnickers downwind

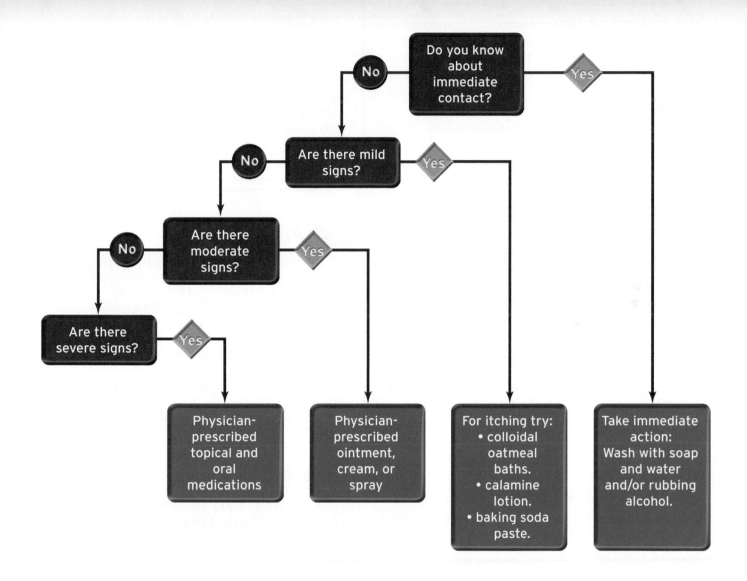

Do you know about immediate contact?

No → Are there mild signs?

Yes → Take immediate action: Wash with soap and water and/or rubbing alcohol.

No → Are there moderate signs?

Yes → For itching try:
• colloidal oatmeal baths.
• calamine lotion.
• baking soda paste.

No → Are there severe signs?

Yes → Physician-prescribed ointment, cream, or spray

Yes → Physician-prescribed topical and oral medications

oily resin or apply rubbing (isopropyl) alcohol liberally (not in swab-type dabs). If too little isopropyl alcohol is used, the oil will be spread to another site and enlarge the injury. Other solvents, such as paint thinner, can be used, but they can irritate or damage the skin. Rinse with water to remove the solubilized material. Water removes urushiol from the skin, oxidizes and inactivates it, and does not penetrate the skin (as solvents do).

2. For a mild reaction, have the victim soak in a lukewarm bath sprinkled with 1 to 2 cups of colloidal oatmeal. Colloidal oatmeal makes a tub slick, so take appropriate precautions. Or, apply one of the following:
   - Wet compresses soaked with aluminum acetate for 20 to 30 minutes three or four times a day
   - Calamine lotion (calamine ointment if the skin becomes dry and cracked) or zinc oxide
   - Baking soda paste: 1 teaspoon of water mixed with 3 teaspoons of baking soda
3. For a mild to moderate reaction, care for the skin as you would for a mild reaction and use a physician-prescribed corticosteroid ointment.
4. For a severe reaction, care for the skin as you would for mild and moderate reactions and use a physician-prescribed oral corticosteroid such as prednisone. Apply a topical corticosteroid ointment or cream, cover the area with a transparent plastic wrap, and lightly bind the area with an elastic or self-adhering bandage.

FYI

Conducting a Black Spot Test

Most victims of poison ivy dermatitis do not recognize the plant. Poison ivy and poison oak leaves have three leaflets; poison sumac has 7 to 13 leaflets per leaf. The mature fruit is an off-white berry. These botanical characteristics explain the axioms, "leaflets three, let it be" and "berries white, poisonous sight!"

The black spot test is another means of identifying these plants. To check a suspicious plant, grasp a leaf and its stem where it attaches to the branch with a folded sheet of white paper (do not touch the leaf). Crush the end of the leaf stalk in the folded sheet of white paper with a rock. The paper needs to be wet with the leaf stem's sap. The clear sap of poison ivy, poison oak, and poison sumac on the paper will turn dark brown within 10 minutes and black within 24 hours. This test is not conclusive but can strongly suggest that the plant is one of the three plants.

Source: Guin JD: The black spot test for recognizing poison ivy and related species. *J Am Acad Dermatol* 2(4):332-333.

FYI

Preventing Poisonous-Plant Dermatitis

To reduce the likelihood of developing poisonous-plant dermatitis, follow these suggestions:

- Avoid the plants.
- Wear protective clothing, and use appropriate commercial barrier preparations.
- Replenish the barrier protection every 4 to 6 hours, if practical.
- Decontaminate after known exposure with liberal amounts of soap and water, and then reapply the barrier preparation.
- Decontaminate at the end of the day with isopropyl alcohol and a water rinse.
- Dispose of all contaminated clothing and equipment.

CAUTION

DO NOT use nonprescription hydrocortisone creams, ointments, and sprays in strengths of less than 1%. They offer little benefit.

DO NOT use over-the-counter anti-itch lotions that also have antihistamines because they can cause further skin irritation. Oral antihistamines often are used in conjunction with prescription creams to help decrease itching.

DO NOT let the victim rub or scratch the rash or itching skin.

▶ Stinging Nettle

The stinging nettle plant has stinging hairs on its stem and leaves. The stinging hair is a fine, hollow tube with a bladder at its base that contains a chemical irritant. When the stinging hair is touched, a fine needlepoint that penetrates the skin and injects an irritating chemical is formed.

Recognizing Stinging Nettle Poisoning

Stinging nettle affects almost all people. Its effects are not an allergic response, as with poison ivy, but rather are due to a direct irritant effect of the plant's sap. The effects are limited to the exposed area, and the response is usually immediate.

Stinging nettle produces some degree of redness, burning, and itching for an hour or more, depending on the area of the body exposed to the plant. For example, the thicker skin on the soles and the palms retards the stinging hairs better than areas of thinner skin, such as the backs of the hands and the arms. Humans vary in sensitivity when the plant actually contacts exposed skin.

The typical response to contact with stinging nettle is a rapid, intense burning sensation at the site of the injection. The area then might itch for an hour or more. Usually, no systemic (whole-body) effects are noted.

Care for Someone With Stinging Nettle Poisoning

Follow these guidelines to care for someone with stinging nettle poisoning:

1. Wash the exposed area with soap and water to remove irritant chemicals.

2. Apply a cold, wet pack to help soothe the painful itching. Other treatments might include a paste of colloidal oatmeal, an over-the-counter hydrocortisone cream (1%), or calamine lotion.

3. Take an over-the-counter antihistamine, if desired. Be sure to follow package directions, and be aware that antihistamines cause drowsiness.

4. The duration of the stinging nettle reaction is measured in hours, rather than days, so little therapy is needed.

▶ Poisoning

What to Look For	What to Do

Ingested (swallowed) poisoning
- Abdominal pain and cramping
- Nausea or vomiting
- Diarrhea
- Burns, odor, or stains around and in mouth
- Drowsiness or unresponsiveness
- Poison container nearby

1. Determine the age and size of the victim, what and how much was swallowed, and when it was swallowed.
2. If victim is responsive, call the poison control center at 1-800-222-1222. If advised, give activated charcoal. The center will advise if medical care is needed.
3. If victim is unresponsive, open airway, check breathing, and treat accordingly. If breathing, place on left side in recovery position. Call 9-1-1.

Alcohol intoxication
- Alcohol odor on breath or clothing
- Unsteadiness, staggering
- Confusion
- Slurred speech
- Nausea and vomiting
- Flushed face

1. If the victim is responsive:
   - Monitor breathing.
   - Look for injuries.
   - Place in recovery position.
   - Call poison control center for advice (1-800-222-1222).
   - If victim becomes violent, leave area and call 9-1-1.
2. If victim is unresponsive, open airway, check breathing, and treat accordingly.

Drug overdose
- Drowsiness, agitation, anxiety, hyperactivity
- Change in pupil size
- Confusion
- Hallucinations

1. If the victim is responsive:
   - Monitor breathing.
   - Look for injuries.
   - Place in recovery position.
   - Call poison control center for advice (1-800-222-1222).
   - If victim becomes violent, leave area and call 9-1-1.
2. If victim is unresponsive, open airway, check breathing, and treat accordingly.

Carbon monoxide poisoning
- Headache
- Ringing in ears
- Chest pain
- Muscle weakness
- Nausea and vomiting
- Dizziness and vision difficulties
- Unresponsiveness
- Breathing and heart stopped

1. Move victim to fresh air.
2. Call 9-1-1.
3. Monitor breathing.
4. Place unresponsive breathing victim in recovery position.

Plant (contact) poisoning
- Rash
- Itching
- Redness
- Blisters
- Swelling

1. For known contact, immediately wash with soap and water.
2. For mild reaction, use one or more:
   - 1–2 cups of colloidal oatmeal in bathwater
   - Calamine lotion
   - Baking soda paste
3. For severe reactions, perform step 2 and seek medical care.

▶ Ready for Review

- A poison is any substance that impairs health or causes death by its chemical action when it enters the body or comes in contact with the skin.
- Poisons are classified by how they enter the body. They can be ingested, inhaled, absorbed, and injected.
- Ingested poisoning occurs when the victim swallows a toxic substance.
- Alcohol is a depressant that affects a person's judgment, vision, reaction time, and coordination.
- Drugs are classified according to their effects on the user:
  - Uppers (stimulants)
  - Downers (depressants)
  - Hallucinogens
  - Volatile chemicals
- Carbon monoxide is the leading cause of poisoning death in the United States each year.
- About 85% of the population is sensitive to poison ivy, poison oak, and poison sumac.

▶ Vital Vocabulary

activated charcoal Powdered charcoal that has been treated to increase its powers of absorption. Used to treat patients who have ingested poisons.

carbon monoxide A colorless, odorless, poisonous gas formed by incomplete combustion, such as in fire.

ingested poisoning Poisoning caused by swallowing a toxic substance.

poison Any substance that impairs health or causes death by its chemical action when it enters the body or comes in contact with the skin; also known as a toxin.

poison control center Medical facility providing immediate, free, expert advice any time. Can be reached by calling 1-800-222-1222.

▶ Assessment in Action

You find your 2-year-old son vomiting. You notice that the top of a nearby medicine bottle is off. The label on the bottle reveals that the medicine inside belongs to your mother, who is visiting. You realize that he must have swallowed some of the highly potent medicine.

Directions: Circle Yes if you agree with the statement, circle No if you disagree.

Yes   No   1. Immediately have him drink water or milk.

Yes   No   2. Call the poison control center immediately.

Yes   No   3. Induce vomiting with syrup of ipecac.

Yes   No   4. Place him on his left side.

Yes   No   5. Give him activated charcoal if advised by a poison control center.

Answers: 1. No; 2. Yes; 3. No; 4. Yes; 5. Yes

▶ Check Your Knowledge

Directions: Circle Yes if you agree with the statement, circle No if you disagree.

Yes   No   1. Swallowing a poison can produce nausea.

Yes   No   2. Activated charcoal can be used for all victims of ingested poison.

Yes   No   3. The best activated charcoal to use is in a capsule form.

Yes   No   4. Carbon monoxide has a unique smell.

Yes   No   5. Everyone who touches a poison ivy, poison oak, or poison sumac plant will have some type of skin reaction.

Yes   No   6. Causing a poisoned victim to vomit is a recommended first aid practice.

Yes   No   7. Some cases of poison ivy, poison oak, or poison sumac require medical care.

Yes   No   8. Calamine lotion can help relieve itching caused by poison ivy, poison oak, or poison sumac.

Yes   No   9. If an intoxicated or drugged person becomes violent, leave the area.

Yes   No   10. Move a carbon monoxide victim to fresh air.

Answers: 1. Yes; 2. No; 3. No; 4. No; 5. No; 6. No; 7. Yes; 8. Yes; 9. Yes; 10. Yes

Bites and Stings

▶ Animal Bites

It is estimated that one of every two Americans will be bitten at some time by an animal or by another person. Dogs are responsible for about 80% of all animal-bite injuries **Figure 19-1**. Of the nearly 5 million dog bites that occur yearly, 80% are trivial or minor, and medical care is not required or sought, which demonstrates the importance of knowing first aid. The remainder account for about 1% of all emergency department and physician office visits. Each year, about 19 bite-related deaths occur in the United States **Table 19-1**.

Animal bites represent a major, largely unrecognized public health problem. Two concerns result from an animal bite: immediate tissue damage and later infection from microorganisms. A dog's mouth can carry more than 60 species of bacteria, some of which are dangerous to humans **Table 19-2**. Two examples of infection—tetanus and rabies—have been almost eradicated by medical advances, but they still pose a potential problem.

Although cat bites are less mutilating than dog bites, cat bites have a much higher rate of infection than dog bites. Cats have very sharp teeth, which can create deep puncture wounds and involve muscle, tendon, and bone.

Another pet especially likely to bite children is the ferret. These animals are often unpredictable and can cause severe facial injury to infants. Ferrets sometimes unleash frenzied, rapid-fire bite-and-slash attacks on infants, usually on their heads and throats, and can inflict hundreds of bites.

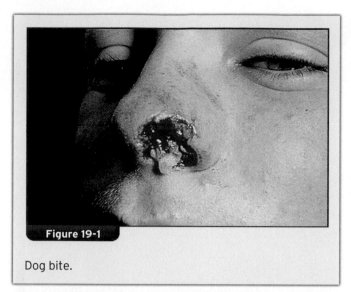

Figure 19-1

Dog bite.

Table 19-1 Animal-Related Human Deaths in the United States (1991–2001)

Animal	Average number of deaths each year
Venomous animals	
Snake	5.2
Spider	6
Scorpion	0.45
Hornet, bee, wasp	48.5
Centipede	0.45
Other specified venomous arthropod	6
Venomous marine animal	0.18
Other specified venomous animal	2.1
Total venomous	68.88
Nonvenomous animals	
Dog	18.9
Rat	0.27
Nonvenomous snake	0
Other animals except arthropod	4
Other specified animal*	76.9
Unspecified animal	4
Total nonvenomous	104.07
Overall total	172.95

*Note that this category includes bitten or struck by other mammals, contact with marine animal, bitten or stung by nonvenomous insect or other nonvenomous arthropods, bitten or struck by crocodile or alligator, bitten or confronted by other reptiles.
Source: Adapted from Langley RL: Animal-related fatalities in the United States: An update. *Wilderness Environ Med* 16(2):67–74.

Besides children, elderly people and people unable to help themselves are especially prone to animal bites because they are sometimes unable to detect or prevent a dangerous situation. Many animal-related deaths occur when the victim is left alone with the offending pet. Contrary to popular belief, wild or stray dogs seldom are involved in fatal attacks.

Damage mostly occurs on the hands, arms, legs, and face. A damaged face presents several problems because the proximity of blood vessels to the skin surface makes it susceptible to copious bleeding. Facial disfigurement and scarring can result in emotional trauma. Complete or partial loss of an eye also is possible.

Rabies

Rabies is one of the most ancient and feared of diseases **Figure 19-2**. Although human rabies rarely occurs in the United States or in other industrialized nations, it remains a scourge in developing countries. A virus found in warm-blooded animals causes rabies, which spreads from one animal to another in the saliva, usually through a bite or by licking. Bites from cold-blooded animals such as reptiles do not carry the danger of rabies.

A bite or a scratch is considered a significant rabies exposure if it penetrates the skin. Unprovoked attacks are more likely to have been inflicted by a rabid animal than are provoked attacks. Nonbite exposure consists of contamination of wounds, including scratches, abrasions, and weeping skin rashes.

Consider an animal as possibly rabid if any of the following applies:

- The animal made an unprovoked attack.
- The animal acted strangely, that is, out of character (for example, a usually friendly dog is aggressive, or a wild fox seems docile and friendly).
- The animal was a high-risk species (skunk, raccoon, or bat).

FYI

Human Rabies

The number of human deaths in the United States attributed to rabies has declined from 100 or more each year to an average of 1 or 2 each year. Two programs have been responsible for this decline. First, animal control and vaccination programs, which were begun in the 1940s; and second, effective human rabies vaccines and immunoglobulins have been developed.
Sources: Centers for Disease Control and Prevention; United States Rabies Surveillance Data.

Table 19-2   Facts About Dog Bites

- Carefully choose your pet dog. Evaluate your environment and lifestyle and speak with a professional to determine the appropriate type of pet.
- Dogs should be neutered to reduce aggressive tendencies.
- Never leave infants or young children alone with a dog. Be sensitive to cues that a child is fearful or apprehensive about a dog.
- Teach children basic safety around dogs, and review regularly.
- Dogs with histories of aggression are inappropriate for families with children.
- Do not play aggressive games with your dog, for example, wrestling.
- Never approach an unfamiliar dog. Immediately report stray dogs or dogs displaying unusual behavior.
- Remain motionless when approached by an unfamiliar dog—never run or scream.
- Do not disturb a dog that is sleeping, eating, or caring for puppies.
- If knocked down by a dog, lie still and remain in a ball.
- If bitten by a dog, immediately report the bite.

Source: Centers for Disease Control and Prevention: Nonfatal dog bite-related injuries treated in hospital emergency departments—United States 2001. *MMWR Weekly,* 2003;52(26):605-610 accessed at *www.cdc.gov/mmwr/preview/mmwrhtml/mm5226a1.htm.*

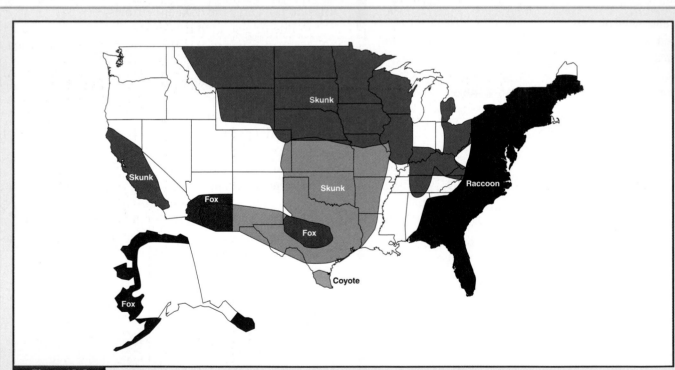

Figure 19-2

Distribution of major terrestrial reservoirs of rabies in the United States.

Source: Centers for Disease Control and Prevention.

Animal Bites

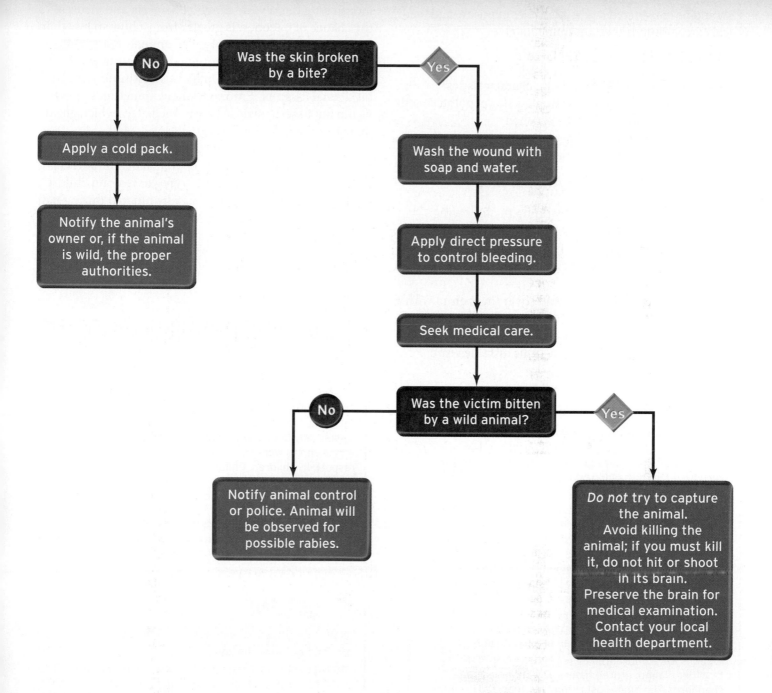

Was the skin broken by a bite?

No → Apply a cold pack. → Notify the animal's owner or, if the animal is wild, the proper authorities.

Yes → Wash the wound with soap and water. → Apply direct pressure to control bleeding. → Seek medical care. →

Was the victim bitten by a wild animal?

No → Notify animal control or police. Animal will be observed for possible rabies.

Yes → *Do not* try to capture the animal. Avoid killing the animal; if you must kill it, do not hit or shoot in its brain. Preserve the brain for medical examination. Contact your local health department.

Report animal bites to the police or animal control officers; they should be the ones to capture the animal for observation. If a healthy domestic dog or cat bit the victim, the animal should be confined and observed for 10 days for any illness. If a wild animal bit the victim, it should be considered a possible rabies exposure and medical care should be sought immediately.

Recognizing an Animal Bite

An animal bite has the following characteristics:
- Puncture wound from animal's sharp, pointed teeth
- Tissue and skin can be crushed
- Open wound on fingers, knuckles, and/or hand
- Animal might be present

Care for Victims of an Animal Bite

Help an animal bite victim by doing the following:
1. If the wound is not bleeding heavily, wash with soap and water. Flush the wound with water under pressure. Avoid scrubbing, which can bruise the tissues.
2. Control the bleeding and cover the wound with a sterile or clean dressing.
3. Seek medical care for further wound cleaning and closure, and possible tetanus or rabies care.

FYI

Dog Bites

During the past few years, there has been a rash of news stories about vicious attacks by pit bull terriers. The public hysteria has spurred some communities to such action as outlawing pit bulls.

The Centers of Disease Control undertook a study of fatalities related to dog bites. The researchers found 157 fatalities during a 10-year period. Pet dogs were responsible for almost 70% of fatalities, strays were involved in 27% of cases, and police or guard dogs in only 2.8% of the deaths. No significant seasonal trends were noted, except that strays seemed to be more involved in the fall, while pets were more involved in the winter. The victims were primarily children under 10 years of age (70%) with a particularly high death rate noted for infants less than one month old.

Pit bulls were implicated in more than 40% of the fatalities, "almost three times more than German shepherds, the next most commonly reported breed." Deaths attributed to pit bulls increased from 20% to 62% during the period. The researchers concluded that dog bite fatalities had been underestimated and suggested "strong animal control laws, public education regarding dog bites, and more responsible dog ownership."
Source: Sacks JJ et al: Dog bite-related fatalities from 1979 through 1988. *JAMA* 262:1489-1492.

Human Bites

After dogs and cats, the animal most likely to bite humans is another human. Human bites can cause severe injury, often more so than other animal bites. The human mouth contains a wide range of bacteria and viruses, so the chance of infection is greater from a human bite than from bites of other warm-blooded animals **Figure 19-3**.

Most human bites are inflicted by fighting youths, by children at play, by people in mental institutions, or during sexual assaults. Embarrassment sometimes causes a victim not to seek medical care immediately, which greatly increases the risk of infection.

Although most human bites occur during acts of violence, about one fourth are accidental or sports-related, sustained by hospital workers trying to restrain children or patients having a seizure, or self-inflicted during nail chewing or thumb sucking. Men are more often victims than women, mostly during aggressive altercations, with

FYI

Dog Bites: Which Breeds Are Most Dangerous?

Researchers who checked Denver records recently found 178 reports of dog bites for a 1-year period to people outside the dog owners' households (this is more common than bites to family members). They also identified 178 nonbiting dogs from the same neighborhoods. Results showed that male dogs (especially unneutered males), German shepherds, and chow chows were the most likely to bite outsiders, especially children. Children under age 12 were the victims in 51% of cases. Too few pit bulls, Akitas, and collies were involved in this study to rate their risks.
Source: Gershman KA et al: Which dogs bite? A case-control study of risk factors. *Pediatrics* 93(6):913-917.

CAUTION

DO NOT try to capture the animal yourself.

DO NOT get near the animal.

DO NOT kill the animal unless absolutely necessary. If it must be killed, protect the head and brain from damage so they can be examined for rabies. Transport a dead animal intact to limit exposure to potentially infected tissues or saliva. The animal's remains should be refrigerated to prevent decomposition.

DO NOT handle the animal without taking appropriate precautions. Infected saliva might be on the animal's fur, so wear heavy gloves or use a shovel if you have to move a dead animal.

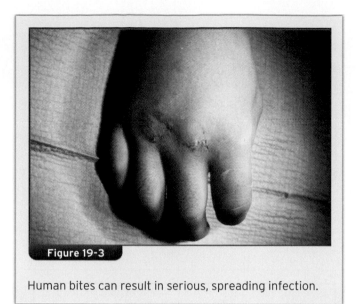

Figure 19-3

Human bites can result in serious, spreading infection.

the peak age being 25 years. The most common injury location is the hand, sustained on a closed fist as the result of a punch.

Recognizing Human Bites

There are two types of human bites. True bites occur when any part of the body's flesh is caught between teeth, usually deliberately. True bites happen during fights and in cases of abuse. Mandatory reporting laws apply if spousal or child abuse is involved. A schoolyard bite, with one child biting another, generally is not reportable.

Much worse than a true bite is the clenched-fist injury, which results from cutting a fist on teeth. It is associated with a high likelihood of infection. The injury is usually a laceration over the knuckles. Although clenched-fist injuries usually result from a fight, unintentional injury can happen during sports and play.

Care for Victims of Human Bites

Help someone with a human bite in the following manner:

1. If the wound is not bleeding heavily, wash it with soap and water for 5 to 10 minutes. Avoid scrubbing, which can bruise tissues.
2. Flush the wound thoroughly with running water under pressure.
3. Control bleeding with direct pressure.
4. Cover the wound with a sterile dressing. Do *not* close the wound with tape or butterfly bandages. Closing the wound traps bacteria in the wound, increasing the chance of infection.
5. Seek medical care for possible further wound cleaning, a tetanus shot, and sutures to close the wound, if needed.

▶ Snakebites

Throughout the world, about 50,000 people die of snakebites each year. Each year in the United States, 40,000 to 50,000 people are bitten by snakes, 7,000 to 8,000 of them by venomous snakes **Figure 19-4**. Amazingly, fewer than a dozen Americans die each year of snakebites. Victims who die of snakebites in the United States usually do so during the first 48 hours after the bite. Only four snake species in the United States are poisonous: rattlesnakes (which account for about 65% of all venomous snakebites and nearly all the snakebite deaths in the United States), copperheads, water moccasins (also known as cottonmouths), and coral snakes **Figure 19-5**, **Figure 19-6**, **Figure 19-7**, and **Figure 19-8**.

The first three are pit vipers, which have three characteristics in common:

- Triangular, flat heads wider than their necks
- Elliptical pupils (cat's eyes)
- A heat-sensitive pit between the eye and the nostril on each side of the head

The coral snake is small and colorful, with a black snout and a series of bright red, yellow, and black bands around its body (every other band is yellow). It also has a black snout. At least one species of venomous snakes is found in every state except Alaska, Hawaii, and Maine

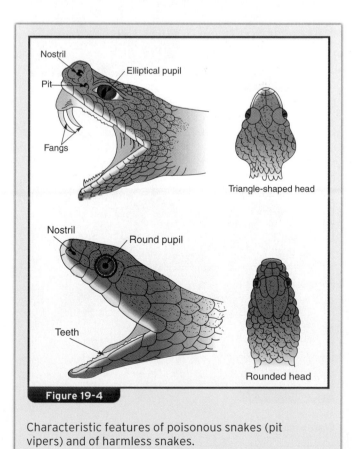

Nostril

Elliptical pupil

Pit

Fangs

Triangle-shaped head

Nostril

Round pupil

Teeth

Rounded head

Figure 19-4

Characteristic features of poisonous snakes (pit vipers) and of harmless snakes.

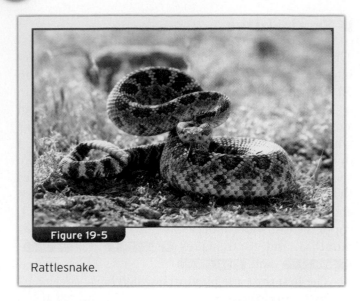

Figure 19-5

Rattlesnake.

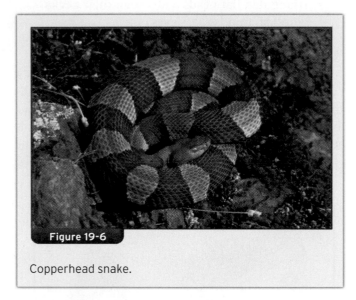

Figure 19-6

Copperhead snake.

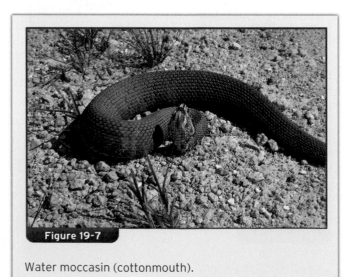

Figure 19-7

Water moccasin (cottonmouth).

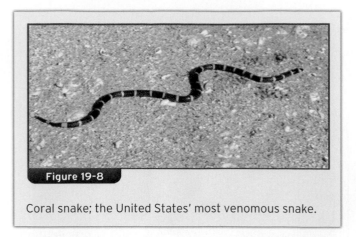

Figure 19-8

Coral snake; the United States' most venomous snake.

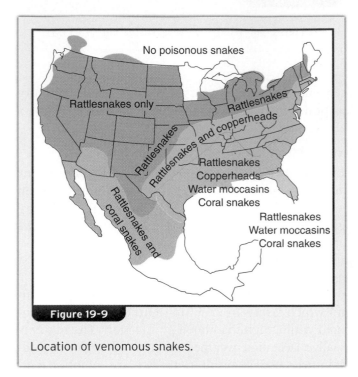

Figure 19-9

Location of venomous snakes.

Figure 19-9. Exotic snakes, whether imported legally or smuggled into the United States, can be found in zoos, schools, snake farms, and amateur and professional collections, and account for at least 15 bites a year. Some of the exotic snakes can be poisonous.

A legitimate snakebite is one in which the victim was bitten before the encounter with a snake was recognized or while trying to move away from the snake. They most often involve the lower extremities and are accidental **Table 19-3**.

An illegitimate snakebite is one in which, before being bitten, the victim recognized the encounter with a snake but did not attempt to move away from the snake. Most illegitimate bites occur on the upper extremities. Most bites of this type occur when the victim tries to kill, capture, play with, or move a snake. Adult snakes deliver

Snakebites

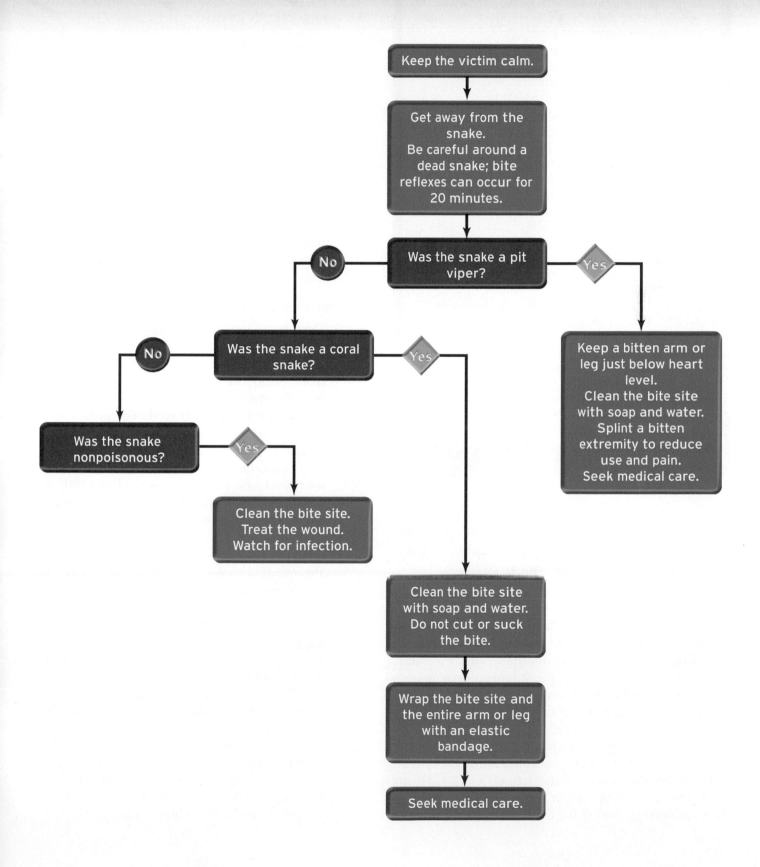

Keep the victim calm.

Get away from the snake.
Be careful around a dead snake; bite reflexes can occur for 20 minutes.

Was the snake a pit viper?

No — Was the snake a coral snake?

Yes → Keep a bitten arm or leg just below heart level.
Clean the bite site with soap and water.
Splint a bitten extremity to reduce use and pain.
Seek medical care.

No — Was the snake nonpoisonous?

Yes → Clean the bite site.
Treat the wound.
Watch for infection.

Yes → Clean the bite site with soap and water. Do not cut or suck the bite.

Wrap the bite site and the entire arm or leg with an elastic bandage.

Seek medical care.

Table 19-3   Preventing Snakebites

Follow these guidelines to prevent snakebites:

- Do not handle venomous snakes.
- Avoid hiking and camping in snake-infested areas; avoid exploring caves, rock crevices, dens, lairs, stone walls, and wood piles.
- Know the outdoor terrain, and be alert for snakes in thick foliage.
- Watch where you sit, step, and stretch; do not reach into holes or hidden ledges.
- Wear protective gear such as boots, trousers, long pants, long-sleeved shirts, and gloves when you are in possible snake habitats.
- Take a friend with you; it could save your life.
- Do not alarm a sleeping snake (even a newborn snake) or tease or molest a snake that is awake.
- Do not keep poisonous snakes as pets; zoos are better qualified to care for them. A 16% reduction in bites from rattlesnakes would occur if they were not kept as pets.
- Do not sit on or step over logs until you closely scrutinize the area.
- Do not handle a dead venomous snake. The reflex action of the jaws can still inflict a wound 20 minutes or more after the snake has died.
- Do not surprise or corner a snake. Use a walking stick to prod uncleared ground and make noise so a snake can sense you coming.
- Researchers suggest that more than one half of all rattlesnake bites would be eliminated if people simply moved away from the snake.

more serious bites because they inject more venom than do young snakes, even though a young snake's venom is two to three times more toxic than an adult's.

Pit Vipers

Pit vipers are found in every state but Alaska, Maine, and Hawaii. Despite their sinister reputation, snakes are almost always more scared of you than you are of them. Snakes benefit us by keeping the rodent population from exploding out of control. They consume hundreds of thousands of mice and rats every year. Few snakes act aggressively toward a human unless provoked. The vast majority of bites are not deadly and can be effectively treated.

Ninety-eight percent of snakebites are on the extremities. Alcohol intoxication of the victim is a factor in many bites. The majority of bites in the United States occur in the southwestern part of the country—partly due to the

near-extinction of pit vipers in the eastern United States. The eastern and western diamondback rattlesnakes account for almost 95% of the deaths that usually occur most often in children, in the elderly, and in victims to whom **antivenin** (also known as antivenom) is not given or is inappropriately given.

Recognizing Pit Viper Bites

Signs of a pit viper bite include:

- Severe burning pain at the bite site
- Two small puncture wounds about ½ inch apart (some cases have only one fang mark)
- Swelling (occurs within 10 to 15 minutes and can involve an entire extremity)
- Discoloration and blood-filled blisters possibly developing in 6 to 10 hours
- In severe cases, nausea, vomiting, sweating, and weakness
- In about 25% of poisonous snake bites, there is no venom injection, only fang and tooth wounds (known as a dry bite).

Care for Victims of Pit Viper Bites

The Wilderness Medical Society lists these guidelines for dealing with pit viper bites:

1. Get the victim and bystanders away from the snake. Snakes have been known to bite more than once. Pit vipers can strike about one half of their body length. Be careful around a decapitated snake head—head reactions can persist for 20 minutes or more.
2. Do not attempt to capture or kill the snake. It wastes valuable time, there is a risk of additional bites, and identification of the snake is not usually needed because the same antivenin is used for all pit viper bites.
3. Keep the victim quiet. Activity increases venom absorption. If possible, carry the victim or have the victim walk very slowly to help to minimize exertion.
4. Gently wash the bitten area with soap and water **Figure 19-10**. Any ring(s) or jewelry that might reduce blood circulation if swelling occurs should be removed.
5. Stabilize the bitten extremity (arm or leg) with a sling or a splint as you would for a fracture. Keep the extremity below heart level despite the fact that swelling might occur.
6. Seek medical care *immediately*. This is the most important thing to do for the victim. Antivenin must be given within 4 hours of the bite (not every venomous snake bite requires antivenin).

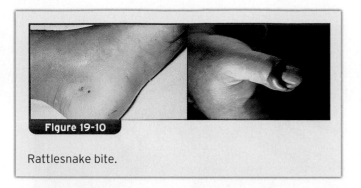

Figure 19-10

Rattlesnake bite.

CAUTION

DO NOT apply cold or ice to a snakebite. It does not inactivate the venom and poses a danger of frostbite.

DO NOT use the cut-and-suck procedure—you could damage underlying structures (for example, blood vessels, nerves).

DO NOT apply mouth suction. Your mouth is filled with bacteria, increasing the likelihood of wound infection.

DO NOT use any form of suction—it removes no venom.

DO NOT apply electric shock. No medical studies support this method.

DO NOT apply a constriction band—their use remains controversial.

FYI

Dead Snakes Can Still Bite

Data collected at the Good Samaritan Regional Medical Center in Phoenix show that fatal injuries do not prevent rattlesnakes from biting humans. Of the 34 patients admitted to the Phoenix Center for Rattlesnake Bites in a recent 11-month period, five were bitten by snakes that had been fatally injured and were presumed dead. One patient was bitten on the index finger after picking up a snake he had bludgeoned in the head and assumed was dead. Another was bitten after picking up a snake he had shot, then decapitated.
Source: Suchard JR, LoVecchio F: Envenomations by rattlesnakes thought to be dead. *N Engl J Med* 34(24):1930.

Coral Snake Bites

The coral snake is America's most venomous snake, but it rarely bites people. The coral snake has short fangs and tends to hang on and chew its venom into the victim rather than to strike and release, like a pit viper. Coral snake venom is a neurotoxin, and symptoms can begin 1 to 5 hours after the bite.

Recognizing Coral Snake Bites

Someone who has been bitten by a coral snake might exhibit the following symptoms:

- Minimal pain
- Sagging or drooping of upper eyelids
- Weakness
- Pricking, tingling of skin (often numb at bite site)
- Double vision (seeing two of a single object)
- Difficulty in swallowing
- Sweating
- Abnormal flow of saliva

Care for Victims of Coral Snake Bites

You can help a coral snake bite victim in the following manner:

1. Keep the victim calm.
2. Gently clean the bite site with soap and water.
3. Apply mild pressure by wrapping several elastic bandages over the bite site and the entire arm or leg. Applying mild pressure is recommended only for bites from elapid snakes like the coral snake, not pit vipers. The technique originated in Australia, where it has been very successful. Do not cut the victim's skin, suck on the wound, or use a suction device.
4. Seek medical care for antivenin.

Nonpoisonous Snake Bites

Nonvenomous snakes inflict most snake bites. If you are not positive about a snake, assume it was venomous. Some so-called nonpoisonous North American snakes such as the hognose and garter snakes have venom that can cause painful local reactions but no systemic (whole-body) symptoms.

Recognizing Nonpoisonous Snake Bites

A nonpoisonous snake bite results in the following:

- Feeling of a mild to moderate pinch
- Curved lines (horseshoe shaped) of tiny pinpricks on the skin that correspond with the rows of sharp, pointy teeth
- Bleeding
- Mild itching

Care for Victims of Nonpoisonous Snake Bites

A victim of a nonpoisonous snake bite should be treated thusly:

1. Gently clean the bite site with soap and water.
2. Care for the bite as you would a minor wound.
3. Seek medical care.

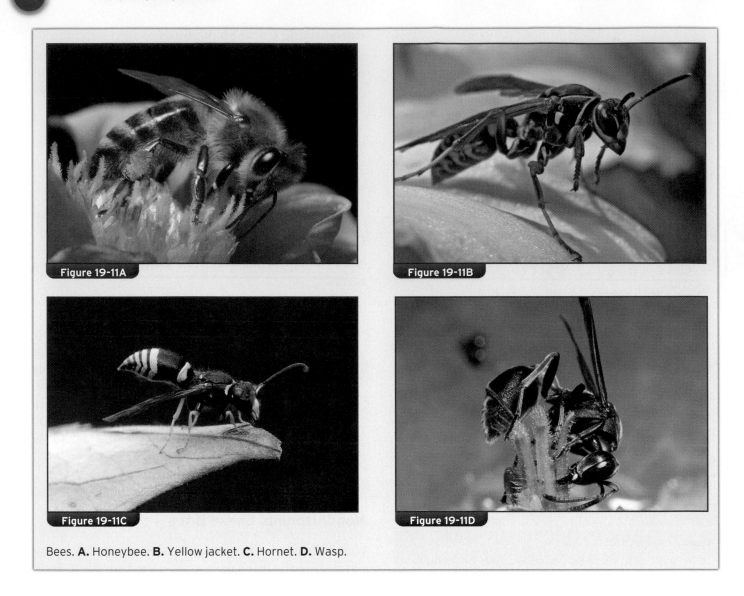

Bees. **A.** Honeybee. **B.** Yellow jacket. **C.** Hornet. **D.** Wasp.

▶ Insect Stings

The stinging insects belonging to the order of *Hymenoptera* include honeybees, bumblebees, yellow jackets, hornets, wasps, **Figure 19-11** and fire ants. These insects account for more deaths and illnesses each year than all other venomous animals combined. About 1 in every 200 people is dangerously allergic to *Hymenoptera* venom. Fortunately, localized pain, itching, and swelling—the most common consequences of an insect bite—can be treated with first aid.

Generally, venomous flying insects are aggressive only when threatened or when their hives or nests are disrupted. Under such conditions, they sting, sometimes in swarms. Honeybees and some yellow jackets have barbed stingers that become embedded in the victim's skin during the sting. After injecting its venom, the bee flies away, tearing and leaving behind the embedded stinger and venom sac, which causes it to die. Honeybees and bumblebees do not release all their venom during the initial injection; some remains in the stinger embedded in the

victim's skin. If the stinger and venom sac are not removed properly, additional venom can be released and worsen the victim's reaction.

In contrast, the stingers of wasps, yellow jackets, hornets, and fire ants are not barbed and do not become embedded in the victim. Thus, these insects can sting multiple times, and most species (with a few exceptions, such as some yellow jacket species) do not die as a result of the stinging. There are two types of yellow jackets, one is a wasp and can sting multiple times. The other is a ground-nesting bee that stings once then dies, sometimes leaving an embedded stinger like other bees. These bees are smaller than yellow jacket wasps.

Most stings cause only self-limited, local inflammatory reactions consisting of pain, itching, redness, and swelling. These reactions are usually more a nuisance than a medical emergency. However, local reactions can be extensive, for example, involving the victim's entire arm. In an extensive reaction, the swelling and redness might peak 2 to 3 days after the sting and last a week or longer. Signs and symptoms of life-threatening reactions include nausea, vomiting, wheezing, fever, and drippy nose. A victim might go into anaphylaxis almost immediately or after experiencing a variety of symptoms. Most people who have anaphylactic reactions have no history of them. In a study of 400 fatal bee stings, only 15% of the victims had a known sensitivity.

Reactions generally occur within a few minutes to 1 hour after the sting. Bee-sting victims who have anaphylactic reactions develop throat swelling and bronchospasm, which are manifested by difficulty speaking, tightness in the throat or chest, wheezing, shortness of breath, and chest pain. Respiratory-tract obstruction accounts for the majority of deaths among victims of flying-insect stings.

For the severely allergic person, a single sting could be fatal within minutes. Although there are accounts of people who have survived some 2,000 stings at one time, 500 stings will usually kill even people who are not allergic to stinging insects.

Massive numbers of stings are rare. They might occur if a person stumbled into a hive or a truck carrying a load of hives crashed. With the slow migration of Africanized bees (so-called killer bees) from South and Central America into the United States, the number of multiple-sting cases is likely to increase. The venom of the Africanized bee is no more potent than that of the European type; it is just that the African type is extremely

aggressive and, thus, more likely to be involved in multiple stings. A number of child deaths have resulted from the multiple stings of fire ants, which are common in the southeastern United States.

Recognizing Insect Stings

A rule of thumb is that the sooner symptoms develop after a sting, the more serious the reaction will be.

- Usual reactions are instant pain, redness around the sting site, and itching.
- Worrisome reactions include hives, swelling of lips or tongue, a tickle in the throat, and wheezing.
- Life-threatening reactions are bluish or grayish skin color, seizures, unresponsiveness, and an inability to breathe because of swelling and spasm of the airway.

About 60–80% of anaphylactic deaths are caused by the victim's not being able to breathe because swollen airway passages obstruct airflow to the lungs. The second most common cause of death is shock, caused by collapse of blood circulation through the body.

One of the difficulties in dealing with stings is the lack of uniformity in victims' responses. One sting is not necessarily equivalent to another, even within the same species, because the amount of venom injected varies from sting to sting. A person who experiences anaphylactic shock after being stung by a hornet might respond to a bee sting with only a small amount of swelling. One person might have a local reaction involving an entire limb, although the more typical response is a small circle of redness and swelling that disappears without incident in a few days. In beekeepers, for whom stings are an accepted occupational hazard, the response is likely to be even less than in most other people, because they have become tolerant to the toxins in the venom from having been stung many times on different occasions. There seems to be no easy way to predict how a person will react. Most people who are stung, however, have local reactions: redness, swelling, and pain.

Stings to the mouth or eye tend to be more dangerous than stings to other body areas. Also, victims tend to react more severely to multiple stings, especially 10 or more. The most dangerous single stings in nonallergic individuals are those inside the throat, which can result from swallowing an insect that has dropped into a soft drink can or from inhaling one that flies into the victim's open mouth. A sting in the mouth or throat can cause swelling that obstructs the airway even in a person who is not allergic to insect stings. If the sting is not life threatening, have the victim suck on ice or flush his or her mouth with cold water. For a bee sting, dissolve a teaspoon of baking soda in a glass of water. Have the victim rinse his or her mouth and then hold the water in the mouth for several minutes.

FYI

Preventing Insect Stings

People who know they are allergic to insect stings need to exercise extra care to avoid being stung. They should carry a bee-sting kit and follow these guidelines:

- Wear long pants and long-sleeved shirts.
- Because insects are attracted to bright colors and floral patterns, wear white, green, tan, and khaki—the least attractive colors to insects.
- Wear shoes outdoors.
- Avoid yard work and other activities in which insect contact is frequent.
- Keep garbage cans away from the house.
- Remove insect-attracting plants from inside as well as the immediate proximity of the house.
- Do not use scented soaps, lotions, or perfumes.
- Keep car windows closed.
- If an insect confronts you, avoid quick movements and do not provoke it. Turn away, lower your face, and walk away slowly. Do not run about wildly or move erratically when bees are nearby.
- Do not eat when bees are nearby.
- Have insect nests around the house removed by professional exterminators.

Insect Stings

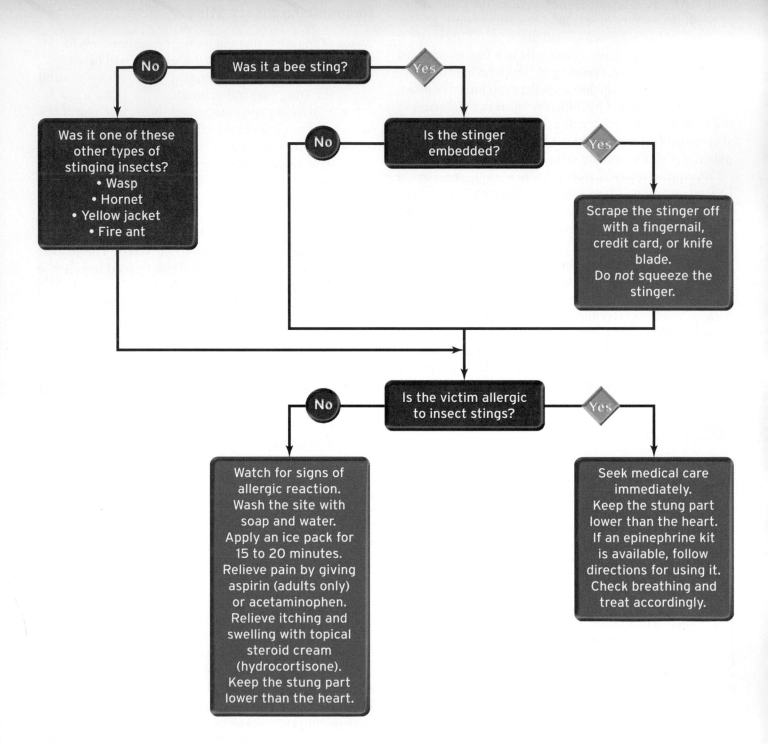

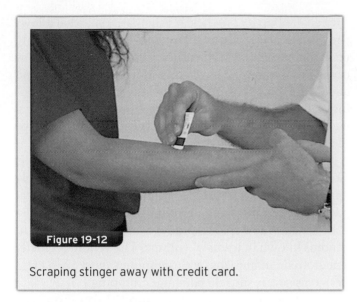
Figure 19-12

Scraping stinger away with credit card.

Care for Someone Who Has Insect Stings

The following outlines how to assist someone who has been bitten or stung by an insect.

1. Most people who have been stung can be treated on site, and everyone should know what to do if a life-threatening allergic reaction (anaphylaxis) occurs. In particular, people who have had a severe reaction to an insect sting should be instructed about what they can do to protect themselves. They also should be advised to wear a medical-alert identification tag identifying them as allergic to insect stings.
2. Look at the sting site for a stinger and venom sac embedded in the skin. Bees are the only stinging insects that leave their stingers and venom sac behind. If the stinger is embedded, remove it or it will continue to inject poison for 2 or 3 minutes. Scrape the stinger and venom sac away with a hard object such as a long fingernail, credit card, scissor edge, or knife blade **Figure 19-12** .
3. Wash the sting site with soap and water to prevent infection.
4. Apply an ice pack over the sting site to slow absorption of the venom and relieve pain. Use a commercial sting stick containing a topical anesthetic such as Xylocaine (unless the victim is known to be allergic to the drug). Because bee venom is acidic, a paste made of baking soda and water can help. Sodium bicarbonate is an alkalinizing agent that draws out fluid and reduces itching and swelling. Wasp venom, on the other hand, is alkaline, so apply vinegar or lemon juice. A paste made of unseasoned meat tenderizer can help a bee sting victim if the paste comes in direct con-

tact with the venom. That generally is not possible, however, because the bee will have injected the venom through too small a hole and too deeply into the victim's skin.

5. To further relieve pain and itching, use aspirin (adults only), acetaminophen, or ibuprofen. A topical steroid cream, such as hydrocortisone, can help combat local swelling and itching. An antihistamine can prevent some local symptoms if given early, but it works too slowly to counteract a life-threatening allergic reaction.
6. Observe the victim for at least 30 minutes for signs of an allergic reaction. For a person having a severe allergic reaction, a dose of epinephrine is the only effective treatment. A person with a known allergy to insect stings should have a physician-prescribed emergency kit that includes a prefilled, spring-loaded device that automatically injects epinephrine. The allergic person should take the kit whenever he or she is going someplace where stinging insects are known to exist. Because epinephrine is short-acting, watch the victim closely for signs of returning anaphylaxis. Another dose of epinephrine as often as every 15 minutes might be needed.
7. Do not use epinephrine to treat a sting unless the victim has a severe allergic reaction. Epinephrine has a shelf life of 1 to 3 years or until it turns brown.
8. Watch for signs and symptoms of a delayed allergic reaction, especially during the first 6 to 24 hours. If the victim develops difficulty breathing, facial swelling, fever, chills, or dizziness, call 9-1-1.

▶ Spider and Insect Bites

Most spiders are venomous, which is how they paralyze and kill their prey. However, most spiders lack an effective delivery system—long fangs and strong jaws—to bite a human. About 60 species of spiders in North America are capable of biting humans, although only a few species have produced significant poisonings **Figure 19-13** .

Most bites are by female spiders. Male spiders are almost always smaller than females and have fangs that are too short and fragile to bite humans. Death rarely occurs and only from bites by brown recluse and black widow spiders.

The number of deaths from spider bites is not accurately known. A spider bite is difficult to diagnose, especially when the spider was not seen or recovered, because the bites typically cause little immediate pain. In a study of 600 suspected spider bites, 80% were caused by other

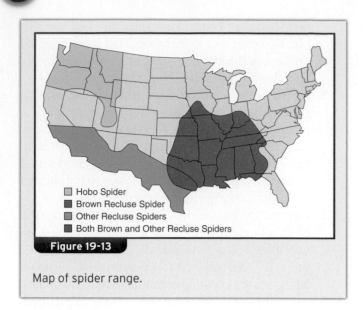

Figure 19-13

Map of spider range.

Hobo Spider
Brown Recluse Spider
Other Recluse Spiders
Both Brown and Other Recluse Spiders

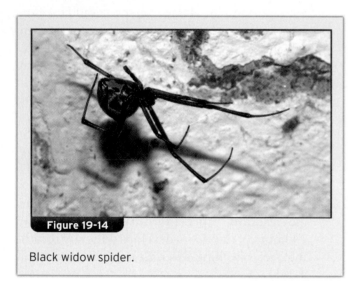

Figure 19-14

Black widow spider.

arthropods (for example, kissing bugs, ticks, fleas, mites, and bedbugs) and 10% by disease states (for example, poison ivy, diabetic ulcer, bedsore, Lyme disease, and gonococcus). Spiders rarely bite more than once, and they do not always release venom.

Black Widow Spiders

Black widow spiders are also commonly known as brown widow spiders and red-legged spiders, depending on the species **Figure 19-14**. The term black widow is actually inaccurate, because only three of the five species of widow spider are actually black; the others are brown and gray. Newly hatched spiders are almost entirely red. Males have white stripes along the outside of the abdomen.

The female black widow spider is one of the largest spiders, with a body that ranges up to ½ inch in length and a leg span of up to 2 inches. It is her large size that allows the female black widow's fangs to be large and strong enough to penetrate human skin. The female black widow can live as long as 3 years. Black widow spiders have round abdomens that vary from gray to brown to black, depending on the species. In the female black widow, the abdomen is shiny black with a red or yellow spot (often in the shape of an hourglass) or white spots or bands.

The male is only one third of the size of the female. Contrary to popular myth, the male usually mates safely with the female. Because he is small, his fangs are incapable of penetrating human skin, so bites are from the female. Black widow spiders produce one of the most potent venoms known in terms of volume. The venom is chiefly a neurotoxin in humans, with symptoms most often manifested as severe muscle pain and cramping.

Black widow spiders are found throughout the world. In the Western Hemisphere, they are found from southern Canada, throughout every state in the continental United States, to the tip of South America, and in Hawaii.

The web of the black widow spider is an extensive, irregular, shaggy trap for the insects she normally eats. The black widow rarely leaves the web and stays close to her egg mass. She aggressively defends the egg mass and bites if it is disturbed. When she is not guarding eggs, the spider often attempts to escape rather than bite.

Frequent cleaning to remove spiders and their webs from buildings, outbuildings, and outdoor living areas decreases the chance of accidental contact with black widow spiders. Insecticides could decrease the population of the food for the black widows but do not usually affect the spiders themselves.

Recognizing Black Widow Spider Bites

The following could indicate a black widow spider bite:
- If the spider is trapped against the skin or crushed, it will bite. It is difficult to determine if a person has been bitten by a black widow spider or by any spider.
- The victim might feel a sharp pinprick when the spider bites, but some victims are not aware of the bite. Within 15 minutes, a dull, numbing pain develops in the bite area.
- Two small fang marks might be seen as tiny red spots.
- Within 15 minutes to 4 hours, muscle stiffness and cramps occur, usually affecting the abdomen when the bite is on a lower part of the body and the shoulders, back, or chest when the bite is on an upper part. Victims often describe the pain as the most severe they have ever experienced.

- Headache, chills, fever, heavy sweating, dizziness, nausea, and vomiting occur next. Severe pain around the bite site peaks in 2 to 3 hours and can last 12 to 48 hours.

Care for Victims of Black Widow Spider Bites

To care for someone who has been bitten by a black widow spider, do the following:

1. If possible, catch the spider to confirm its identity. Even if the body has been crushed, save it for identification (although most spider-bite victims never see the spider). The species helps determine the treatment, so the dead spider (if it can be found) should be taken with the victim to the hospital.
2. Clean the bite area with soap and water or rubbing alcohol.
3. Place an ice pack over the bite to relieve pain and delay the effects of the venom.
4. Give aspirin (adults only), ibuprofen, or acetaminophen.
5. Monitor breathing.
6. Seek medical care immediately. For black widow spider bites, an antivenin exists. It is usually reserved for children younger than 6 years, people older than 60 years and with high blood pressure, pregnant women, and victims with severe reactions. The antivenin will give relief within 1 to 3 hours.

Brown Recluse Spiders

Brown recluse spiders are also known in North America as fiddle-back and violin spiders **Figure 19-15**. They have a violin-shaped figure on their backs (several other spider species have a similar configuration on their backs). Color varies from fawn to dark brown, with darker legs. Male and female spiders are venomous. Brown recluse spiders are found primarily in the southern and midwestern states, with other less toxic but related spiders throughout the rest of the country. They are absent from the Pacific Northwest.

Recognizing Brown Recluse Spider Bites

If you suspect a brown recluse spider bite, remember the following:

- The brown recluse spider bites only when it is trapped against the skin.
- A local reaction usually occurs within 2 to 8 hours with mild to severe pain at the bite site and the development of redness, swelling, and local itching.
- In 48 to 72 hours, a blister develops at the bite site, becomes red, and bursts. During the early stages,

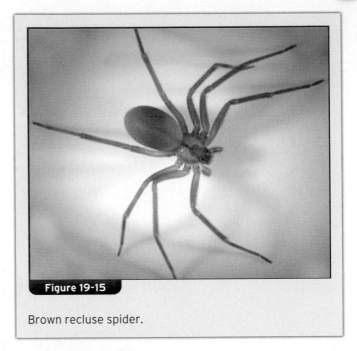

Figure 19-15

Brown recluse spider.

the affected area often takes on a bull's-eye appearance, with a central white area surrounded by a reddened area, ringed by a whitish or blue border. A small, red crater remains, over which a scab forms. When the scab falls away in a few days, a larger crater remains. That too scabs over and falls off, leaving a larger crater. The craters are known as *volcano lesions*. This process of slow tissue destruction can continue for weeks or months. The ulcer sometimes requires skin grafting.

- Fever, weakness, vomiting, joint pain, and a rash could occur.
- Stomach cramps, nausea, and vomiting might occur. Death is rare.

Care for Victims of Brown Recluse Spider Bites

This is how you can care for someone who has been bitten by a brown recluse spider:

1. If possible, catch the spider to confirm its identity. Even if the body has been crushed, save it for identification (although most spider-bite victims never see the spider). The species helps determine the treatment, so the dead spider (if it can be found) should be taken with the victim to the hospital.
2. Clean the bite area with soap and water or rubbing alcohol.
3. Place an ice pack over the bite to relieve pain and delay the effects of the venom.
4. Give aspirin (adults only), ibuprofen, or acetaminophen.
5. Seek medical care immediately.

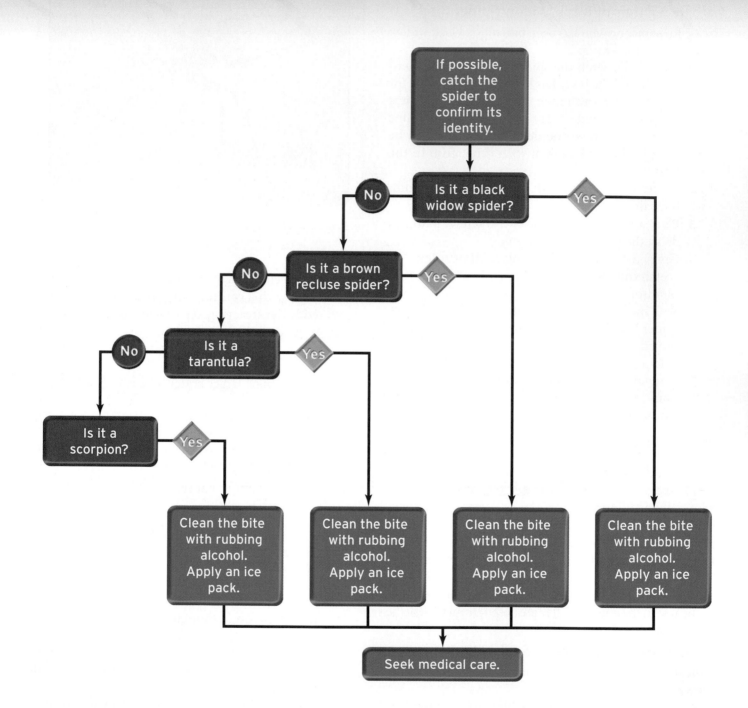

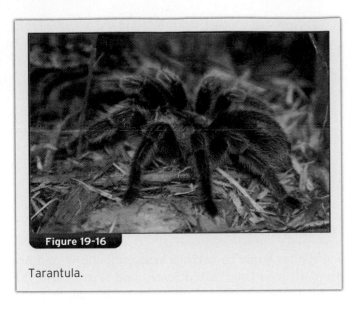

Figure 19-16

Tarantula.

Tarantulas

Tarantulas bite only when vigorously provoked or roughly handled **Figure 19-16**. The bite varies from almost painless to a deep throbbing pain lasting up to 1 hour. The tarantula, when upset, will roughly scratch the lower surface of its abdomen with its legs and flick hairs onto a person's skin.

Recognizing Tarantula Bites and Embedded Hairs

Tarantula bites and embedded hairs have the following characteristics:
- The bite causes pain—aching or stinging.
- The hairs cause itching and inflammation that can last several weeks.

Care for Victims of Tarantula Bites and Embedded Hairs

To care for a victim of a tarantula bite:
1. If possible, catch the spider to confirm its identity. Even if the body has been crushed, save it for identification (although most spider-bite victims never see the spider). The species helps determine the treatment, so the dead spider (if it can be found) should be taken with the victim to the hospital.
2. Clean the bite area with soap and water or rubbing alcohol.
3. Place an ice pack over the bite to relieve pain and delay the effects of the venom.
4. Give aspirin (adults only), ibuprofen, or acetaminophen.
5. Seek medical care immediately.

To care for a victim of embedded tarantula hairs:
1. Remove the hairs from the skin with sticky tape (repeating as necessary).
2. Wash the area with soap and water.
3. Apply hydrocortisone cream.
4. Give the victim pain medication (aspirin—for adults only—or ibuprofen or acetaminophen)
5. Give the victim an antihistamine.

Common Aggressive House Spider (Hobo Spider)

Another biter is the common aggressive house spider, or hobo spider. It arrived in the Pacific Northwest in 1936 and slowly made its way across Washington State and into surrounding states. In those areas, the hobo spider is the most common large spider.

Recognizing Common Aggressive House Spider Bites

The signs and symptoms of the common aggressive house spider bite are similar to those of the brown recluse spider.
- Redness, blisters, and later, gangrene (dead tissue)
- Headache, visual problems, weakness

Care for Victims of Common Aggressive House Spider Bites

If someone has been bitten by a common aggressive house spider, you can help by doing the following:
1. If possible, catch the spider to confirm its identity. Even if the body has been crushed, save it for identification (although most spider-bite victims never see the spider). The species helps determine the treatment, so the dead spider (if it can be found) should be taken with the victim to the hospital.
2. Clean the bite area with soap and water or rubbing alcohol.
3. Place an ice pack over the bite to relieve pain and delay the effects of the venom.
4. Give aspirin (adults only), ibuprofen, or acetaminophen.
5. Seek medical care immediately.

Scorpion Stings

Scorpions look like miniature lobsters, with lobsterlike pincers and a long, up-curved taillike appendage with a poisonous stinger **Figure 19-17**. Several species of scorpions inhabit the southwestern United States, but only the bark scorpion poses a threat to humans. Severe cases, which usually appear only in children, could include paralysis, spasms, or breathing difficulties. Death due to scorpion stings in the United States is rare.

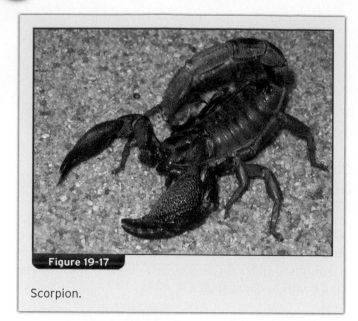

Figure 19-17

Scorpion.

The bark scorpion is found primarily in Arizona. Rare stings have been reported in other parts of the United States, after the scorpions traveled from Arizona as stowaways in luggage or in car trunks. The bark scorpion is pale tan and is ¾ to 1¼ inches long, not including the so-called tail.

Stings to adult victims usually are not life threatening. Stings to small children, however, are often dangerous. When a child is stung, every effort should be made to get the victim to medical care as quickly as possible. Pay close attention to make sure the victim's airway is open and that he or she is breathing.

Recognizing Scorpion Stings

The most frequent symptom of a scorpion sting, especially to an adult victim, is local, immediate pain and burning around the sting site. Later, numbness or tingling occurs. There is no swelling or blanching. Tapping a finger over the sting site can cause pain (the tap test) and could serve to indicate a scorpion sting. More severely affected people will experience pain along the stung arm or leg, even paralysis. In more serious stings, uncontrolled jerking movements of the legs or arms and facial twitching might occur.

Victims with a severe reaction will have a fast heart rate, salivate, and experience breathing distress. Symptoms begin from within minutes to half an hour and reach their height within the first few hours. Symptoms usually last from 6 to 24 hours.

Care for Victims of Scorpion Stings

Care for a scorpion bite victim by doing the following:
1. Monitor breathing.
2. Gently clean the sting site with soap and water or rubbing alcohol.

3. Apply an ice pack over the sting site to reduce pain and venom absorption.
4. Give aspirin (adults only), ibuprofen, or acetaminophen.
5. Seek medical care. Recently, bark scorpion antivenin production has been discontinued. Its use was controversial. The US Food and Drug Administration has given approval for clinical trials to evaluate a Mexican antivenin for use in the United States.

Centipede Bites

Centipedes come in various sizes and colors and are found all over the United States and throughout the world. The giant desert centipede, which can be up to 8 inches long, is the only US centipede that is dangerous to humans.

Like spiders, any centipede with fangs that can penetrate human skin can inject venom. These arthropods inject toxic substances into the skin from a pair of hollow jaws that act like fangs. Contrary to popular belief, centipedes do not inject venom with their feet. Exaggerated stories about the deadly effects of their bites and reports that the tip of each leg carries a poisonous spur have caused many people to have an unreasonable fear of centipedes. Their venom is relatively weak.

Recognizing Centipede Bites

Generally, bite indications are burning pain and local inflammation of the wound site, with mild swelling of the lymph nodes. The bite of the giant desert centipede causes inflammation, swelling, and redness that last 4 to 12 hours. Swelling and tenderness can last as long as 3 weeks or can disappear and recur.

Care for Victims of Centipede Bites

Centipedes, which have one pair of legs per body segment, are sometimes confused with millipedes, which have two pairs of legs per body segment. Millipedes cannot inject venom, but their secretions can irritate the skin. Treat those who have been exposed to millipede secretions by washing the area of contact with soap and water and applying a cortisone cream or ointment.

Care for a centipede bite victim in the following manner:
1. Clean the wound with soap and water.
2. Apply an ice pack at the bite site.
3. For pain, give aspirin (adults only), acetaminophen, or ibuprofen.
4. Seek medical care for severe reactions.

FYI

Preventing Mosquito Bites

To minimize being bitten by mosquitoes, follow these guidelines:

- Wear protective clothing: pants, long-sleeved shirt, and full-brimmed hat. Mosquito netting draped over a hat will protect the face and neck. Mosquito bed nets should be used when sleeping in unscreened rooms.
- Use insect repellents on exposed skin. DEET (diethyltoluamide)-containing repellents are most effective against mosquitoes and, to a lesser extent, helpful in repelling ticks and black flies.
- DEET is considered to have low toxicity. However, it is absorbed through the skin, and hives, skin rashes, and blisters can result when it is used for prolonged periods or in excessive amounts. The long-acting 35% solution has a polymer that prevents evaporation and skin absorption.
- Products that contain 100% DEET are available but unnecessary, especially for children. Long-acting formulations of 35% DEET seem equally effective in protecting against mosquitoes and have far less potential for toxic effects.
- DEET products can be applied over other creams such as sunscreens and moisturizers. Use DEET only on exposed skin, and avoid the hands of young children because they often put their hands in their mouths. Keep DEET out of the reach of small children because ingestion could be fatal. Children younger than 5 years should not be exposed to concentrations greater than 10%, according to the American Academy of Pediatrics. Children under 2 months of age should not have DEET applied to their skin. For children ages 5 or older, the DEET concentration should not exceed 30%.
- Other nontoxic insect repellents seem to be less effective than DEET. They might be only 25% as effective as DEET and might need to be reapplied every half hour. Mixed opinions exist about whether 100 mg of vitamin B_1 (thiamine) taken daily for 1 week before being exposed is an effective preventive agent. Some experts believe that a diet high in garlic will make a person undesirable to a mosquito.
- Permethrin is a pesticide, not a repellent. It should be applied to clothing and not the skin.

Mosquito Bites

Mosquitoes bite millions of people. Mosquitoes are not only a nuisance, but they also carry many diseases. In developing countries, mosquitoes transmit malaria, yellow fever, and dengue fever; in the United States, they carry encephalitis. There is no evidence that mosquitoes transmit HIV, the virus that causes acquired immunodeficiency syndrome, or AIDS.

Female mosquitoes need blood to lay their eggs. Because they breed in water, mosquitoes are most often found in marshes, wetlands, and wooded areas. Mosquitoes usually can be separated into daytime and nighttime biters, but most bite at twilight.

Care for Victims of Mosquito Bites

You can care for someone who has mosquito bites in the following manner:

1. Wash the bitten area with soap and water.
2. Apply an ice pack.
3. Apply calamine lotion or hydrocortisone ointment to decrease redness and itching.
4. For a victim with a number of bites or a delayed allergic reaction, an antihistamine every 6 hours or a physician-prescribed cortisone might be useful.

FYI

Mosquito Bites

In tropical climates, mosquitoes are important carriers of infectious diseases such as malaria and yellow fever. Mosquito bites can also provoke unpleasant skin lesions. In many areas of the world, massive and disturbing mosquito infestations occur. For example, in Alaska it is possible to be bitten by mosquitoes as many as 1,000 times in one hour. Under such conditions, complete avoidance of bites is impossible without use of effective repellents and protective clothing. Topical treatment with over-the-counter sticks, creams, and lotions containing antihistamines, hydrocortisone, or other antipruritic agents is common. However, only a few studies have been made on the effectiveness of these products.

Source: Reunala T, et al: Treatment of mosquito bites with cetirizine. Clin Exp Allergy 23 (1):72-75.

Embedded Ticks

Ticks are not insects but are close relatives of mites and spiders. They have eight legs and are classified as hard ticks and soft ticks **Figure 19-18**. Hard ticks are more familiar because of their wide distribution and common

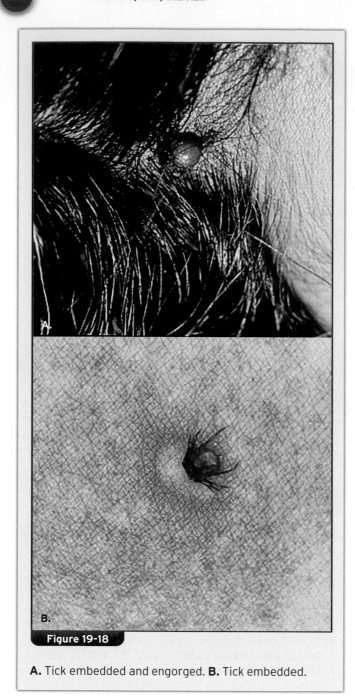

A. Tick embedded and engorged. **B.** Tick embedded.

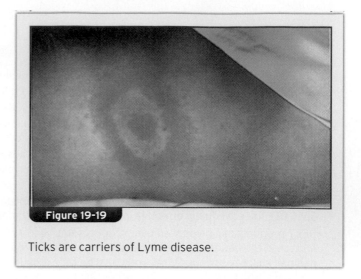

Ticks are carriers of Lyme disease.

occurrence on domestic animals. Soft ticks are found mainly in western states (Figure 19-19). In the United States, seven kinds of hard ticks and five kinds of soft ticks carry diseases (for example, Lyme disease), are a nuisance (causing itching and swelling), or cause paralysis (toxin injected). Ticks hatch from eggs and grow through three distinct stages: nymph (too small to see), larva (just visible), and adult (ready to lay eggs).

The adult is most likely to be seen. Ticks at any stage of development can use humans for food; at each stage, they need a blood meal before they can grow to the next stage. Ticks are limited in their ability to find their meals. They cannot fly, they crawl very slowly, and, without some

help, they cannot travel more than a few yards from where they were hatched. When they are ready for their next meal, they might wait months, years, or even decades for the right host to come along. Bites are nearly painless, so the tick attachment is not noticed until later.

The front part of a tick consists of the head area and the mouthparts. The mouthparts have a central structure, the hypostome, which is shaped like a blunt harpoon. A tick makes a hole in the victim's skin with the sharp teeth (barbs) on the front of the hypostome and inserts its hypostome. The barbs anchor the tick to the skin and make it difficult to pull the tick out. Some ticks produce a substance that helps cement them to the host. As they feed, some ticks increase in size 20 to 50 times.

Care for Victims of Embedded Ticks

Remove ticks as soon as possible. If a tick is carrying a disease, the longer it stays embedded, the greater the chance of the disease being transmitted. Because its bite is painless, a tick can remain embedded for days before the victim realizes it. Most tick bites are harmless, although ticks can carry Lyme disease, Rocky Mountain spotted fever, and other serious diseases.

To pull a tick off:

1. Use tweezers or a specialized tick-removal tool.
2. Grasp the tick as close to the skin as possible, and lift it with enough force to tent the skin surface. Hold it in this position until the tick lets go (about one minute). Pull the tick away from the skin. Do not pull hard enough to break the tick apart because this will leave parts of the tick behind, which will cause infection (Figure 19-20).

After the tick has been removed:

1. Wash the area with soap and water. Apply rubbing alcohol to further disinfect the area.
2. Apply an ice pack to reduce pain.
3. Apply calamine lotion to relieve itching. Keep the area clean.

Tick Removal

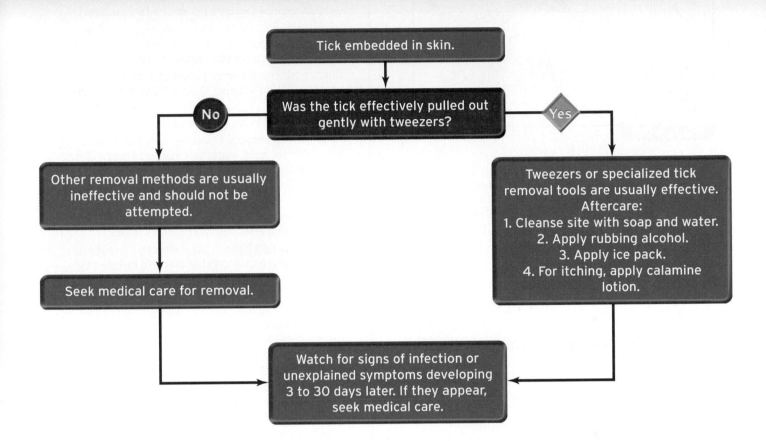

Tick embedded in skin.

Was the tick effectively pulled out gently with tweezers?

No

Yes

Other removal methods are usually ineffective and should not be attempted.

Tweezers or specialized tick removal tools are usually effective.
Aftercare:
1. Cleanse site with soap and water.
2. Apply rubbing alcohol.
3. Apply ice pack.
4. For itching, apply calamine lotion.

Seek medical care for removal.

Watch for signs of infection or unexplained symptoms developing 3 to 30 days later. If they appear, seek medical care.

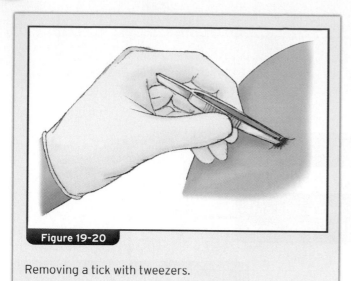

Figure 19-20

Removing a tick with tweezers.

4. For 1 month, continue to watch the bite site for a rash. If a rash appears, seek medical care. Watch for other signs such as fever, muscle aches, sensitivity to bright light, and paralysis that begins with leg weakness.

FYI

The Knot Method of Tick Removal

An embedded tick should be removed as soon as possible. The longer an infected tick stays embedded, the more likely it is to transmit a disease. An alternative to using tweezers and special commercial tick removal devices, especially when they are not available, is the knot method.

Use cotton thread or dental floss and tie an overhand knot (similar to a shoelace knot without the bows). The open overhand knot is placed over the tick as close as possible to the skin surface and then gently closed to form a loop around the tick. Lift the tick's body over its head in a somersault-type fashion to remove the tick. This method removes the entire tick and is simple and effective.

Source: Celensa A: The knot method of tick removal. *Wilderness Environ Med* 13(2):181.

FYI

Preventing Tick Bites

- Wear light-colored clothing so you can see any ticks on your clothes.
- Wear a long-sleeved shirt that fits tightly at the wrists and neck and tuck the shirt into your pants.
- Wear long pants and tuck the pant legs into your boots or socks, or use masking tape to tape the pant legs tightly to your socks, shoes, or boots.
- Check your clothes while you are outdoors and before entering a house. Wash your clothes as soon as possible.
- Inspect your pets for ticks before they come inside.
- After coming indoors, shower or bathe and check your body for ticks, especially in areas that have hair or where clothing was tight. Another person could do the checking.
- Treat your body and clothing with a repellent. The most common, Environmental Protection Agency–approved, and effective tick repellent is DEET.
- You can buy DEET and apply it directly to your skin. Ticks crawling on the treated area are irritated by the repellent and drop off. DEET is most effective against ticks when applied to clothing from a spray can.
- There have been a few reports of adverse toxic reactions to DEET, such as seizures, allergic responses, and skin irritation. To minimize reactions, do the following:
  - Apply DEET sparingly to your skin.
  - Avoid applying high-concentration products (more than 35% DEET) to the skin.
  - Do not inhale or ingest DEET-containing products or get them in your eyes.
  - Do not apply DEET to wounds or irritated skin.
  - Wash your skin after coming indoors.
  - Do not use products with more than 10% DEET on infants and small children (younger than 5 years).
- You can also use 0.5% preparations of permethrin (a pesticide). Permethrin should be applied only to clothing (especially shirt sleeves, pants legs, and collars), never directly on the skin.

CAUTION

DO NOT use the following popular methods of tick removal, which are useless:
- Applying petroleum jelly
- Applying fingernail polish
- Applying rubbing alcohol
- Touching a hot match to the tick
- Applying a petroleum product, such as gasoline

DO NOT grab a tick at the rear of its body. The internal organs could rupture, and the contents could be squeezed out, causing infection.

DO NOT twist or jerk the tick, which could result in incomplete removal.

FYI

Commercial Tick Removal Tools

Original Ticked Off, Pro-Tick Remedy, and Tick Plier, also called the Tick Nipper, three commercially available tick removal tools, were compared against medium-tipped tweezers. All tools removed adult ticks of both the American dog and lone star species successfully. American dog ticks proved easier to remove than the lone star ticks, whose mouthparts often remained in the skin. The researchers concluded that commercial tick removal tools could remove nymphs (too small to see with the human eye), as well as adults. A magnifying glass is necessary to see the nymph. Some of the tools have a built in magnifying glass.

Source: Stewart RL, et al: Evaluation of three commercial tick removal tools. *Wilderness Environ Med* 9(4):137-142.

FYI

Fire Ants

Fire ants are aggressive, will defensively attack anything that disturbs them, and can sting repeatedly **Figure 19-21**. The fire ant bites its victim by securing itself to the skin with its mandibles, causing pain, then, using its head as a pivot, the ant swings its abdomen in an arc, repeatedly stinging the victim with an abdominal stinger. Up to 40% of the people who live in infested urban areas are stung each year, and more than 30 deaths have been attributed to these insect bites.

The fire ant sting usually produces immediate pain and a red, swollen area, which disappears within 45 minutes **Figure 19-22**. A blister then forms, rupturing in 30 to 70 hours, and the area often becomes infected. In some cases, a red, swollen, itchy patch develops instead of a blister. Although the stings are not usually life threatening, they are easily infected and can leave permanent scars.

Some people become sensitive to fire ant stings and should seek the advice of an allergist. Anaphylaxis (a life-threatening allergic reaction) occurs in about 1-2% of people stung by fire ants. Therefore, if a sting leads to shortness of breath, tightness and swelling in the throat, tightness in the chest, increased pulse rate, swelling of the tongue and mouth, dizziness, or nausea, the person should be taken to a hospital emergency department immediately. Some people lapse into a coma from even one sting.

First aid for fire ant stings includes placing an ice cube over the sting to reduce the pain and to slow absorption of the venom. A topical corticosteroid cream can help combat local swelling and itching. An antihistamine can prevent some local symptoms if given early, but it works too slowly to counteract a life-threatening allergic reaction. People who are allergic to stings should always carry a kit with antihistamine tablets and a preloaded syringe of epinephrine.

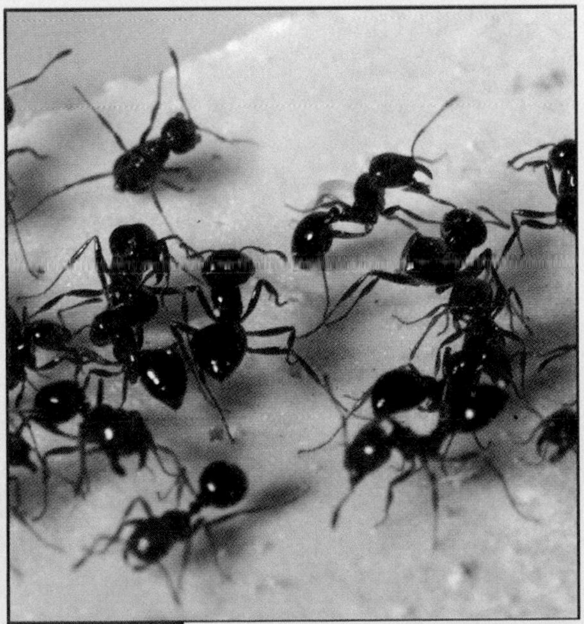

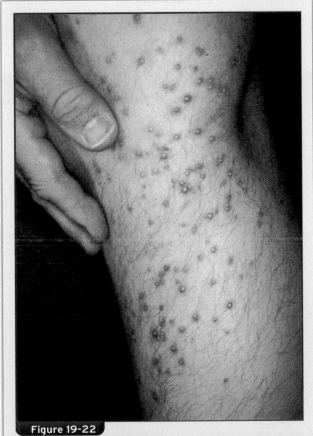

Figure 19-22

Fire ant stings.

Figure 19-21

Fire ant.

▶ Marine Animal Injuries

Most marine animals bite or sting in defense, rather than attack. Marine venoms are similar to many venoms found in reptiles and arthropods and can cause anaphylaxis or other types of reactions. The general first aid guidelines are similar to those for any disorder involving trauma, allergy, or cardiopulmonary failure. Serious allergic reactions require primary attention to keeping the airway open.

Sharks

Sharks are the most feared of all marine animals, but the chance of being attacked by a shark along the North American coastline is less than 1 in 5,000,000 Table 19-4. Although exact figures are unavailable, it is estimated that, worldwide, more than 50 attacks and fewer than a dozen deaths occur each year. The number of unprovoked shark attacks has grown at a steady rate over the past century.

Most attacks occur within 100 feet of shore, and most victims are attacked by a single shark without warning. In the majority of attacks, the victim does not see the shark before the attack Figure 19-23. The leg is the most frequently bitten part. Sharks are clearly more attracted to people on the surface than to underwater scuba divers.

Table 19-4	Preventing Shark Attacks

No shark repellents are universally effective. Explosive and electronic devices could threaten diver safety instead of sharks. The following guidelines can help prevent shark attacks:

- Avoid swimming in areas frequented by sharks or where shark attacks have occurred. (In the United States, the greatest concentration of great white shark attacks is off the northern California coast.)
- Do not swim or dive alone.
- Do not swim far offshore, in murky water, or incautiously along deep drop-offs.
- People with open wounds and menstruating women should avoid swimming in areas where there is risk of a shark attack.
- Avoid swimming in the vicinity of seal or sea lion colonies or turtle habitats.
- Do not spear fish for an extended period in the same area, and do not attach fish to your body.
- Avoid swimming at dawn, dusk, or night in potentially dangerous waters.

The greatest attraction for sharks seems to be chemicals found in fish blood—sharks can detect them in quantities as small as one part per million parts of water. Shark bite wounds, among the most devastating of all animal bites, are similar to injuries caused by boat propellers and chainsaws. Immediate control of bleeding and treatment for shock are essential.

Recognizing a Shark Bite

Most victims are attacked by single sharks, violently and without warning. In most attacks the victim does not see the shark before the attack. Signs include:

- Severe bleeding
- Large, open wounds, most often on the legs
- Abrasions caused by contact with sharkskin

Care for Victims of a Shark Bite or Puncture

To care for a victim of shark bite or puncture:

1. Control bleeding.
2. Treat for shock.
3. Seek medical care.

Barracudas and Moray Eels

Barracudas have a fearsome appearance, but they have an undeserved reputation as attackers of humans. The risk of a barracuda bite is exceedingly small. First aid for a barracuda bite is identical to that for a shark bite.

Moray eels also have a fierce appearance. They are not infrequent biters of divers who handle or tease them, usually in competition for food or in pursuit of lobsters. The multiple puncture wounds created by moray eel bites have a high infection risk. Treat these wounds as you would shark bites.

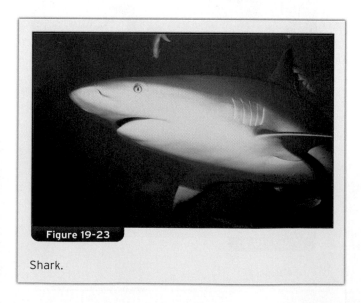

Figure 19-23

Shark.

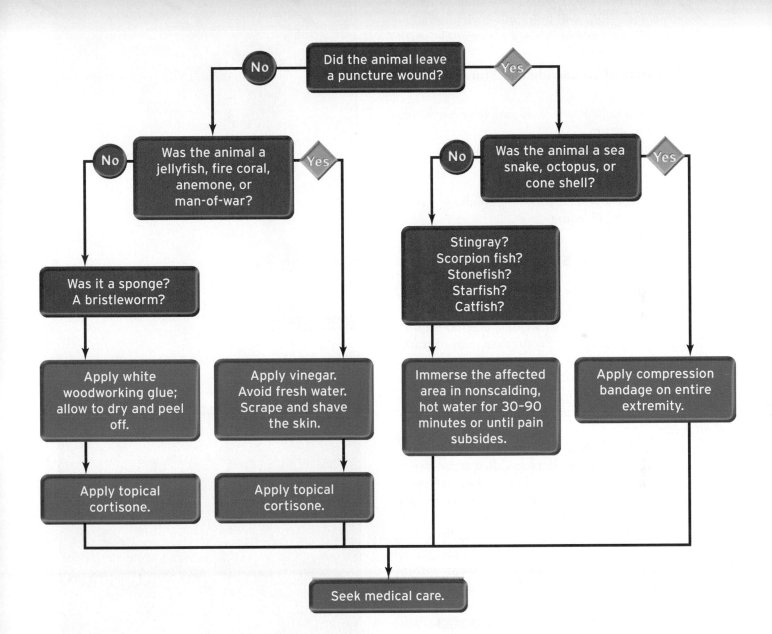

Recognizing Barracuda and Moray Eel Bites

Barracuda and moray eel bites have the following characteristics:

- Barracuda lacerations are similar to those of a shark.
- Eel bites involve severe puncture wounds with their narrow jaws. Eels will hold onto a victim, rather than strike and release. They leave multiple, small puncture wounds.

Care for Victims of Barracuda and Moray Eel Bites

The following list indicates how to care for a barracuda or moray eel bite victim.

- Care for a barracuda bites as you would a shark bite.
- Care for an eel bite by:
  - Flushing the wound with water under pressure.
  - Controlling bleeding.

Marine Animals That Sting

Stings from marine animals lead the list of adverse marine animal encounters. It is important to identify the offending animal, because in many cases, first aid is quite specific. Each year, jellyfish, Portuguese man-of-wars, corals, and anemones that lie along the shallow ocean waters of the United States sting more than 1 million people. Reactions to being stung vary from mild dermatitis to severe reactions. Most victims recover without medical attention.

Jellyfish and Portuguese man-of-wars have long tentacles equipped with stinging devices called *nematocysts*. When cast ashore or onto rocks, detached nematocysts retain their ability to sting for a long time, usually until they are completely dried out.

The Portuguese man-of-war sting is usually in the form of well-defined linear welts or scattered patches of welts with redness, which usually disappear within 24 hours **Figure 19-24**. The jellyfish sting produces severe muscle cramping with multiple, thin lines of welts crossing the skin in a zigzag pattern **Figure 19-25**. Pain usually is a burning type that lasts 10 to 30 minutes. The welts on the skin usually disappear within an hour. Anemones are beautiful but potentially dangerous **Figure 19-26**. Many anemone stings result from the improper handling of aquarium animals.

Recognizing Marine Stings

Marine stings cause the following symptoms:

- stinging
- severe itching, burning
- prickling, tingling
- blisters

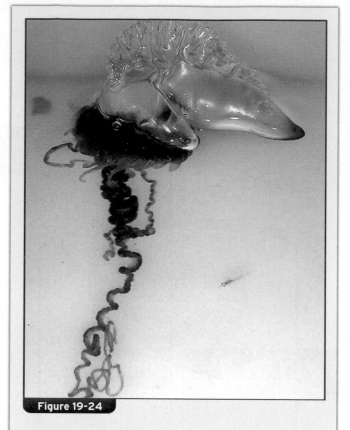

Figure 19-24

Portuguese man-of-war.

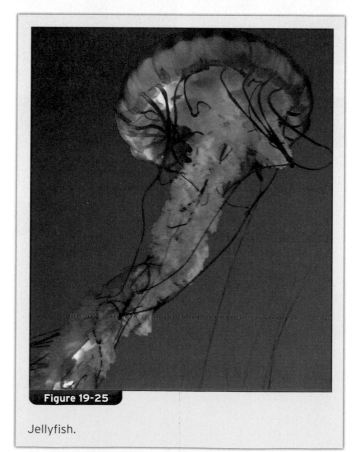

Figure 19-25

Jellyfish.

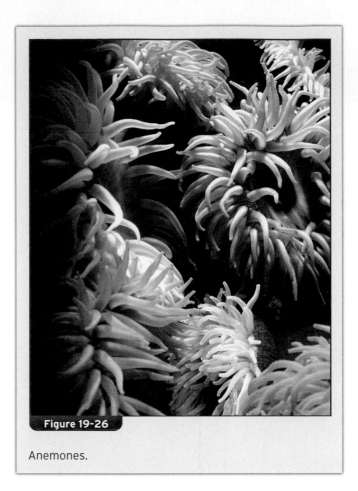

Figure 19-26

Anemones.

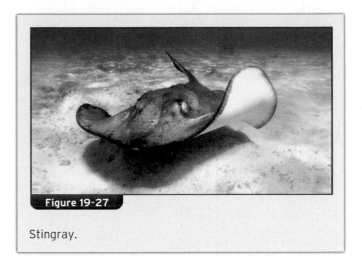

Figure 19-27

Stingray.

- severe allergic reaction
- difficulty breathing
- muscle cramping
- nausea, vomiting

Care for Victims of Marine Stings

Follow these steps to care for a victim of a marine sting:

1. Apply vinegar or alcohol to the sting area; it deactivates the nematocysts.
2. Immediately scrape off any tentacles remaining on the skin by using a credit card, stick, comb, knife blade, or similar object, or apply shaving cream or a baking soda paste and shave the area. For large tentacles, use tweezers or pliers.
3. Reapply vinegar or alcohol, and soak the area for 15 minutes.
4. Monitor breathing.

Stingrays

Stingrays, commonly found in tropical and subtropical waters, are peaceful, reclusive bottom feeders that generally lie buried in the sand or mud **Figure 19-27**. Most wounds inflicted by stingrays are produced on the ankle or foot when the victim steps on a ray. The ray reacts by thrusting its barbed tail upward and forward into the victim's leg or foot. At least 1,500 stingray injuries occur each year in coastal US waters. The stingray's venomous tail barb easily penetrates human skin. The sting usually is more like a laceration because the large tail barb can do significant damage. The venom causes intense burning pain at the site.

Recognizing a Stingray Puncture

A stingray puncture results in the following:

- Sudden, intense pain
- An open wound
- Swelling

Care for Stingray Puncture Victims

You can care for stingray puncture victims by doing the following:

1. Relieve pain by immersing the injured body part in hot water (110° F) for 30 to 90 minutes. Make sure the water is not hot enough to cause a burn.
2. Wash the wound with soap and water.
3. Irrigate the area with water under pressure to wash out as much of the toxin and foreign material as possible.
4. Treat the wound like any puncture wound.

▶ Bites and Stings

What to Look For	What to Do
Animal and human bites • Torn tissue • Bleeding	1. Wash wound with soap and water with water. 2. Flush wound thoroughly under pressure. 3. Control bleeding. 4. Seek medical care.
Poisonous snake bites • Severe, burning pain • Small puncture wounds • Swelling • Nausea, vomiting, sweating, weakness • Discoloration and blood-filled blisters developing hours after the bite	1. Get away from the snake. 2. Limit victim's movement and keep bitten extremity below heart level. 3. Call 9-1-1. 4. Gently wash area with soap and water. 5. For a coral snake bite, apply mild pressure by wrapping the entire affected arm or leg with an elastic bandage.
Insect stings • Pain • Itching • Swelling • Severe allergic reaction, including breathing problems	1. Scrape away any stinger. 2. Wash with soap and water. 3. Apply an ice or cold pack. 4. Give pain medication, hydrocortisone cream, and an antihistamine. 5. Observe for at least 30 minutes for signs of severe allergic reaction. Call 9-1-1 if a severe allergic reaction occurs. If victim has an epinephrine auto-injector, help victim use it.

Spider bites
• Black widow
  • May feel sharp pain
  • Two small fang marks
  • Severe abdominal pain
  • Headache, chills, fever, sweating, dizziness, nausea
• Brown recluse and hobo
  • Blister developing several days later
  • Ulcer in skin
  • Headache, fever, weakness, nausea
	1. Catch spider for identification.
	2. Wash bitten area with soap and water.
	3. Apply an ice or cold pack.
	4. Seek medical care.

Scorpion stings • Pain and burning at sting site • Later, numbness or tingling	1. Wash sting site with soap and water. 2. Apply an ice or cold pack. 3. Seek medical care.
Tick bites • Tick still attached • Rash (especially one shaped like a bull's-eye) • Fever, joint aches, weakness	1. Remove tick. 2. Wash bitten area with soap and water. 3. Apply rubbing alcohol. 4. Apply an ice or cold pack. 5. Watch bitten area for 1 month for rash. Seek medical care if rash or other signs such as fever or muscle joint aches appear.

▶ Marine Animal Injuries

What to Look For	What to Do
Bites, rips, or punctures from marine animals (for example, sharks, barracudas, moray eels)	1. Control bleeding. 2. Care for shock. 3. Call 9-1-1.
Stings from marine animals (for example, jellyfish, Portuguese man-of-war)	1. Scrape off tentacles. 2. Apply vinegar.
Punctures from marine animal spines (for example, stingray)	1. Immerse injured part in hot water for 30 to 90 minutes. 2. Wash with soap and water. 3. Flush with water under pressure. 4. Care for wound.

▶ Ready for Review

- Almost half of all Americans will suffer a bite from either an animal or human.
- Throughout the world, about 50,000 people die each year of snake bites.
- The stinging insects belonging to the order of *Hymenoptera* include honeybees, bumblebees, yellow jackets, hornets, wasps, and fire ants.
- Most spiders are venomous, which is how they paralyze and kill their prey. However, most spiders lack an effective delivery system—long fangs and strong jaws—to bite a human.
- Most marine animals bite or sting in defense, rather than attack.

▶ Vital Vocabulary

<u>antivenin</u> An antiserum containing antibodies against reptile or insect venom.

<u>nematocysts</u> Stinging cells found on certain marine animals.

<u>rabies</u> An acute viral infection of the central nervous system transmitted by the bite of an infected animal.

▶ Assessment in Action

A child has been attacked by a large dog at a local park. The dog has run off into the woods. At least one bystander recognized the dog and believes she knows the owner. You find several dog bite marks on the child's legs and arms.

Directions: Circle Yes if you agree with the statement, circle No if you disagree.

Yes   No   1. Seek medical care for the child.

Yes   No   2. You should call animal control or the police.

Yes   No   3. The dog should be observed for possible rabies.

Yes   No   4. You should control bleeding and care for shock.

Yes   No   5. Dogs account for most animal bite injuries.

Answers: 1. Yes; 2. Yes; 3. Yes; 4. Yes; 5. Yes

▶ Check Your Knowledge

Directions: Circle Yes if you agree with the statement, circle No if you disagree.

Yes   No   1. Severe abdominal pain is a sign of a black widow spider bite.

Yes   No   2. Apply an ice or cold pack over a snake bite.

Yes   No   3. Use the cut and suck method for a snake bite.

Yes   No   4. Remove a bee's stinger by using tweezers to pull it out.

Yes   No   5. Apply an ice or cold pack over an insect sting or a suspected spider bite.

Yes   No   6. A baking soda paste can help reduce the itching and swelling from an insect sting.

Yes   No   7. A victim's prescribed auto-injector might have to be used if the victim has a life-threatening reaction to an insect sting.

Yes   No   8. Care for stings from marine animals (for example, jellyfish) by pouring hydrogen peroxide on the affected area.

Yes   No   9. Covering an embedded tick with petroleum jelly causes the tick to back out because of the lack of oxygen.

Yes   No   10. Ticks can transmit disease.

Answers: 1. Yes; 2. No; 3. No; 4. No; 5. Yes; 6. Yes; 7. Yes; 8. No; 9. No; 10. Yes

Cold-Related Emergencies

Cold-Related Emergencies

Heat flows from an area with a higher temperature to an area with a lower temperature. When a person is surrounded by air or water cooler than body temperature, the body loses heat. If heat escapes faster than the body produces heat, the body temperature falls. Normal body temperature is 98.6° F, and if the body temperature falls much below that, cold injuries can result.

► How Cold Affects the Body

Humans protect themselves from cold primarily by avoiding or reducing cold exposure through the use of clothing and shelter. When that protection proves inadequate, the body has biologic defense mechanisms to help maintain correct body temperature. The internal mechanisms to maintain body temperature during cold exposure include vasoconstriction and shivering. Triggering of these responses is a signal that clothing and shelter are inadequate.

__Vasoconstriction__ is the tightening of blood vessels. During cold exposure, vasoconstriction occurs in the exposed skin. The reduced blood flow in the skin conserves body heat but can lead to discomfort, numbness, loss of dexterity in the hands and fingers, and, eventually, cold injuries.

Cold triggers shivering, which increases internal heat production and helps offset the heat lost. Shivering is the body's main involuntary defense against the cold. Shivering produces body heat by forcing muscles to contract and relax rapidly. About 80% of the muscle energy used in shivering is turned into body heat. When the core temperature rises, shivering is no longer needed and is shut down by the brain. When the core temperature falls to about 86–90° F, the shivering reflex stops. Likewise, when there is no further fuel for the body, shivering stops. Several drugs suppress the shivering response, including barbiturates, narcotics, beta-blocking agents, and alcohol.

Internal heat production is also increased by physical activity; the more vigorous the activity, the greater the heat production. In fact, heat production during intense exercise or strenuous work usually is sufficient to completely compensate for heat loss, even when it is extremely cold. However, high-intensity exercise and hard physical work are fatiguing, and cannot be sustained indefinitely. If clothes become wet with sweat, heat loss is markedly increased after exertion.

Susceptibility to cold injuries can be minimized by maintaining proper hydration and nutrition; avoiding alcohol, caffeine, and nicotine; and limiting periods of inactivity in cold conditions. Humans do not acclimatize to cold weather nearly as well as they acclimatize to hot weather.

The colder the surrounding temperature, the greater the potential for body heat to escape. When the skin is exposed to cold, the brain signals the blood vessels in the skin to tighten, and blood flow to the skin decreases. This is the body's attempt to prevent heat inside the body from being carried to the skin, where it will be lost. However, because of reduced blood flow to the skin, the skin temperature falls.

When cold exposure lasts more than an hour, cooling of the skin and reduced blood flow to the hands will blunt sensation, touch, and pain, and will cause a loss of dexterity and agility. These changes can impair a person's ability to perform manual tasks and, because symptoms could go unnoticed, can lead to more severe cold injuries.

Heat Loss From the Body

Normal body temperature is maintained by a balance of heat production and heat loss. Heat is produced by food metabolism and muscle activity, and shivering can increase heat production up to 500%. Shivering causes a large increase in heat production, but it rapidly consumes calories stored in the liver and muscles as glycogen. Lack of food limits the body's ability to produce heat; when glycogen stores are depleted, heat output decreases.

Heat loss occurs primarily through the skin. Blood flow to the skin varies in different parts of the body, and some areas lose more heat than others. Thermograms demonstrate high losses from the head and neck (up to 50%), axillary area (armpits), and groin area. The constriction of blood vessels caused by cold conserves heat.

Body heat can be lost by four mechanisms:

- Conduction, or direct contact with a colder object (for example, lying on the snow), normally accounts for only a small fraction of heat loss. The exception is immersion in cold water, in which heat loss can be 25 to 30 times greater than in air and even more in moving water.
- Convection is the loss of heat from the body by air blowing over the skin or through porous clothing. **Windchill** is the combined effect of the ambient temperature and wind speed.
- Evaporation, or conversion of liquid on the skin to a vapor, normally accounts for about 20% of heat loss (two thirds through sweating and one third through respiration).
- Radiation is the primary method of heat loss, accounting for about 65% of the body's heat loss. A warm object gives off (radiates) heat to cooler air. It has been demonstrated that up to 50% of the body's total heat production can be lost by radiation through a person's unprotected head **Figure 20-1** .

Susceptibility to Cold Injury

A person's susceptibility to cold injury is affected by many factors. Physically unfit people are more susceptible to cold injury. They tire more quickly and are unable to stay active to keep warm as long as people who are physically fit.

Dehydration reduces blood flow in the skin, which increases susceptibility to cold injury. Fat functions as an

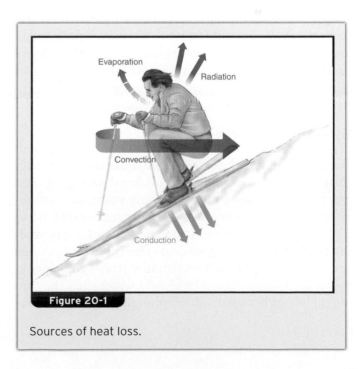

Figure 20-1

Sources of heat loss.

insulator against heat loss because it has less blood flow than muscle and loses less heat. Therefore, a very lean person may can be susceptible to the effects of cold, if clothing is inadequate or wet, or if the person is relatively inactive. Elderly people are less tolerant of the cold than younger people because of the decline in physical fitness that often occurs with aging.

Alcohol and, to a lesser extent, caffeine cause the blood vessels in the skin to open, which can accelerate body heat loss. Also, alcohol and caffeine both increase urine formation, leading to dehydration, which can further degrade the body's defenses against cold. Most important, alcohol blunts the senses and impairs judgment, so a person may might not feel the signs and symptoms of developing cold injury.

Because nicotine decreases blood flow to the skin, smoking and chewing tobacco can increase susceptibility to frostbite. Inadequate nutrition, illness, and injury compromise the body's responses to cold and a person's ability to recognize and react appropriately to the symptoms of developing cold injury. People who have experienced a cold injury are at greater risk of experiencing another cold injury.

Effects of Altitude

Assessing weather conditions in mountainous regions must include altitude considerations, especially if the assessment is based on weather measurements obtained at lower elevations. Temperatures, windchill, and the risk of cold injury at high altitudes can differ considerably from those at lower elevations.

In general, it can be assumed that air temperature drops 3.6° F every 1,000 feet above the original measurement site. Winds usually are more severe at high altitudes, and there is less cover above the tree line. People are more susceptible to frostbite and other cold injuries at altitudes above 8,000 feet than at sea level because of lower temperatures, higher winds, and less oxygen.

Effects of Water

Water can conduct heat away from the body much faster than air of the same temperature. When clothing becomes wet because of snow, rain, splashing water, or accumulated sweat, the body's loss of heat is accelerated, up to 25 times faster. Swimmers and people working or wading in water can lose a great deal of body heat, even when the water temperature is only mildly cool. People working in cold water should be closely watched as they enter the water because sudden plunging into cold water

can produce an irregular heartbeat, gasping, and hyperventilation, which can cause inhalation of water, heart failure, and drowning.

Effects of Wind

For any given air temperature, the potential for body heat loss, skin cooling, and decreased internal temperature is increased by wind. Wind increases heat loss from skin exposed to cold air, in effect lowering the temperature. The windchill index integrates wind speed and air temperature to provide an estimate of the cooling power of the environment and the associated risk of cold injury.

Windchill temperatures obtained from weather reports do not take into account artificial wind, which worsens the windchill effect of natural wind. For example, riding in an open vehicle can subject the passengers to dangerous windchill, even when natural winds are low.

Effects of Metals and Liquid Fuels

Metal objects and liquid fuels that have been left outdoors in the cold pose a serious hazard. Both can conduct heat away from the skin rapidly. Fuels and solvents remain liquid at very low temperatures. Skin contact with fuel or metal at below-freezing temperatures can result in nearly instantaneous freezing. Fuel handlers must use great care and not allow exposed skin to come into contact with spilled fuels or metals.

Minimizing Effects of Cold on the Body

When adequately protected, humans can tolerate temperatures as low as −72° F. Adequate clothing maintains the microclimate surrounding the body. Air is an excellent insulator, and the basis for most clothing is to trap a layer of air around the body. Layering, which has been used for centuries, allows the removal or opening of a garment to vent excess heat during times of greater activity or changes in environment, and it accommodates individual needs and preferences. Wearing layered clothing is especially important for people who frequently change environments by going in and out of buildings or who periodically undertake vigorous physical activity.

Three important layers are recommended for most outdoor activities. The first layer (undergarments) removes perspiration from the skin, the middle layers insulate, and the outer layer or outer shell protects against wind. By understanding this principle, people can vary their clothing for protection and comfort.

For the first layer, use underwear that wicks away perspiration, that is, it stays dry by drawing moisture away from the skin to the next layer of clothing. Wet clothing transfers heat away from the body. Cotton holds moisture next to the skin, so the person feels cold and clammy. Silk feels warm and soft, but it also retains moisture. Fabrics such as polypropylene or one of the new types of polyesters such as Capilene or Thermax should be considered.

The middle layer can be a synthetic pile or fleece jacket that is warm and dries quickly or a wool or synthetic sweater. Synthetic insulating materials, unlike down or wool, provide warmth without bulk or heavy weight. Insulation should be effective even when wet. In that respect, synthetics are clearly superior to natural fibers and natural products. Duck or goose down, for example, is virtually useless when wet, and it dries slowly. One exception, however, is the insulating ability of wool, even when wet.

Physically active people can sweat even in extremely cold weather. Therefore, the best choice for an outside layer is a jacket that is waterproof, wind resistant, and "breathable." Materials such as Gore-Tex allow perspiration to evaporate. A zipper is preferable, so the clothing can be opened easily to increase ventilation. Nylon and vinyl are poor choices because they produce a sauna effect by holding in perspiration. Because the head loses more body heat than any other part (up to 50%), heed the admonition, "If the feet are cold, cover the head." A wool or synthetic cap serves well.

▶ Nonfreezing Cold Injuries

Nonfreezing cold injuries can occur when conditions are cold and wet (air temperatures between 32° F and 55° F) and the hands and feet cannot be kept warm and dry. The most prominent nonfreezing cold injuries are chilblain and trench foot.

Chilblain

Chilblain is a nonfreezing cold injury that, while painful, causes little or no permanent damage. Chilblain can develop in 3 to 6 hours in skin exposed to cold and moisture.

Recognizing Chilblain

The signs of chilblain include:
- swollen skin
- tender, hot to the touch, and possibly itchy skin
- blisters might form

- condition can worsen to an aching, prickly (pins and needles) sensation and then numbness

Care for a Victim of Chilblain

To care for a victim of chilblain, get victim out of the cold.

Trench Foot

Trench foot (also called immersion foot) is a serious non-freezing cold injury that develops when the skin on the feet is exposed to moisture and cold for prolonged periods (12 hours or longer). Wearing wet boots or shoes and socks causes trench foot; prolonged immersion of the feet in cold water causes immersion foot. The combination of cold and moisture softens the skin, causing tissue loss and, often, infection. The risk of this potentially crippling

FYI

If a Blizzard Traps You in Your Car
- Pull off the road. Turn on hazard lights and hang a distress flag from the radio aerial or window.
- Remain in your vehicle, where rescuers are most likely to find you. Do not set out on foot unless you can see a building close by where you know you can take shelter. Be careful: distances are distorted by blowing snow. A building might seem close but be too far to walk to in deep snow.
- Run the engine and heater about 10 minutes each hour to keep warm. When the engine is running, open a window slightly for ventilation. This will protect you from possible carbon monoxide poisoning. Periodically clear snow from the exhaust pipe.
- Exercise to maintain body heat, but avoid overexertion. In extreme cold, use road maps, seat covers, and floor mats for insulation. Huddle with passengers and use your coat for a blanket.
- If others are with you, take turns sleeping. One person should be awake at all times to look for rescue crews.
- Drink fluids to avoid dehydration.
- Be careful not to waste battery power. Balance electrical energy needs—the use of lights, heat and radio—with supply.
- At night, turn on the inside light so work crews or rescuers can see you.
- If stranded in a remote area, spread a large cloth over the snow to attract attention of rescue personnel who might be surveying the area by airplane.
- Once the blizzard passes, you might need to leave the car and proceed on foot.

Source: Federal Emergency Management Agency.

injury is high during wet weather. People who wear rubberized or tight-fitting boots are at risk for trench foot regardless of weather conditions, because sweat accumulates inside the boots and keeps the feet wet.

Recognizing Trench Foot (also called Immersion Foot)

Signs of trench foot include:
- itching, numbness, or tingling pain
- swollen feet and pale skin that feels cold when touched
- red or bluish blotches on the skin, sometimes with open weeping or bleeding

Care for Someone With Trench Foot (also called Immersion Foot)

Care for someone with trench foot includes these guidelines:
1. Dry the skin.
2. Rewarm the foot gradually.
3. Care for open weeping areas by cleansing with mild soap and water and applying breathable dressings.

▶ Freezing Cold Injuries

Freezing cold injuries can occur whenever the air temperature is below freezing (32° F). Freezing limited to the skin surface is <u>frostnip</u>. Freezing that extends deeper through the skin and into the flesh is <u>frostbite</u>.

Frostbite is prevalent during military campaigns and is a known hazard for mountain climbers and explorers. As more people pursue cross-country skiing, snowmobiling, and other outdoor winter sports, the number of frostbite cases probably will increase. However, it is still thought to be rare in nonmilitary situations.

Frostnip

Frostnip is caused when water on the skin surface freezes. Frostnip should be taken seriously because it could be the first sign of impending frostbite.

Recognizing Frostnip

It is difficult to tell the difference between frostnip and frostbite. Signs of frostnip include:
- Skin appears red and sometimes swollen.
- Painful, but usually no further damage after rewarming.
- Repeated frostnip in the same spot can dry the skin, causing it to crack and become sensitive.

Care for a Frostnip Victim

To care for a frostnip victim:
1. Gently warm the affected area by placing it against a warm body part (for example, put bare hands

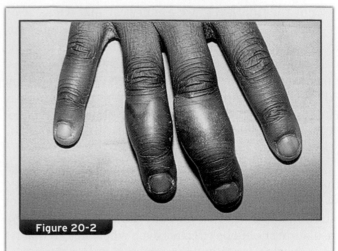

Figure 20-2

Frostbitten fingers, 6 hours after rewarming in 108°F water.

under the armpits or on the stomach) or by blowing warm air on the area. After rewarming, the affected area can be red and tingling.
2. Do not rub the affected area.

Frostbite

Frostbite happens only in below freezing temperatures. Tissue is not composed of water alone, so it will not freeze until it has been cooled to about 28° F. Tissue is damaged in two ways: (1) actual tissue freezing, which results in the formation of ice crystals within the tissue (the ice crystals expand as they freeze, damaging cells), and (2) the obstruction of the blood supply to the tissue, which causes sludged blood clots and further prevents blood from flowing to the tissues. The second type of tissue damage is more extensive than the first. In severely cold temperatures, flesh can freeze in less than a minute **Figure 20-2**.

Frostbite affects mainly the feet, hands, ears, and nose. These areas do not contain large heat-producing muscles and are some distance from the body's heat-generation sources. The most severe consequences of frostbite occur when tissue dies (gangrene), and the affected part might have to be amputated.

Recognizing Frostbite

The severity and extent of frostbite are difficult to judge until hours after thawing. Frostbite can be classified as superficial or deep before thawing.

The signs and symptoms of superficial frostbite are as follows:
- The skin is white, waxy, or grayish yellow.
- The affected part feels very cold and numb. There might be tingling, stinging, or an aching sensation.

CAUTION

DO NOT use water hotter than 108° F—burns can result.

DO NOT use water cooler than 100° F—it will not thaw frostbite rapidly enough.

DO NOT break any blisters.

DO NOT rub or massage the affected part—ice crystals can be pushed into body cells, rupturing them.

DO NOT rub the affected part with ice or snow.

DO NOT rewarm the part with a heating pad, hot-water bottle, stove, sunlamp, radiator, or exhaust pipe or over a fire. Excessive temperatures cannot be controlled, and burns can result.

DO NOT allow the victim to drink alcoholic beverages. Alcohol dilates blood vessels and causes loss of body heat.

DO NOT allow the victim to smoke. Smoking constricts blood vessels, thus impairing circulation.

DO NOT rewarm if there is any possibility of refreezing.

DO NOT allow the thawed part to refreeze because the ice crystals formed will be larger and more damaging. If refreezing is likely or even possible, it is better to leave the affected part frozen.

DO NOT use the dry rewarming technique (putting the victim's hands in your armpits) because that takes three to four times longer than the wet, rapid method to thaw frozen tissue. Slow rewarming results in greater tissue damage than rapid rewarming.

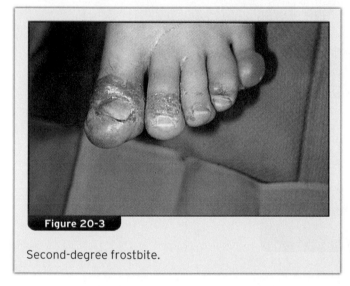

Figure 20-3

Second-degree frostbite.

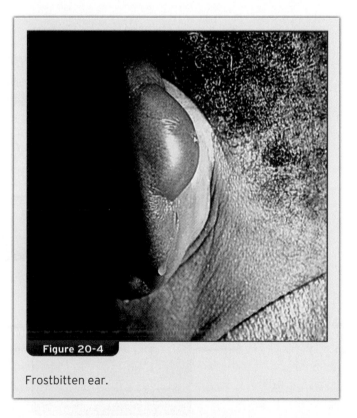

Figure 20-4

Frostbitten ear.

- The skin surface feels stiff or crusty and the underlying tissue soft when depressed gently and firmly.

The following signs and symptoms indicate deep frostbite:

- The affected part feels cold, hard, and solid and cannot be depressed—it feels like a piece of wood or frozen meat.
- Blisters might appear after rewarming.
- The affected part is cold, with pale, waxy skin.
- A painfully cold part suddenly stops hurting.

After a part has thawed, frostbite can be categorized by degrees, similar to the classification of burns. First-degree frostbite is superficial, and second-, third-, and fourth-degree frostbite are deeper.

- First-degree frostbite: The affected part is warm, swollen, and tender.

- Second-degree frostbite: Blisters form minutes to hours after thawing and enlarge over several days **Figure 20-3** and **Figure 20-4**.
- Third-degree frostbite: Blisters are small and contain reddish blue or purplish fluid. The surrounding skin can be red or blue and might not blanch when pressure is applied.
- Fourth-degree frostbite: No blisters or swelling occur. The part remains numb, cold, and white to dark purple.

Frostbite

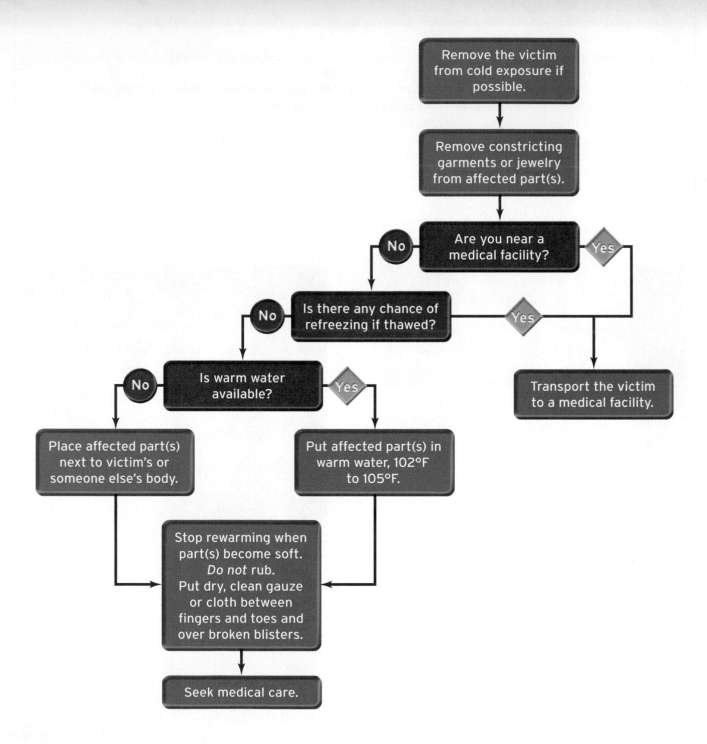

Remove the victim from cold exposure if possible.

↓

Remove constricting garments or jewelry from affected part(s).

↓

Are you near a medical facility? — **No** / **Yes**

No → **Is there any chance of refreezing if thawed?** — **Yes**

Yes → Transport the victim to a medical facility.

Is there any chance of refreezing if thawed? — **No**

No → **Is warm water available?** — **Yes**

No → Place affected part(s) next to victim's or someone else's body.

Yes → Put affected part(s) in warm water, 102°F to 105°F.

Stop rewarming when part(s) become soft. *Do not* rub. Put dry, clean gauze or cloth between fingers and toes and over broken blisters.

↓

Seek medical care.

Care for Frostbite Victims

All frostbite injuries require the same first aid treatment. Seek medical care immediately. Rewarming of frostbite should seldom be attempted outside a medical facility.

1. Get the victim out of the cold and to a warm place.
2. Remove any wet clothing or constricting items such as rings that could impair blood circulation.
3. Seek immediate medical care.
4. If the affected part is partially thawed or the victim is in a remote or wilderness situation (more than 1 hour from a medical facility), and you have warm water, use the following wet, rapid rewarming method. Place the frostbitten part in warm (102° F to 105° F) water. If you do not have a thermometer, pour some of the water over the inside of your arm or put your elbow into it to test that it is warm, not hot. Maintain water temperature by adding warm water as needed. Rewarming usually takes 20 to 40 minutes or until the tissues are soft. To help control the severe pain during rewarming, give the victim aspirin (adults only) or ibuprofen. For ear or facial injuries, apply warm, moist cloths, changing them frequently.
5. After thawing:
   - If the feet are affected, treat the victim as a stretcher case—the feet will be impossible to use after they are rewarmed.
   - Protect the affected area from contact with clothing and bedding.
   - Place dry, sterile gauze between the toes and the fingers to absorb moisture and keep them from sticking together.
   - Slightly elevate the affected part to reduce pain and swelling.
   - Apply aloe vera gel to promote skin healing.
   - Provide aspirin (adults only) ibuprofen or acetaminophen to limit pain and inflammation.

▶ Hypothermia

Body temperature falls when the body cannot produce heat as fast as it is lost. **Hypothermia** is a life-threatening condition in which the body's core temperature falls below 95° F. Generally, the core temperature will not fall until after many hours of continuous exposure to cold air, if the person is healthy, physically active, and reasonably dressed. However, because wet skin and wind accelerate body heat loss and the body produces less heat during inactive periods, the core body temperature can fall even when the air temperature is above freezing if conditions are windy, clothing is wet, or the person is inactive.

Hypothermia can occur year round. Most people think of hypothermia as related only to cold outdoor exposure. It can happen indoors, in the southern states, and even on a summer day. It does not require subfreezing temperatures.

Hypothermia happens when the body loses more heat than it produces. If the body temperature falls to 80° F, most people die. Hypothermia can occur in indoor or outdoor situations. Hypothermia occurs rapidly during cold-water immersion (1 hour or less when the water temperature is less than 45° F). Because water has a tremendous capacity to drain heat from the body, prolonged immersion (several hours) in even slightly cool water (less than 70° F) can cause hypothermia. Hypothermia is a medical emergency. Untreated, it results in death.

Even though hypothermic victims might have no heartbeat, breathing, or response to touch or pain, they may not be dead. Sometimes, the heartbeat and breathing of hypothermic victims will be so faint that they are not detected, because the unresponsiveness may be due to drowning, not hypothermia. When a hypothermic victim is found on land, however, take a little extra time to determine whether CPR really is required. Thus, it is important to take 30 to 45 seconds, instead of the usual 10, to check circulation. If hypothermia has resulted from submersion in cold water, cardiopulmonary resuscitation (CPR) should be started without delay. Hypothermic victims should be treated as gently as possible because rough handling can cause life-threatening disruptions in heart rate. All hypothermic victims, even those who do not seem to be alive, must be evaluated by a physician.

In the past, the people believed most vulnerable to hypothermia have been hunters, hikers, backpackers, careless drinkers, and accident victims. However, disadvantaged urban dwellers exposed to the elements and elderly persons with impaired thermoregulatory mechanisms also are susceptible. Lightly clad persons almost anywhere can quickly become chilled outdoors when it is raining, even though the temperatures are only cool, and people immersed for some time in cool or cold water lose heat even more readily. Even well-conditioned athletes such as long-distance runners can be victims. Hypothermia should be considered whenever the victim's behavior and history and the weather conditions indicate abnormal heat loss. Hypothermia is an underreported cause of death in the United States. In most cases, death is attributed to other factors, with hypothermia considered a secondary cause.

The victim's history may might be sufficient to determine hypothermia has occurred. Hypothermia is likely if a victim is reported by companions to be acting strangely and is shivering after exposure to cold or moisture or if he or she has been suddenly immersed in cold water. Predisposing factors are important: drinking alcoholic beverages is commonly associated with hypothermia. A typical scenario involves one or more people in lightweight garments who drink too much, fall asleep outdoors or in a poorly heated shelter, become chilled by cold air or moisture, and remain exposed for many hours. Certain medications predispose people to hypothermia because they interfere with the hypothalamus, which acts as the brain's thermostat in regulating body heat.

Especially vulnerable to hypothermia are very old and very young people. Infants and children have a small muscle mass, so the shivering response is poor in children and nonexistent in infants. They also have less body fat. Younger children need help to protect themselves against the cold because they cannot put on or take off clothes. People who are less fit are also more likely to become hypothermic.

Types of Exposure

There are three classifications of cold exposure:

- Acute exposure (also known as immersion) occurs when the victim loses body heat very rapidly, usually in water. Acute exposure is considered to be 6 hours or less.
- Subacute exposure (also known as mountain or exhaustion exposure) occurs when exposure is 6 to 24 hours and can be land or water based.
- Chronic exposure (also known as urban exposure) involves long-term cooling. It generally occurs on land and exceeds 24 hours.

Recognizing Hypothermia

Consider hypothermia in all victims who have been exposed to cold and who have altered mental status. Suspect hypothermia in any person who has a temperature less than 95° F. (Keep in mind that some thermometers do not measure below 95° F.) Shivering is a good clue, but it could be suppressed when energy stores (glycogen) are depleted. Suspect hypothermia in people with frostbite and those injured in a cold environment.

Some people die of hypothermia because they or those around them do not recognize the symptoms, which are difficult to recognize in the early stages. Here are some signs to watch for:

- *Change in mental status.* This is one of the first symptoms of developing hypothermia. Examples are disorientation, apathy, and changes in personality, such as unusual aggressiveness.

- *Shivering.* Shivering is the first, and most important, body defense against a falling body temperature. Shivering starts when the body temperature drops 1° F and can produce more heat than many rewarming methods. As the core temperature continues to fall, shivering decreases and usually stops at about 86° F. Shivering also stops as body temperature rises. If shivering stops as responsiveness decreases, assume that the core temperature is falling. If, on the other hand, shivering stops while the victim is becoming more coordinated and feeling better, assume that the core temperature is rising.
- *Cool abdomen.* Place the back of your hand between the clothing and the victim's abdomen to assess the victim's temperature. When the victim's abdominal skin under clothing is cooler than your hand, consider the victim hypothermic until proven otherwise.
- *Low core body temperature.* The best indicator of hypothermia is a thermometer reading of the core body temperature. The ability to reliably measure core temperature depends on the availability of an appropriate thermometer and access to the victim's rectum. Normal thermometers do not register below 94° F and so do not indicate whether the hypothermia is mild or severe. Because first aid for mild hypothermia is different from that for severe hypothermia, it is helpful to have a rectal thermometer that registers below 90° F. Oral and axillary (armpit) temperatures are influenced by too many external factors to make them reliable.

Measuring rectal temperatures in wilderness or remote locations is seldom done, mainly because low-reading rectal thermometers usually are not readily available. Also, taking a rectal temperature can be difficult, inconvenient, and embarrassing to victim and rescuer. If done outdoors, such a procedure can further expose the already cold victim.

Types of Hypothermia

The difference between mild and severe hypothermia is based on the core body temperature, but taking a rectal temperature often is not possible. The second most significant difference is that with severe hypothermia, the victim becomes so cold that shivering stops, which means the victim's body cannot rewarm itself internally and requires external heat for recovery. In fact, 50–80% of all victims of severe hypothermia die.

The National Association of Emergency Medical Service Physicians recommends that CPR not be started on a severe hypothermic victim if one of the following applies:

- The victim's core body temperature is less than 60° F.
- The victim's chest is frozen (cannot be compressed).
- The victim was submerged in water for more than 60 minutes.
- The victim has a lethal injury.
- Transport for controlled rewarming will be delayed.
- Rescuers are endangered.

For CPR to be effective, heart activity must be restored within a short time, which requires defibrillation, oxygen, and medications. Do not start CPR until you have checked the victim's circulation for 30 to 45 seconds. A hypothermic victim will have an extremely slow pulse rate. CPR can cause cardiac arrest in an already beating heart.

Recognizing Mild Hypothermia

Signs of mild hypothermia include the following:

- Vigorous, uncontrollable shivering
- Victim has the "umbles"—grumbles, mumbles, fumbles, stumbles
- Has cool or cold skin on the abdomen, chest, or back
- Victims have a core body temperature above 90° F

Care for Victims of Mild Hypothermia

Do the following to care for victims of mild hypothermia:

1. Stop further heat loss:
   - Get the victim out of the cold.
   - Handle the victim gently.
   - Prevent heat loss by replacing wet clothing with dry clothing and placing insulation (blankets, towels, pillows, wadded-up newspapers) beneath and over the victim. Cover the victim's head (50–80% of the body's heat loss is through the head).
   - Cover the victim with a vapor barrier (such as a tarp, sheet of plastic, or trash bags). If you are unable to remove wet clothing, place a vapor barrier between clothing and insulation. For a dry victim, the vapor barrier can be placed outside of the insulation.
   - Keep the victim in a horizontal (flat) position. Do not raise the legs.
   - Do not let the victim walk or exercise. Do not massage the victim's body. Either activity could drive cold blood from the extremities to the torso and produce what is known as temperature after drop.

2. Call 9-1-1 for immediate medical transportation. Remember that hypothermia is more common in urban settings than in victims found in the wilderness.
3. Allow the victim to shiver—do not stop the shivering by adding heat to the victim. Shivering that generates heat will rewarm mildly hypothermic victims.

Recognizing Severe Hypothermia

The following signs indicate severe hypothermia:

- No shivering
- Skin feels ice cold and appears blue
- Muscles can be stiff and rigid, similar to rigor mortis
- Altered mental status—not alert
- Breathing and pulse slow
- Victim might appear to be dead
- Victim has a core body temperature below 90° F

Care for Severe Hypothermia Victims

Care for someone with severe hypothermia by doing the following:

1. Stop further heat loss:
   - Get the victim out of the cold.
   - Handle the victim gently. Rough handling can cause a cardiac arrest.
   - Prevent heat loss by replacing wet clothing with dry clothing and placing insulation (blankets, towels, pillows, wadded-up newspapers) beneath and over the victim. Cover the victim's head (50–80% of the body's heat loss is through the head).
   - Cover the victim with a vapor barrier (such as a tarp, plastic sheets, or trash bags). If you are unable to remove wet clothing, place a vapor barrier between clothing and insulation. For a dry victim, the vapor barrier can be placed outside of the insulation.
   - Keep the victim in a horizontal (flat) position. Do not raise the legs.
   - Do not let the victim walk or exercise. Do not massage the victim's body. Either activity could drive cold blood from the extremities to the torso and produce what is known as temperature after drop.

2. Call 9-1-1 for immediate medical transportation. Remember that hypothermia is more common in urban settings than in victims found in the wilderness.
3. When the victim is in a remote location and far from medical care, warm the victim by any available external heat source (such as body-to-body contact).

Adding Heat

Adding heat to a victim is extremely difficult. The longer the victim has been exposed to the cold, the longer it will take to raise the core temperature to normal. Trying to rewarm a hypothermic victim could cause cardiac arrest.

Although surface rewarming suppresses shivering, it might be the only option when the victim is far from medical care. In that case, the victim must be warmed by any available external heat source.

There are problems with the commonly recommended rewarming methods.*

Warm water immersion requires a lot of warm water (no hotter than 106°F) and a bathtub—both rarely found in remote locations. Hot baths can produce rapid changes in the blood that can produce cardiac arrest.

*Paton BC: Field treatment of hypothermia. Second World Congress on Wilderness Medicine, Wilderness Medical Society.

Recent studies show that body-to-body contact in an insulated sleeping bag is ineffective for rewarming. Reasons include the following:

- All the heat produced by the rescuer's body is not enough to rewarm a victim. For example, heat loss of adults cooled to 91°F exceeds 300 kcal (kilocalories); heat production of a rescuer is only 100 kcal per hour.
- There usually is only a small amount (less than 50%) of direct skin contact, which is essential for effective heat transfer, between the victim and the rescuer.
- The victim's peripheral blood vessel constriction can impair heat transfer to the body's core.
- Skin warming can slow the victim's shivering response, which effectively rewarms the body.

Because skin rewarming suppresses shivering, which slows the rate of core rewarming, body-to-body rewarming should be used only when there will be a long delay in getting the victim to medical care and when more

FYI

How Cold Is It?

In addition to cold, two other factors account for body heat loss: moisture and wind. Moisture—whether from rain, snow, or perspiration—speeds the conduction of heat away from the body.

Wind causes sizable amounts of body heat loss. If the thermometer reads 20°F and the wind speed is 20 mph, the exposure is comparable to 4°F. This is called the windchill factor. Use the following rough measures of wind speed: if you feel the wind on your face, wind speed is at least 10 mph; if small branches move or if dust or snow is raised, it is 20 mph; if large branches are moving, it is 30 mph; and if a whole tree bends, it is about 40 mph.

To determine the windchill factor:

1. Estimate the wind speed by checking for the aforementioned signs.
2. Look at an outdoor thermometer reading (in degrees Fahrenheit).
3. Match the estimated wind speed with the actual thermometer reading in the following table.

Source: National Weather Service.

Wind Chill Chart

Effective 11/01/01

Wind (mph) \ Calm	40	35	30	25	20	15	10	5	0	-5	-10	-15	-20	-25	-30	-35	-40	-45
5	36	31	25	19	13	7	1	-5	-11	-16	-22	-28	-34	-40	-46	-52	-57	-63
10	34	27	21	15	9	3	-4	-10	-16	-22	-28	-35	-41	-47	-53	-59	-66	-72
15	32	25	19	13	6	0	-7	-13	-19	-26	-32	-39	-45	-51	-58	-64	-71	-77
20	30	24	17	11	4	-2	-9	-15	-22	-29	-35	-42	-48	-55	-61	-68	-74	-81
25	29	23	16	9	3	-4	-11	-17	-24	-31	-37	-44	-51	-58	-64	-71	-78	-84
30	28	22	15	8	1	-5	-12	-19	-26	-33	-39	-46	-53	-60	-67	-73	-80	-87
35	28	21	14	7	0	-7	-14	-21	-27	-34	-41	-48	-55	-62	-69	-76	-82	-89
40	27	20	13	6	-1	-8	-15	-22	-29	-36	-43	-50	-57	-64	-71	-78	-84	-91
45	26	19	12	5	-2	-9	-16	-23	-30	-37	-44	-51	-58	-65	-72	-79	-86	-93
50	26	19	12	4	-3	-10	-17	-24	-31	-38	-45	-52	-60	-67	-74	-81	-88	-95
55	25	18	11	4	-3	-11	-18	-25	-32	-39	-46	-54	-61	-68	-75	-82	-89	-97
60	25	17	10	3	-4	-11	-19	-26	-33	-40	-48	-55	-62	-69	-76	-84	-91	-98

Frostbite Times ■ 30 minutes ■ 10 minutes ■ 5 minutes

Wind Chill (°F) = 35.74 + 0.6215T - 35.75 $(V^{0.16})$ + 0.4275T $(V^{0.16})$

Where, T=Air Temperature (°F) V=Wind Speed (mph)

Hypothermia

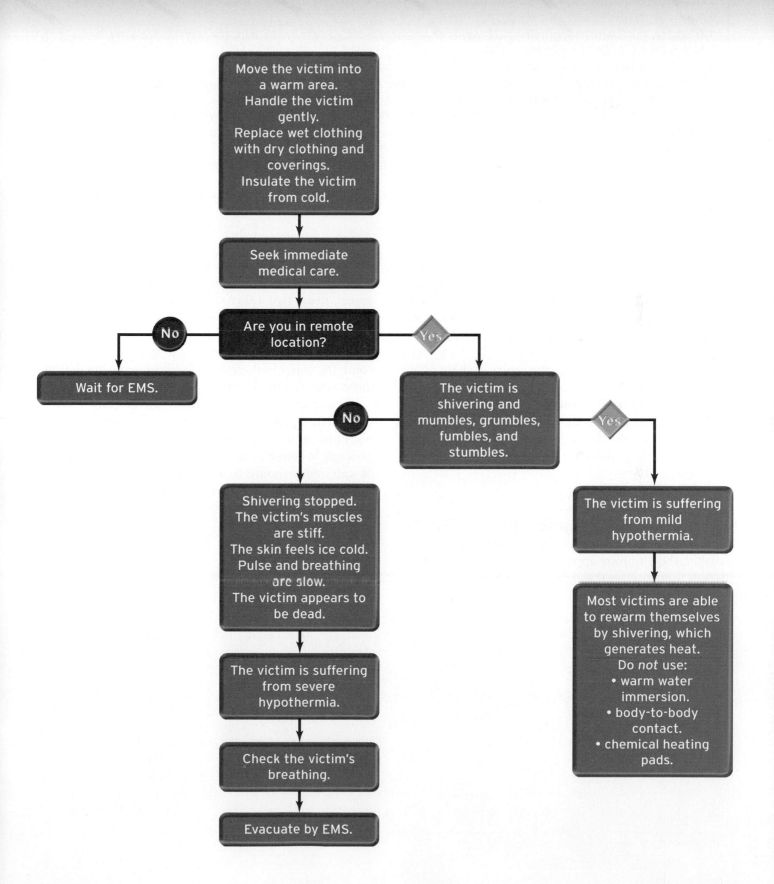

Move the victim into a warm area.
Handle the victim gently.
Replace wet clothing with dry clothing and coverings.
Insulate the victim from cold.

↓

Seek immediate medical care.

↓

Are you in remote location?

No →

Wait for EMS.

Yes →

The victim is shivering and mumbles, grumbles, fumbles, and stumbles.

No ↓

Shivering stopped.
The victim's muscles are stiff.
The skin feels ice cold.
Pulse and breathing are slow.
The victim appears to be dead.

↓

The victim is suffering from severe hypothermia.

↓

Check the victim's breathing.

↓

Evacuate by EMS.

Yes →

The victim is suffering from mild hypothermia.

↓

Most victims are able to rewarm themselves by shivering, which generates heat.
Do *not* use:
• warm water immersion.
• body-to-body contact.
• chemical heating pads.

CAUTION

DO NOT allow the victim to physically exert himself or herself (no walking, no climbing).

DO NOT try to rewarm a hypothermic victim outside a medical facility. External measures to rewarm should not be used, especially on the extremities, because surface rewarming leads to vasodilation (wider blood vessels), which can lead to a drop in blood pressure and after temperature drop.

DO NOT try to rewarm a hypothermic victim outside a medical facility because rewarming the skin will stop shivering, which is the most effective way to rewarm.

DO NOT put an unconscious victim in a bathtub.

DO NOT give the victim alcohol. Alcohol interferes with shivering and accelerates heat loss by dilating the blood vessels in the skin. The victim might feel warmer temporarily, but there is a greater risk of hypothermia.

DO NOT give the victim a caffeine drink. Caffeine has a diuretic effect, and the victim probably is already dehydrated.

DO NOT rub or massage the victim's arms or legs. Rubbing the skin suppresses shivering, dilates the blood vessels in the skin (resulting in more heat loss), and produces temperature after drop.

DO NOT raise the victim's legs, which allows cold blood from the legs to flow into the body core and adversely affect the heart. Keep the victim in a flat position.

appropriate methods of adding heat are unavailable. Several types of chemical heating pads are available. Although they might be effective for warming hands and feet, there is no evidence that they are capable of rewarming a hypothermic victim. For example, one type of heating pad is 7 inches by 9 inches and provides 14.5 kcal of total heat, with a maximum temperature of about 125° F. A minimum of 20 pads would be needed to provide enough heat to rewarm a victim with a temperature of 91° F, even if heat transfer were 100% efficient. This method can stop the desirable effects of shivering, leaving the victim hypothermic.

▶ Dehydration

Dehydration occurs because of unperceived fluid loss combined with inadequate fluid intake. In very cold weather, the humidity approaches zero, and large quantities of fluid are lost through exhaled breath.

People in a cold environment must drink even when they are not thirsty. Inactive people in comfortable climates need two quarts of water a day to prevent dehydration.

A person's hydration status can be monitored by noting the color and the volume of the urine. The lighter the color, the better hydrated; dark yellow urine is a definite indication that fluid consumption should be increased.

Unmelted snow and ice should not be consumed for water. Eating snow and ice irritates the mouth, wastes body heat, and, if enough is consumed, lowers body temperature. When snow and ice are the only available sources of water, they should be melted before being consumed. Melted snow or ice should not be considered drinkable until it has been appropriately disinfected (by boiling, filtering, or using chemicals).

▶ Cold-Related Emergencies

What to Look For

What to Do

Frostbite

- White, waxy-looking skin
- Skin feels cold and numb (pain at first, followed by numbness)
- Blisters, which may appear after rewarming

1. Move victim to warm place.
2. Remove tight clothing or jewelry from injured part(s).
3. Place dry dressings between toes and/or fingers.
4. Seek medical care.

Hypothermia

- Mild
  - Uncontrollable shivering
  - Confusion, sluggishness
  - Cold skin even under clothing
- Severe
  - No shivering
  - Muscles stiff and rigid
  - Skin ice cold
  - Appears to be dead

All victims:

1. Move victim to warm place.
2. Prevent heat loss by
   - Replacing wet clothing with dry clothing
   - Covering victim's head

Mild

1. Give warm, sugary beverages.
2. Do not add anything warm to the skin—let the shivering rewarm the body.

Severe

1. Do not rewarm unless in a very remote location.
2. Call 9-1-1.

prep kit

▶ Ready for Review

- When a person is surrounded by air or water cooler than body temperature, the body loses heat.
- Humans protect themselves from cold primarily by avoiding or reducing cold exposure through the use of clothing and shelter.
- Nonfreezing cold injuries can occur when conditions are cold and wet and the hands and feet cannot be kept warm and dry.
- Freezing cold injuries can occur whenever the air temperature is below freezing.
- Hypothermia is a life-threatening condition in which the body's core temperature falls below 95° F.
- Dehydration occurs because of unperceived fluid loss combined with inadequate fluid intake.

▶ Vital Vocabulary

<u>frostbite</u> The damage to tissues as a result of prolonged exposure to extreme cold.

<u>frostnip</u> The superficial local tissue destruction caused by freezing; it is limited in scope and does not destroy the full thickness of skin.

<u>hypothermia</u> Decreased body temperature.

<u>vasoconstriction</u> The narrowing of the diameter of a blood vessel.

<u>windchill</u> The relationship of wind velocity and temperature in determining the effect of cold on living organisms.

▶ Assessment in Action

It is a cold winter weekend, and you feel the need to check on an elderly relative who lives alone. The front door is unlocked, and upon entering her home you notice that it is not much warmer inside the house than outside. You find her wrapped in a blanket lying on the couch. You speak to her, but she only mumbles. She is shivering severely.

Directions: Circle Yes if you agree with the statement, circle No if you disagree.

Yes   No   1. Add insulation (blankets) around and under her.

Yes   No   2. Shivering can rewarm a victim suffering mild hypothermia.

Yes   No   3. Apply a heating pad immediately.

Yes   No   4. It is too warm in the house for hypothermia to develop.

Yes   No   5. Call 9-1-1 if the condition does not improve in minutes.

Answers: **1.** Yes; **2.** Yes; **3.** No; **4.** No; **5.** Yes

▶ Check Your Knowledge

Directions: Circle Yes if you agree with the statement, circle No if you disagree.

Yes   No   1. Shivering is a signal that clothing and shelter are inadequate to protect the body from the cold.

Yes   No   2. Up to 100% of the body's total heat production can be lost by radiation through a person's unprotected head.

Yes   No   3. Physically unfit people are more susceptible to cold injury.

Yes   No   4. Frostnip is caused when water on the skin surface freezes.

Yes   No   5. Shivering produces body heat.

Yes   No   6. Rub a frostbitten part to rewarm it.

Yes   No   7. Rewarm a hypothermic victim quickly in a hot shower or with chemical heat packs.

Yes   No   8. Replace any wet clothing with dry clothing for a hypothermic victim.

Yes   No   9. Seek medical care for a severe hypothermic victim.

Yes   No   10. Hypothermia requires below freezing temperatures for it to occur.

Answers: **1.** Yes; **2.** No; **3.** Yes; **4.** Yes; **5.** Yes; **6.** No; **7.** No; **8.** Yes; **9.** Yes; **10.** No

Heat-Related Emergencies

Heat-Related Emergencies

When the temperature goes up, a multitude of problems can—and do—arise. Given the right (or wrong) conditions, anyone can develop heat illness. Some victims are lucky enough to have only **heat cramps**, but less fortunate people could be laid low by heat exhaustion or devastated by heatstroke.

▶ How the Body Stays Cool

The human body is constantly engaged in a life-and-death struggle to disperse the heat that it produces. If allowed to accumulate, the heat would quickly increase your body temperature beyond its comfortable 98.6° F. That does not normally happen, because your body is able to lose enough heat to maintain a steady temperature. Usually, you are aware of this struggle only during hard labor or exercise in a hot environment, when your body produces heat faster than it can lose it. In certain circumstances, your body can build up too much heat, your temperature might rise to life-threatening levels, and you can become delirious or lose consciousness. This condition is called **heatstroke** and is a serious medical emergency. If you do not rid your body of excess heat fast enough, it cooks the brain and other vital organs. It is often fatal, and people who survive might have permanent damage to their vital organs. Before your temperature reaches heatstroke level, however, you might experience heat exhaustion with its flulike symptoms. By treating the symptoms of **heat exhaustion**, you avoid heatstroke.

How does the body dispose of excess heat? Humans lose heat largely through their skin, much as a car loses heat through its radiator. Exercising muscles warms the blood, just as the car's hot engine warms its radiator fluid. Warm blood travels through the skin's dilated blood vessels, losing heat by evaporating sweat to the surrounding air, just as the car loses engine heat through the radiator.

When blood delivers heat to the skin, the body loses heat primarily in two ways: radiation and evaporation (vaporization of sweat). When the air temperature is 70° F or less, the body releases heat into its surroundings by radiation. As the environmental temperature approaches the body's temperature, however, heat loss through radiation is greatly reduced. In fact, people working or exercising on a hot summer day actually gain heat through radiation from the sun, leaving evaporation as the only way to effectively control body temperature.

Water Loss

Water makes up about 50–60% of an adult's body weight. You lose about 2 quarts every day through breathing, urinating, bowel movements, and sweat. The lost fluid must be replaced. Although the amount of water used each day varies from person to person, an adult requires about 2 quarts a day from water, other beverages, and food (about 70% of most food is water). A working adult can produce 2 to 3 quarts of sweat an hour for short periods and up to 10 to 15 quarts a day. When the body's water absorption rate of 1.5 quarts per hour is pitted against a sweat loss of 2 quarts per hour, dehydration results—drinking water cannot keep up with sweat losses.

When you are thirsty, you are already dehydrated. Thirst is not a good guide for when to drink water. In fact, in hot and humid conditions, people could be so dehydrated by the time they become thirsty that they have trouble catching up with their fluid losses. One guideline regarding water intake is to monitor urine output. You are getting enough water if you are producing clear urine at least five times a day. Cloudy or dark urine or urinating fewer than five times a day probably means you should drink more.

If possible while working, especially in hot weather, drink 1 cup (8 ounces) of water every 20 minutes. Usually, 1 pint (16 ounces) is the most a person can comfortably drink at once. It takes time for water to pass from the stomach into the blood, so you cannot catch up by drinking extra water later; about 1 quart of water per hour can pass out of the stomach.

Cool water (50° F) is easier for the stomach to absorb than warm water, and a little flavoring can make the water more tasty. The best fluids are those that leave the stomach fast and contain little sodium and less than 8% sugar. Coffee and tea should be avoided because they contain caffeine, a diuretic that increases water loss through urination. Alcoholic beverages also dehydrate by increasing urination. Soda pop contains about 10% sugar and, therefore, is not absorbed as well as water or commercial sports drinks (which contain about 5–8% sugar). Fruit juices range from 11–18% sugar and have an even longer absorption time.

Electrolyte Loss

Sweat and urine contain potassium and sodium, essential electrolytes that control the movement of water in and out of the cells. These electrolytes can be found in many everyday foods. Bananas and nuts are rich in potassium, and most American diets have up to 10 times as much sodium as the body needs. Acclimatizing to heat can reduce sodium loss tenfold. Getting enough salt (sodium chloride) is rarely a problem in the typical American diet. In fact, most Americans consume an excessive amount of sodium, averaging 5 to 10 grams of sodium per day, although humans probably require only 1 to 3 grams. Sodium loss, therefore, is seldom a problem, unless a person is sweating profusely for long periods and drinking large amounts of water (more than 1 quart an hour).

Most people require only water most of the time. Commercial sports drinks can be useful for participants in vigorous physical activity for longer than 1 hour. The human body needs water more than it needs salt. Whenever extra sodium is added to a diet, more water should be consumed. Otherwise, excessive sodium can draw water out of the cells, accelerating dehydration.

Drinking large amounts of water (more than 1 quart an hour) and profuse sweating for long periods can lead to a condition called water intoxication, in which electrolytes are flushed from the body. Symptoms of water intoxication include frequent urination and behavior changes (irrationality, combativeness, seizures, and coma).

FYI

Water Intoxication in Recreational Hikers

Water intoxication (hyponatremia), often seen in endurance athletes, has been reported in recreational hikers. Water intoxication results when people replace sweat loss with plain water instead of an enhanced product that more nearly resembles sweat. Differentiating water intoxication from heat exhaustion is difficult. Recreational wilderness hikers performing sustained exercise in the heat might require electrolyte replacement similar to endurance athletes.

Source: Backer H, et al: Hyponatremia in recreational hikers in Grand Canyon National Park. *J Wilderness Med* 4(4)391-406.

Effects of Humidity

Sweat can cool the body only if it evaporates (vaporizes). In dry air, you will not notice sweat evaporating. In high humidity, no sweat can evaporate. It drips off the skin, without cooling the body. At about 75% humidity, sweating is ineffective in cooling the body.

Because humidity can significantly reduce evaporative cooling, a very humid but mildly warm day can be more stressful than a very hot, dry day. The higher the humidity, the lower the temperature at which heat risk begins, especially for people generating heat with vigorous work.

Who Is at Risk?

Everyone is susceptible to heat illness if environmental conditions overwhelm the body's temperature-regulating mechanisms. Heat waves can set the stage for a rash of heatstroke victims. For example, in the 1995 Chicago heat wave, the death toll reached 591 in 5 days. Several groups are at particular risk, including people who are obese, people with a chronic illness, and people with alcoholism.

Elderly people are at higher risk because of impaired cardiac output and decreased ability to sweat. Infants and young children are also susceptible to heatstroke. Children (and pets) are especially vulnerable when they are left in automobiles. The temperature in a parked car can soar to 150° F, even when a window is open. The fluid loss and dehydration resulting from physical activity put outdoor laborers and athletes at particular risk.

Certain medications predispose to heatstroke. They include drugs that alter sweat production (for example, antihistamines, antipsychotics, and antidepressants) and those that interfere with <u>thermoregulation</u>.

▶ Heat Illnesses

Heat illnesses include a range of disorders `Table 21-1`. Some of them are common, but only heatstroke is life threatening. Untreated heatstroke victims always die.

Heat Cramps

Heat cramps are painful muscle spasms that occur suddenly during or after vigorous exercise or activity. They usually involve the muscles in the back of the leg (calf and hamstring muscles) or the abdominal muscles. Some experts state they are caused by water and electrolyte losses during times of excessive sweating. Victims might be drinking fluids without adequate salt content. However, other experts disagree because the typical American diet is heavy with salt.

Table 21-1	Heat Illnesses		
Condition	**Symptoms**	**What to do**
Heat cramps	Painful muscle spasms Sweaty skin Normal body temperature	1. Sit or lie down in the shade. 2. Drink cool, lightly salted water or a sports drink. 3. Stretch affected muscles.
Heat exhaustion	Profuse sweating Flulike symptoms Clammy or pale skin Dizziness Nausea, vomiting Rapid pulse Thirst Normal or slightly above normal body temperature	1. Treat mild cases the same way as heat cramps (but do not stretch the muscles). 2. If persistent, gently apply wet towels and call 9-1-1.
Heatstroke	Unresponsiveness (if responsive, victim will be confused, stagger, be agitated) Hot skin, which can be dry or wet	1. Move person to a half-sitting position in the shade. 2. Call 9-1-1. 3. If humidity is below 75%, spray victim with water and vigorously fan. If humidity is above 75%, apply ice packs on neck, armpits, and groin.

Recognizing Heat Cramps

Heat cramps have the following characteristics:

- painful muscle spasms that happen suddenly
- affects the muscle in the back of the leg or abdomen
- occurs during or after physical exertion

Care for Someone With Heat Cramps

To relieve heat cramps (it could take several hours), follow these steps:

1. Have the victim rest in a cool place.
2. Have the victim drink lightly salted, cool water (dissolve ¼ teaspoon salt in 1 quart of water) or a commercial sports drink. (A commercial sports drink is easier to absorb if diluted to half strength to reduce the sugar content.)
3. Stretch the cramped calf muscle. Also, try an acupressure method: pinch the upper lip just below the nose.

Heat Exhaustion

Heat exhaustion is characterized by heavy perspiration with a normal or slightly above-normal body temperature. Heavy sweating causes water and electrolyte losses. Some experts believe that a better term would be severe dehydration. Heat exhaustion affects workers and athletes who do not drink enough fluids while working or exercising in hot environments. Symptoms include severe thirst, heavy sweating, fatigue, headache, nausea, vomiting, and sometimes diarrhea. The affected person often mistakenly believes he or she has the flu. Uncontrolled heat exhaustion can evolve into heatstroke.

Recognizing Heat Exhaustion

Heat exhaustion differs from heatstroke by having (1) no altered mental status and (2) skin that is not hot, but clammy. Heat exhaustion causes the following symptoms:

- sweating
- thirst
- fatigue
- flulike symptoms (headache and nausea)
- shortness of breath
- fast heart rate

Care for Heat Exhaustion Victims

Use the following guidelines to care for a victim of heat exhaustion:

1. Move the victim immediately out of the heat to a cool place.
2. Give cool liquids, adding electrolytes (lightly salted water or a commercial sports drink) if plain water does not improve the victim's condition in 20 minutes. Do not give salt tablets; they can irritate the stomach and cause nausea and vomiting.

3. Raise the victim's legs 6 to 12 inches (keep the legs straight).
4. Remove excess clothing.
5. Sponge the victim with cool water and fan him or her.
6. If no improvement is seen within 30 minutes, seek medical care.

Heatstroke

Two types of heatstroke exist: classic and exertional ⬤Table 21-2⬤. Classic heatstroke, also known as the slow cooker, can take days to develop. It is often seen during summer heat waves and typically affects poor, elderly, chronically ill, alcoholic, and obese people. Because elderly people, who often have medical problems, are frequently afflicted, this type of heatstroke has a 50% death rate, even with medical care. It results from a combination of a hot environment and dehydration ⬤Table 21-3⬤. Exertional heatstroke is also more common in the summer. It is frequently seen in athletes, laborers, and military personnel, all of whom often sweat profusely. This type of heatstroke is known as the fast cooker. It affects healthy, active people who are strenuously working or playing in a warm environment. Because its rapid onset does not allow enough time for severe dehydration to occur, 50% of exertional heatstroke victims usually are sweating. (Classic heatstroke victims are not sweating.)

There are several ways to tell the difference between heat exhaustion and heatstroke.

- If the victim's body feels extremely hot when touched, suspect heatstroke.

Table 21-2	Classic or Exertional Heatstroke?	
Characteristics	Classic	Exertional
Age group usually affected	Elderly	Males 15-45 years
Claims many victims at the same time	During heat waves	During athletic competition
Health status of victims	Chronically ill	Healthy and physically fit
Activity at the time of incident	Sedentary	Strenuous exercise
Medication use	Common	Usually none
Sweating	Absent	Often present (50% of victims)

- Altered mental status (behavior) occurs with heatstroke, ranging from slight confusion and disorientation to coma. Between those extreme conditions, victims usually become irrational, agitated, or even aggressive, and they might have seizures.
- In severe heatstroke, a coma can occur in less than an hour. The longer a coma lasts, the lower the chance for survival.
- Rectal temperature can also distinguish heatstroke from heat exhaustion, although obtaining a rectal temperature is usually not practical. A responsive heatstroke victim might not cooperate, taking a rectal temperature can be embarrassing to the victim and the rescuer, and rectal thermometers are seldom available.

Recognizing Heatstroke

Signs of heatstroke include:
- extremely hot skin when touched—usually dry, but can be wet.
- altered mental status ranging from slight confusion, agitation, and disorientation to unresponsiveness.

Care for Heatstroke Victims

Heatstroke is a medical emergency and must be treated rapidly! Every minute delayed increases the likelihood of serious complications or death. Do the following:

1. Move the victim immediately to a cool place.
2. Remove clothing down to the victim's underwear.
3. Keep the victim's head and shoulders slightly elevated.

4. Call 9-1-1 immediately even if the victim seems to be recovering.
5. The only way to prevent damage is to cool the victim quickly and by any means possible. Cooling methods include the following:
   - Spraying the victim with water and then fanning **Figure 21-1**. This method is *not* as effective in high-humidity (more than 75%) conditions.
   - Applying cool, wet sheets or towels.
   - Placing ice bags against the large veins in the groin, armpits, and sides of the neck; this cools the body, regardless of humidity.
   - Placing the victim in an ice bath; this cools a victim quickly, but it requires a great deal of ice—at least 80 pounds—to be effective. The need for a big enough tub also limits this method.
   - Placing the victim in a cool water bath (less than 60° F) can be successful if the water is stirred to prevent a warm layer from forming around the body. This is the most effective method in high-humidity (greater than 75%) conditions.

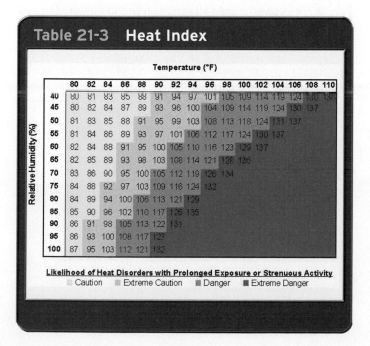

Table 21-3   Heat Index

Temperature (°F)

Relative Humidity (%)	80	82	84	86	88	90	92	94	96	98	100	102	104	106	108	110
40	80	81	83	85	88	91	94	97	101	105	109	114	119	124	130	136
45	80	82	84	87	89	93	96	100	104	109	114	119	124	130	137	
50	81	83	85	88	91	95	99	103	108	113	118	124	131	137		
55	81	84	86	89	93	97	101	106	112	117	124	130	137			
60	82	84	88	91	95	100	105	110	116	123	129	137				
65	82	85	89	93	98	103	108	114	121	128	136					
70	83	86	90	95	100	105	112	119	126	134						
75	84	88	92	97	103	109	116	124	132							
80	84	89	94	100	106	113	121	129								
85	85	90	96	102	110	117	126	135								
90	86	91	98	105	113	122	131									
95	86	93	100	108	117	127										
100	87	95	103	112	121	132										

Likelihood of Heat Disorders with Prolonged Exposure or Strenuous Activity
■ Caution ■ Extreme Caution ■ Danger ■ Extreme Danger

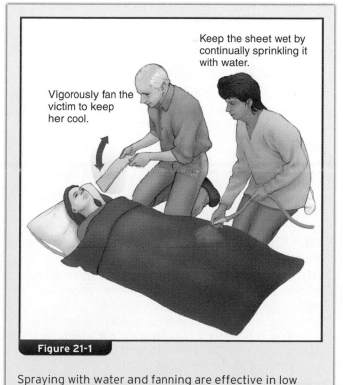

Keep the sheet wet by continually sprinkling it with water.

Vigorously fan the victim to keep her cool.

Figure 21-1

Spraying with water and fanning are effective in low humidity conditions.

FYI

Hot-Weather Precautions

These simple preventive measures can reduce heat stress:

1. Keep as cool as possible.
   - Avoid direct sunlight.
   - Stay in the coolest available location (usually indoors).
   - Use air-conditioning, if available.
   - Use electric fans to promote cooling.
   - Place wet towels or ice bags on the body or dampen clothing.
   - Take cool baths or showers.
2. Wear lightweight, loose-fitting clothing.
3. Avoid strenuous physical activity, particularly in the sun and during the hottest part of the day.
4. Increase intake of fluids, such as water and fruit or vegetable juices. Thirst is not always a good indicator of adequate fluid intake. Fluid intake in hot weather should be one and a half times the amount that quenches thirst. People who are overweight or have a large build or who engage in strenuous activities, such as sports, can require more than a gallon of fluid intake daily in very hot weather. People for whom salt or fluid is restricted should consult their physicians for instructions on appropriate fluid and salt intake.
5. Do not take salt tablets unless instructed to do so by a physician.
6. Avoid alcoholic beverages (beer, wine, and liquor).
7. Stay in contact with other people.

CAUTION

DO NOT delay initiating cooling while waiting for an ambulance. The longer the delay, the greater the risk of tissue damage and prolonged hospitalization.

DO NOT continue cooling after the victim's mental status has improved. Unnecessary cooling could lead to hypothermia.

DO NOT use rubbing alcohol to cool the skin. It can be absorbed into the blood and cause alcohol poisoning. Also, the vapors are a potential fire hazard.

DO NOT give the victim aspirin or acetaminophen. The brain's control center is not elevated, as it is with fever caused by diseases, so these products are not effective for lowering body temperature.

FYI

Other Heat Illnesses

Less serious heat illnesses include heat syncope, heat edema, and prickly heat.

- **Heat syncope**, in which a person becomes dizzy or faints after exposure to high temperatures, is a self-resolving condition. Victims should lie down in a cool place and, if not nauseated, drink water. Syncope may be associated with heat exhaustion.
- **Heat edema**, which is also a self-resolving condition, causes the ankles and feet to swell from heat exposure. It is more common in women who are not acclimatized to a hot climate. It is related to salt and water retention and tends to disappear after acclimatization. Wearing support stockings and elevating the legs could help reduce the swelling.
- **Prickly heat**, also known as a heat rash, is an itchy rash that develops because of unevaporated moisture on skin wet from sweating. Treat by drying and cooling the skin.

FYI

Heat-Related Deaths of Young Children in Parked Cars

Each year, many young children die in the Unites States of heat stroke caused by being enclosed in parked motor vehicles. Researchers located and analyzed 171 heat-related deaths in children under five years of age:

- 39% involved a child "forgotten by a caregiver
- 27% involved a child playing in an unattended vehicle
- 20% involved a child intentionally left in a vehicle by an adult
- 14% involved unclear circumstances

Source: Guard, A. and S.S. Gallagher, "Heat-Related Deaths to Young Children in Parked Cars: An Analysis of 171 Fatalities in the United States" Injury Prevention 11 (1):33-37.

FYI

How Hot It Feels

Under normal conditions, temperature and humidity are the most important elements influencing body comfort. The heat index (Table 21-3) compiled by the National Weather Service lists apparent temperatures—how hot it feels—at various combinations of temperature and humidity.

Heat-Related Emergencies

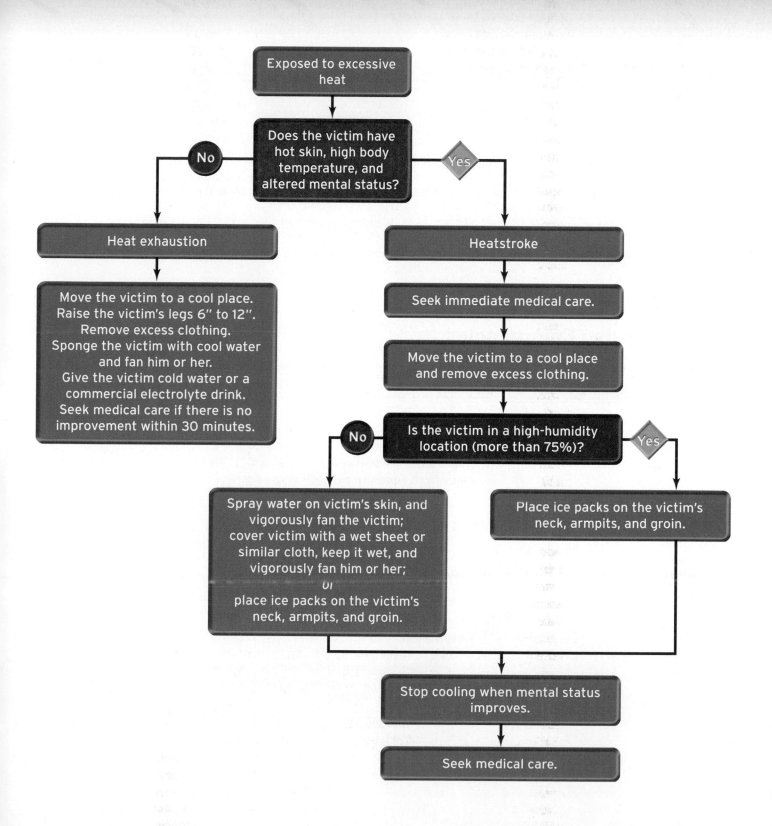

FYI

Heat-Related Deaths

Case 1

A 92-year-old man's family, had not been running the air conditioner in their residence in an attempt to conserve electricity. The daytime heat index recorded at the local airport during the 5 days preceding his death ranged from 102° F to 109° F (38.9° C to 42.8° C).

Case 2

A 4-year-old girl was found in a locked car in front of a child-care center. The temperature inside the car at the time of her death was unknown; however, the estimated heat index in the area that day was 93° F (33.9° C).

Case 3

A 70-year-old woman was found dead in a mobile home. When she was discovered, the air conditioner was blowing hot air, and the temperature inside the mobile home was about 115° F (46° C).

Case 4

A 52-year-old man walked from the lawn he was mowing to a nearby residence and knocked on the back door. When the homeowner opened the door, the man collapsed onto the porch. He died at the hospital. His core temperature was 107.1° F (41.7° C), which, before his death, was reduced to 101° F (38.3° C). The outside temperature at the time he collapsed was 109° F (42.8° C).

Source: Centers for Disease Control and Prevention (CDC). Heat-related illnesses and deaths: Missouri, 1998, and United States, 1979–1996 [correction appears in *MMWR Morb Mortal Wkly Rep* 49:474]. *MMWR Morb Mortal Wkly Rep* 48:469–472.

▶ Heat-Related Emergencies

 What to Look For

 What to Do

Heat cramps
- Painful muscle spasm during or after physical activity
- Usually lower leg affected

1. Move victim to cool place.
2. Stretch the cramped muscle.
3. Remove excess or tight clothing.
4. If the victim is responsive, give water or sports drink.

Heat exhaustion
- Heavy sweating
- Severe thirst
- Weakness
- Headache
- Nausea and vomiting

1. Move victim to cool place.
2. Have victim lie down and raise legs 6 to 12 inches.
3. Apply cool, wet towels to head and body.
4. If victim is responsive, give water or sports drink.
5. Seek medical care if no improvement within 30 minutes.

Heatstroke
- Extremely hot skin
- Dry skin (may be wet at first)
- Confusion
- Seizures
- Unresponsiveness

1. Move victim to cool place.
2. Call 9-1-1.
3. If unresponsive, open airway, check breathing, and provide appropriate care.
4. Rapidly cool victim by whatever means possible (cool, wet sheets; ice or cold packs against armpits, side of neck, and groin).

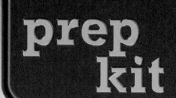

prep kit

▶ Ready for Review

- Given the right conditions, anyone can develop heat illness.
- The human body is constantly dispersing the heat that it produces.
- Heat illnesses include a range of disorders from heat cramps to heatstroke. Only heatstroke is life threatening.

▶ Vital Vocabulary

<u>heat cramp</u> A painful muscle cramp resulting from excessive loss of salt and water through sweating.

<u>heat exhaustion</u> A prostration caused by excessive loss of water and salt through sweating; characterized by clammy skin and a weak, rapid pulse.

<u>heatstroke</u> A life-threatening condition of severe hyperthermia caused by exposure to excessive natural or artificial heat.

<u>thermoregulation</u> The body's ability to maintain a normal body temperature despite the weather.

▶ Assessment in Action

It is a hot and humid summer day. It's your first day off in a week, so you convince your brother to get up off of the couch, leave the air-conditioned house, and play a few rounds of tennis with you. You and your brother are having so much fun that you don't notice the time quickly passing by. After you hit an ace off of your brother, he complains that he feels nauseous. At first you think that he is joking, but as you approach him, you see that he is sweating heavily and looks a bit ill.

Directions: Circle Yes if you agree with the statement, circle No if you disagree.

Yes　No　1. You should immediately move your brother out of the heat into a cool place.

Yes　No　2. Give your brother some salt tablets to increase the rate of hydration.

Yes　No　3. Elevate his legs 6 to 12 inches.

Yes　No　4. Cover your brother with a light blanket so that he does not lose heat too rapidly.

Yes　No　5. Your brother still feels the same after 30 minutes, so you should seek medical care.

Answers: 1. Yes; 2. No; 3. Yes; 4. No; 5. Yes

▶ Check Your Knowledge

Directions: Circle Yes if you agree with the statement, circle No if you disagree.

Yes　No　1. For heat cramps in the legs, stretch the cramped muscle.

Yes　No　2. Commercial sport drinks can be given to victims of heat-related emergencies.

Yes　No　3. Move victims of heat-related illness to a cool place.

Yes　No　4. Victims of heatstroke need immediate medical care—it is a life-threatening condition.

Yes　No　5. Cool heatstroke victims rapidly, including the use of ice packs applied to the neck, armpits, and groin.

Yes　No　6. Fruit juices are digested quickly and rehydrate the body most rapidly.

Yes　No　7. You can drink too much water and cause water intoxication.

Yes　No　8. Humidity cannot significantly reduce evaporative cooling.

Yes　No　9. Certain medications predispose to heatstroke.

Yes　No　10. Heat exhaustion can feel like the flu.

Answers: 1. Yes; 2. Yes; 3. Yes; 4. Yes; 5. Yes; 6. No; 7. Yes; 8. No; 9. Yes; 10. Yes

Childbirth and Gynecologic Emergencies

Childbirth and Gynecologic Emergencies of Pregnancy

Handling childbirth and gynecologic situations of pregnancy requires that a first aider be familiar with the terminology used to describe female reproductive anatomy and physiology.

- The <u>birth canal</u> includes the vagina and the lower part of the uterus.
- The <u>cervix</u> is the small opening at the lower end of the uterus through which the baby passes.
- The <u>placenta</u> (afterbirth) is the organ through which the mother and the fetus exchange nourishment and waste products during pregnancy. It is expelled after the baby's birth.
- The <u>umbilical cord</u> is the extension of the placenta through which the fetus receives nourishment while in the uterus.
- The <u>amniotic sac</u> (bag of waters) surrounds the fetus inside the uterus. Amniotic fluid in the sac cushions the fetus and helps protect it from injury.
- <u>Crowning</u> occurs when the fetus's head presses against the vaginal opening and begins to bulge out.
- <u>Bloody show</u> is the mucus and blood that might be discharged from the vagina as labor begins.
- <u>Labor</u> is the process of childbirth (defined in three stages), from the first regular uterine-muscle contractions until delivery of the placenta.

- A <u>miscarriage</u> (medical term is spontaneous abortion) is the delivery of a fetus before it can live independent of the mother.

Predelivery Emergencies

▶ Miscarriage

Miscarriages usually occur during the first 3 months (first trimester) of pregnancy. Most occur because the fetus was not developing properly and was not able to survive. The woman will be emotionally upset. She might be hesitant about confiding in a stranger, especially a man, and therefore, help from a woman if possible, might be wise.

Recognizing Miscarriage

Signs of a miscarriage include the following:
- Cramping pain in lower abdomen resembling menstrual cramps
- Aching in the lower back
- Vaginal bleeding, which could be sudden and heavy
- Passage of tissue from the vagina

Care for a Woman Having a Miscarriage

Follow these guidelines to care for a woman having a miscarriage:
1. Reassure the woman.
2. Help her into a comfortable position with legs bent.
3. Have the woman place a sanitary pad over the outside of the vagina.
4. Any tissue that passes through the vagina should be transported with the woman to the hospital. Do not try to pull tissue out of the vagina; instead, cover it with a sterile pad.
5. Transport the woman to medical care.
6. Call 9 1 1 if bleeding is heavy or there are signs of shock.

▶ Vaginal Bleeding During Late Pregnancy

A woman experiencing vaginal bleeding late in her pregnancy (third trimester, or last 3 months) usually constitutes an emergency. Find out how long she has been bleeding and how many sanitary pads she has used so that you can report the information to medical personnel. An increase in pulse rate of more than 20 beats per minute when the victim goes from a lying-down to a sitting position suggests blood loss of more than 1 pint. The woman might feel embarrassed. She might be hesitant about confiding in a stranger, especially a man, and therefore, help from a woman might be wise.

Recognizing Vaginal Bleeding During Late Pregnancy

If heavy bleeding occurs, signs of shock could be seen.

Care for a Woman With Vaginal Bleeding During Late Pregnancy

To care for someone with vaginal bleeding during late pregnancy, do the following:
1. Place the woman on her left side to relieve pressure from the fetus on the inferior vena cava (large vein between the spine and the abdominal organs).
2. Have the woman place a sanitary pad over the outside of the vagina.
3. Call 9-1-1 immediately.

▶ Vaginal Bleeding Caused by Injury

It is difficult to determine the source of the bleeding. Vaginal bleeding can be difficult to care for because of the woman's modesty and pain.

Recognizing Vaginal Bleeding Caused by Injury

The following signs could indicate vaginal bleeding caused by injury:
- Injuries of the external female genitalia, including all types of soft-tissue injuries (such as wounds or contusions)
- Severe pain
- Blood in the vaginal area
- Massive internal vaginal bleeding

Care for a Woman With Injury-Related Vaginal Bleeding

To assist a woman with injury-related vaginal bleeding, follow these guidelines:
1. Use direct pressure over a bulky dressing or sanitary pad to control external bleeding from a laceration or other injury.
2. Apply an ice pack to reduce swelling and pain.
3. Never place or pack dressings into the vagina. It is useless and dangerous to introduce packs blindly into the vagina in an attempt to control bleeding.
4. Place the victim on her left side to help prevent vomiting, to prevent aspiration of vomitus, and,

if the woman is pregnant, to relieve pressure on the vena cava from the fetus.

5. Seek medical care.

▶ Non–Injury-Related Vaginal Bleeding

Bleeding from the vagina is most likely to be menstrual bleeding. However, such bleeding can indicate more serious conditions (such as miscarriage, childbirth, infection).

Recognizing Non-Injury-Related Vaginal Bleeding

Abdominal cramps can be a sign of non-injury-related vaginal bleeding.

Care for Victims of Non-Injury-Related Vaginal Bleeding

Non-injury-related vaginal bleeding can result from various causes, but treatment is similar. Here is what you can do:

1. Reassure the woman.
2. Help her into a comfortable position with legs bent.
3. Have the woman place a sanitary pad over the outside of the vagina.
4. Seek medical care.

Delivery

Emergency childbirth occurs when a baby is born at an unplanned time or at an unplanned place. Most babies in the United States are delivered in a hospital. Occasionally, the birth process moves along faster than expected. Because of the infrequency, taking care of an anxious mother and her newborn infant is a stressful event for a first aider. On the other hand, assisting in the birth of a baby is one of the few situations in which first aiders have the opportunity to participate in a happy event rather than an unpleasant one.

▶ Imminent Delivery

Consider transporting the woman to a hospital only if she is not straining or crowning and this is her first pregnancy. Making a hasty decision to transport the woman means that the delivery could take place under the worst possible circumstances. When there is enough time to transport the woman to a hospital, place her on her left side. This position prevents a possible drop in blood pressure caused by pressure on the inferior vena cava, which reduces venous blood returning to the heart.

If the woman is straining or crowning, has had previous pregnancies, and there is not enough time to get to the hospital, you must prepare to assist in the delivery. First, call (or have a bystander call) the EMS. Then, if the woman is in a crowded or public place, try to find a private, clean area. The mother might find it reassuring to have a companion, such as her husband, a friend, or a relative, present. Follow these guidelines:

- Wear medical examination gloves. If available, wear a mask, a gown, and eye protection.
- Do not touch the vaginal area except during delivery and, if possible, with a witness present.
- Do not let the mother use the toilet.
- Do not hold the mother's legs together.

If the baby's head is not the presenting part (the first part to come out of the birth canal), the delivery will be complicated. Tell the mother not to push and attempt to calm and reassure her. Call 9-1-1 if you have not already done so.

> ### CAUTION
> DO NOT allow the mother to go to the toilet if delivery seems imminent.
>
> DO NOT attempt to delay or restrain delivery in any way (for example, holding the mother's legs together).

Stages of Labor

Labor is a three-stage process that begins with the first regular uterine contractions, includes delivery of the baby, and ends with delivery of the placenta. The first stage usually lasts several hours (possibly 12 hours or more for a first baby), from the first contraction until the cervix is fully open (dilated). The cervix gradually stretches until it is large enough to let the baby pass through. (Outside a hospital setting, rescuers cannot safely check for dilation of the cervix.) The contractions usually begin as acutely aching sensations in the small of the back; in a short time, they turn into cramplike pains recurring regularly in the lower abdomen. At first, the contractions are 10 to 15 minutes apart, are not very severe, and last less than 1 minute. Gradually, the intervals between contractions grow shorter, and the contractions increase in intensity. A slight, watery, blood-stained discharge (bloody show) from the vagina might accompany contractions or might occur before labor begins.

At the end of the first stage of labor, the amniotic sac breaks, and a pint or more of watery fluid, the amniotic fluid, discharges. Sometimes the amniotic sac breaks during the first stage of labor, but this is no cause for concern because it usually does not affect labor. If the amniotic sac breaks prematurely and labor does not begin within 12 hours, the risk of infection to mother and baby is great, and medical care should be obtained.

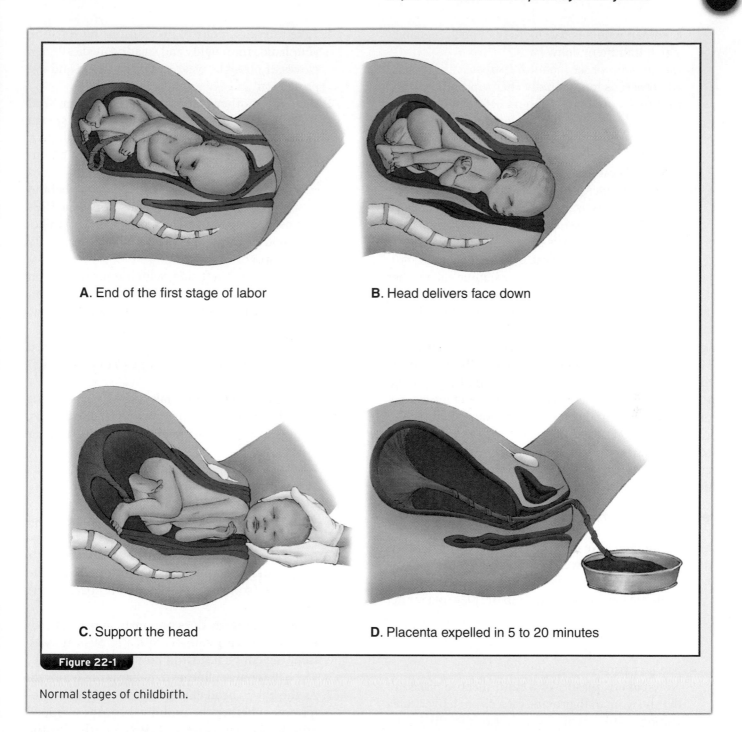

A. End of the first stage of labor

B. Head delivers face down

C. Support the head

D. Placenta expelled in 5 to 20 minutes

Figure 22-1

Normal stages of childbirth.

The second stage lasts from 30 minutes to 2 hours. It begins when the neck of the cervix is fully open and ends with the actual birth of the baby. The baby is normally head down; once the head gets through the pelvis, the rest of the body should follow easily. During the third stage, which lasts about 15 minutes or more, the afterbirth (placenta) is expelled **Figure 22-1**.

Recognizing Signs of Impending Delivery

At the scene of a woman in labor, you will need to determine whether delivery is imminent or whether there is time to transport the woman to the hospital. To make that decision, answer the following questions:

- *Has the woman had a baby before?* Labor during a first pregnancy is usually longer than in subsequent pregnancies. If this is her first pregnancy, there might be more time for transport to a hospital.
- *How frequent are the contractions?* Contractions more than 5 minutes apart are a good indication that there will be enough time to get the mother to a nearby hospital. Contractions less than 2 minutes apart that last 45 to 60 seconds, especially in

a woman who has had more than one pregnancy, signal imminent delivery.

- *Has the amniotic sac ruptured? If so, when?* Labor usually proceeds more rapidly after rupture. If the sac ruptures more than 18 hours before birth occurs, the likelihood of fetal infection increases, and the hospital staff should be alerted. Delivery might be more difficult when the amniotic sac ruptures prematurely because amniotic fluid serves as a lubricant.
- *Does the mother feel as though she has to move her bowels?* That sensation is caused by the fetal head in the vagina pressing against the rectum and indicates that delivery is imminent.

Only if the answers to these questions seem to indicate an imminent birth should you examine the mother for crowning. Look to see if there is bulging at the vaginal opening or if part of the baby is visible. Crowning indicates that the baby is about to be born and that there is no time to get to a hospital before delivery. Because this step might be embarrassing to the mother, the father, bystanders, or even you, it is important that you explain fully what you are doing and why. Make every effort to protect the woman from embarrassment during such an examination by removing only enough clothing to expose the vaginal area. Use something to shield the woman from prying eyes, for example, a blanket used to make a tent, or even a human shield, with people standing with their backs toward her.

Delivery Procedures

Ideally, you should have the following supplies for delivery:
- Clean sheets, towels, and blankets to cover the mother and baby
- A plastic bag or towel to wrap the placenta for delivery to the hospital
- Clean, unused, medical exam gloves to reduce the likelihood of infection
- Sanitary pads
- Newspapers, plastic, or a cloth sheet to place under the woman to provide for a clean delivery area
- Rubber bulb syringe for suctioning the baby's mouth and nostrils
- Sterile gauze pads for wiping blood and mucus from the baby's mouth and nose
- Strips of gauze, new or clean shoelaces, or similar materials to tie the cord (Do not use thread, wire, or string because they might cut through the cord.) Gauze bandages or pads opened into strips can be used.

Care for a Woman During Delivery

If you are faced with an imminent delivery, follow the steps in **Skill Drill 22-1** :

1. Take infection-control precautions by washing your hands thoroughly and wearing medical exam gloves. If possible, wear a mask, a gown, and eye protection.
2. Have the mother lie on her back with her head slightly elevated, knees drawn up and legs spread apart. The mother might want to be in a different position. Other safe positions for childbirth include the following:
   - Sitting up or squatting, with someone behind supporting her. These two positions place less tension on the vaginal tissues, reducing the likelihood of a tear, and allow the force of gravity to help.
   - Lying on her left side, which improves blood return to her heart and prevents aspiration should she vomit. Have someone hold the woman's right leg up out of the way.
   - Kneeling in a knee-chest position, which is used in many countries and in cases of breech presentations.
   - Remind the woman to take short, quick breaths during each contraction. Between contractions, she should rest and breathe deeply through her mouth.
3. Place absorbent, clean materials (such as sheets or towels) under the mother's buttocks.
4. Elevate her buttocks with blankets or a pillow.
5. When the baby's head appears, place the palm of your hand on top of the head and exert very gentle pressure, to prevent explosive delivery. Have the woman stop pushing. Do not push on the fontanels (soft spots on the top and back of the infant's head).
6. If the amniotic sac does not break or has not broken, tear it with your fingers and push it away from the baby's head and mouth as they appear. The baby could suffocate if the sac is not removed.
7. As the baby's head emerges from the vagina, determine whether the umbilical cord is wrapped around the baby's neck. If it is, gently slip the cord over the baby's shoulder. If you cannot do that, attempt to alleviate pressure on the cord. (See number 17 for instructions on how to cut the cord).
8. Support the baby's head as it emerges.
9. Suction the baby's mouth and then the nostrils two or three times with the bulb syringe. Use caution to avoid contact with the back of the baby's mouth. If a bulb syringe is not available, wipe the baby's mouth and then the nose with gauze (Step ❶).

10. As the torso and full body emerge, support the baby with both hands—he or she will be slippery (**Steps ❷** and **❸**).

11. Do not pull on the baby, which could cause cervical spine damage. Do not put your fingers in the baby's armpits; pressure on the nerve centers there could cause paralysis.

12. Keep the baby level with the vagina slightly head down, to improve drainage from the mouth and nose.

13. Wipe blood and mucus from the baby's mouth and nose with sterile gauze; suction the mouth, and then suction the nose again.

14. Dry the infant to reduce heat loss and help stimulate breathing. Rub the baby's back or flick the soles of its feet to stimulate breathing. The baby should breathe within 30 seconds, especially after the cord stops pulsating (**Step ❹**). (Do not hold the baby up by the feet and slap its buttocks, which could cause an increase in intracranial pressure.) If breathing does not start within 30 seconds, begin CPR.

15. Wrap the infant in a warm blanket and place on his or her side, head slightly lower than the trunk. Keep the infant level with the mother's vagina until the cord is cut. Raising the baby above the mother's abdomen (location of the placenta) while the umbilical cord is intact will allow the baby's blood to drain out and might result in shock in the baby. Holding the baby below the mother's abdomen allows her blood to run into the baby, and the extra blood cells can cause serious problems such as jaundice.

16. When the umbilical cord stops pulsating, tie it with gauze (or similar material) or a clean shoelace between the mother and the newborn.

17. If the mother is going to the hospital soon after the birth, and it was a normal delivery, there is no need to cut the cord. Keep the infant warm and wait for the EMS personnel, who will have the proper equipment to clamp and cut the cord. If you are in a remote location, you might have to cut the cord yourself. In such a situation and after cord pulsations stop, tie the cord about 4 inches away from the baby and make a second tie 2 inches from the first tie. Cut the cord between the two ties.

18. Watch for delivery of the placenta, which usually takes a few minutes, but could take as long as 30 minutes. Do not pull on the end of the umbilical cord to speed the placenta's delivery (**Step ❺**).

19. When the placenta is delivered, wrap it in a towel with three quarters of the umbilical cord and place the towel in a plastic bag. Keep the bag at the level of the infant. Take the placenta to the hospital, where it will be examined for completeness. This procedure is necessary because pieces of placenta retained in the uterus can cause persistent bleeding or infection.

20. Place a sterile pad over the vaginal opening, lower the mother's legs, and help her hold them together.

21. Gently massage the woman's abdomen, just below the navel, to help control bleeding.

Delivery Aftercare

After delivery, monitor the mother's breathing and pulse. Replace any blood-soaked sheets and blankets while awaiting transport. A woman can be expected to lose from 1 to 2 cups (300 to 500 mL) of blood after delivery. You should be aware of this amount of blood loss so it does not cause undue psychological stress to the new mother or to you. If blood loss continues, massage the uterus. Uterine massage stimulates the uterus to contract, thus constricting blood vessels within its walls and decreasing bleeding.

1. Use your hand with your fingers fully extended.
2. Place the palm of your hand on the lower abdomen, where you should be able to feel a grapefruit-sized mass.
3. Massage (knead) over the area.
4. If bleeding continues, check your massage technique.
5. The mother can also breast-feed the baby following delivery of the placenta to stimulate uterine contractions and, thus, help control bleeding.

Initial Care of the Newborn

Normal findings in a newborn are a pulse rate of more than 100 beats per minute (feel the brachial artery) and a respiratory rate of more than 40 breaths per minute. The baby often will be crying. The most important care is positioning, drying, keeping warm, and stimulating the newborn to breathe. Wrap the newborn in a blanket, making sure the head is covered. Repeat suctioning if necessary, and continue to stimulate the newborn if he or she is not breathing (flick the soles of the feet and rub the infant's back).

If the newborn does not begin to breathe within 30 seconds or continues to have difficulty breathing after 1 minute, you must begin CPR which includes the following:

1. Ensure that the airway is open.
2. Give one rescue breath every 3 seconds.
3. Reassess after 1 minute.

skill drill

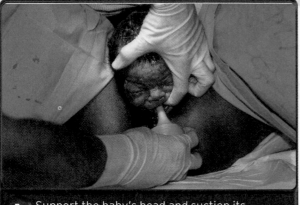

1 Support the baby's head and suction its mouth and nose.

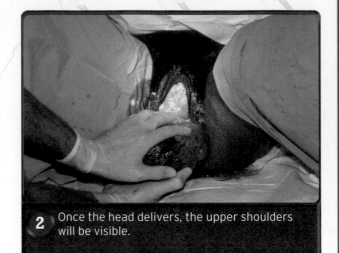

2 Once the head delivers, the upper shoulders will be visible.

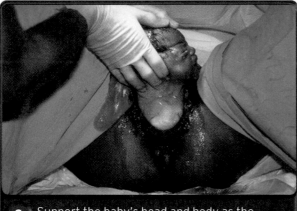

3 Support the baby's head and body as the shoulders deliver.

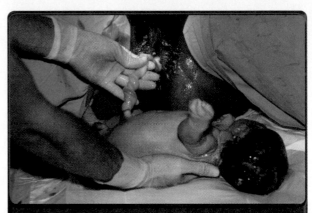

4 Clean and dry the infant to reduce heat loss and stimulate breathing.

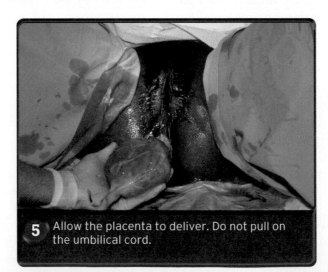

5 Allow the placenta to deliver. Do not pull on the umbilical cord.

▶ Abnormal Deliveries

Most childbirths are normal and natural. Sometimes, however, complications arise. It is essential that you be calm, deliberate, and gentle in a situation that becomes even more stressful because of complications. Call 9-1-1 for all of these situations.

Prolapsed Cord

A prolapsed cord is a condition in which the umbilical cord comes through the birth canal before delivery of the head. The cord is squeezed between the baby's head and the mother's body (vaginal wall), and oxygen supply to the baby could be stopped. This puts the baby in danger of suffocation **Figure 22-2** . This situation is rare and very dangerous.

Recognizing a Prolapsed Cord

If the umbilical cord can be seen before the baby's head, the cord is prolapsed.

Care for an Infant With a Prolapsed Cord

1. Position the woman with her head down or buttocks raised to use gravity to lessen pressure in the birth canal.
2. Insert fingers of your gloved hand into the vagina, placing fingers on either side of the cord to hold pressure from the presenting part (most often the head) of the fetus away from the pulsating cord. Continue until the EMS arrives. Do *not* push the cord back into the vagina. This is one of only two circumstances for putting your fingers into the vagina.
3. Call 9-1-1 immediately.

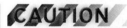

DO NOT attempt to push the cord back into the vagina.

Breech Birth Presentation

A breech presentation occurs when the baby's buttocks or lower extremities emerge before the head or shoulders. Breech presentation is the most common type of abnormal delivery and occurs in 3–4% of all deliveries. Place the mother in a kneeling, head-down position, with her pelvis elevated, and seek medical care immediately **Figure 22-3** .

In a breech presentation, if the baby's head is not delivered within 3 minutes of the body, you must act to prevent suffocation of the baby. Suffocation can occur when

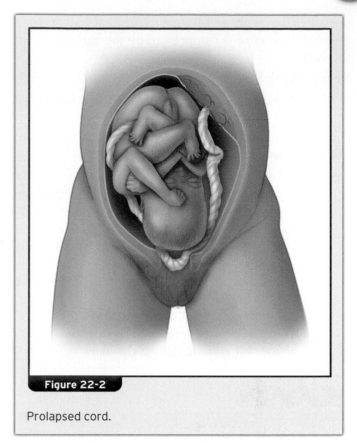

Figure 22-2

Prolapsed cord.

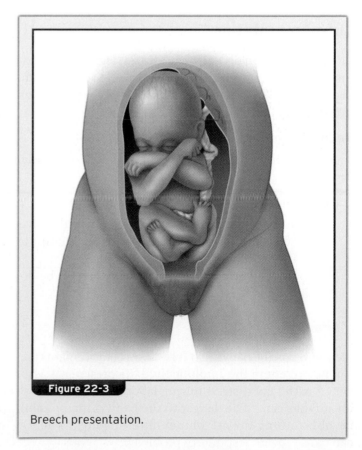

Figure 22-3

Breech presentation.

the baby's face is pressed against the vaginal wall or when the umbilical cord is compressed by the baby's head in the vagina.

Recognizing Breech Birth Presentation

In a breech birth, the baby's buttocks come out first (most babies are born head first).

Care for an Infant With Breech Birth Presentation

To establish an airway, do the following:

1. Place one hand in the vagina, positioning the palm toward the baby's face. This is one of only two circumstances for putting your fingers into the vagina.
2. Form a V with your fingers on either side of the baby's nose.
3. Push the vaginal wall away from the baby's face until the head is delivered.
4. Have someone call 9-1-1 immediately.
5. Have the woman continue to push with contractions and attempt to deliver the baby.

CAUTION

DO NOT pull the baby's head out during a breech delivery.

Limb Presentation

Limb presentation occurs when an arm, leg, or foot of the infant protrudes from the birth canal. A foot more commonly presents when the infant is in breech presentation 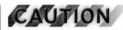 .

Recognizing Limb Presentation

In a case of limb presentation, arm, leg, or foot appears first.

Care for an Infant With Limb Presentation

1. Place mother in head-down position with pelvis elevated. Do *not* pull on the baby or attempt to push the limb back into the vagina.
2. Call 9-1-1 immediately. The baby cannot be delivered in this position.

Meconium

Meconium is the baby's first feces (bowel movement) and can be present in the amniotic fluid. Its presence is associated with fetal distress during labor and a greater risk for infant death. The danger to the baby is the possibility of breathing the meconium into the lungs, where it can cause severe respiratory problems.

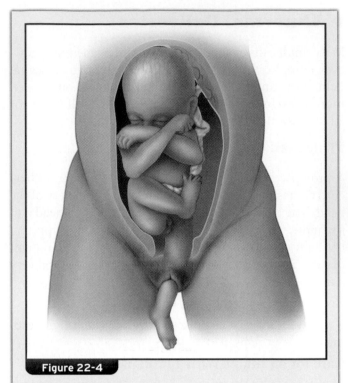

Figure 22-4

Limb presentation.

FYI

Emergencies During Pregnancy
What Medical Specialties Take Care of Women?

A gynecologist specializes in treating conditions related to the female reproductive tract. An obstetrician specializes in treating pregnant women. A pediatrician specializes in treating newborn babies, toddlers, and young teens.

How Is Emergency Care for a Pregnant Woman Different?

There are two people involved—the mother and fetus. Even minor trauma to the mother's abdomen can result in life-threatening consequences. All pregnant women with trauma to the abdomen need a medical examination in a hospital emergency department and often need fetal monitoring. Fetal viability is determined by maternal viability. Position the mother on her left side to help venous blood return to the heart. Care for the pregnant woman the same way you would treat a non-pregnant woman.

What Are Some Indications of Pregnancy Problems?

- The big three warning signs of a serious problem are bleeding, abdominal cramps, and weakness.
- Morning sickness, swollen ankles, and urinary tract infections are not usually dangerous, but call the physician anyway.
- If a pregnant woman is spotting (small amount of vaginal bleeding), have her lie down immediately. Call for medical attention. Spotting can signal the onset of a miscarriage.

Recognizing Meconium

Amniotic fluid containing meconium is greenish or brownish-yellow in color rather than clear. It is tarry and almost odorless.

Care for Baby in Danger of Inhaling Meconium

Follow these steps to prevent a newborn infant from inhaling meconium:

1. Keep the infant in a moderately head-down position to aid with drainage.
2. Suction the mouth and nostrils thoroughly, or the baby will inhale meconium with its first breath into the lungs. Clear amniotic fluid, however, is harmlessly absorbed through the baby's lungs. Try not to stimulate the infant to breathe before suctioning.
3. Maintain the baby's open airway.
4. Call 9-1-1 immediately.

Premature Birth

Any baby weighing less than 5.5 pounds or one who is born before 7 months of pregnancy is defined as premature and needs special care. Premature babies develop problems because they are smaller and less developed than full-term infants. For example, their cardiovascular and respiratory systems are often immature.

Recognizing Signs of Premature Birth

It is difficult without scales to weigh an infant. Signs of premature birth include:

- Premature infant will be smaller and thinner than a full-term infant.
- Premature infant has a head proportionately larger in comparison with the rest of the body.
- The cheesy, white coating on the skin (*vernix caseosa*) of a full-term infant will be minimal or absent on the premature infant.

Care for Premature Babies

Care for a premature baby in the following manner:

1. Keep the baby warm. Premature babies are always at risk for hypothermia.
2. Keep the mouth and nose clear of mucus.
3. Monitor breathing and perform CPR, if necessary.

Gynecologic Emergencies

Gynecologic emergencies are reproductive-system problems that occur in nonpregnant females.

▶ Sexual Assault and Rape

Perhaps one of the most difficult emergency situations that a first aider might have to deal with is sexual assault.

Rape is the fastest growing violent crime in the United States. Authorities suspect that 80–90% of rape cases are not reported to authorities. In most cases, the rape victim is a woman. An estimated 1 in 3 American women will be sexually assaulted at some point in their life. It should be noted, however, that men, heterosexual and homosexual, also can be raped.

There are many definitions of rape, but in general, rape involves attempted or actual sexual intercourse, against the will of the victim. Related physical injury is common, but the psychological trauma is more damaging. It is essential that you be calm and sympathetic when dealing with a victim of sexual assault.

Recognizing Sexual Assault and Rape

A first aider should provide care for the victim and not focus on obtaining evidence (although you should try to *preserve* evidence). Confine your questions to an assessment of the victim's injuries, not a detailed description of the events. Ask questions based on the SAMPLE survey (see Chapter 4).

A sexual assault victim might display:

- headaches
- sleeplessness, nightmares
- nausea and/or muscle spasms
- confusion
- depression
- anxiety, jumpiness

Care for a Victim of Sexual Assault and Rape

The following list outlines what you should do and not do for a victim of sexual assault and rape.

1. Don't ask a lot of questions. Don't blame the survivor in any way or talk about what might have been done or what you would have done. Be supportive. Remind him or her that he or she is safe now.
2. Determine which injuries require immediate care. Whenever it is necessary that a female victim disrobe, try to have another woman present.
3. Do not expose the genitalia unless an injury there requires immediate care (for example, severe bleeding). Examining genitalia, except when childbirth is imminent, has serious legal implications and, therefore, usually should not be done.
4. Try, if possible, to preserve evidence but leave the actual investigation to the police. To preserve evidence, encourage the victim not to change clothes, wash, urinate, defecate, or douche. Explain to the victim in a sympathetic way that it would be best not to clean up. Keep in mind that a rape victim,

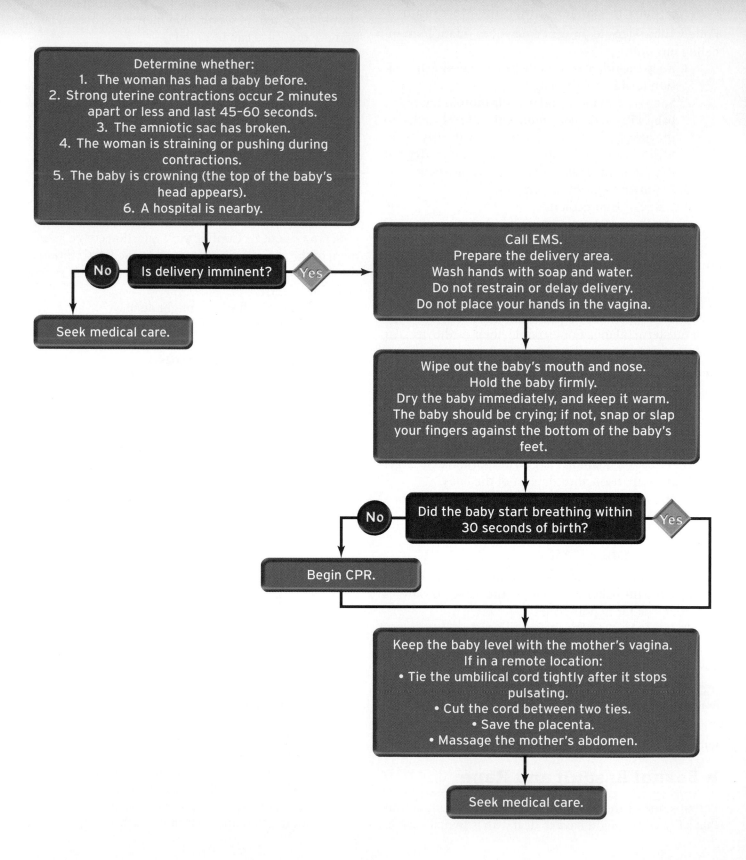

Determine whether:
1. The woman has had a baby before.
2. Strong uterine contractions occur 2 minutes apart or less and last 45–60 seconds.
3. The amniotic sac has broken.
4. The woman is straining or pushing during contractions.
5. The baby is crowning (the top of the baby's head appears).
6. A hospital is nearby.

No — Is delivery imminent? — **Yes**

Seek medical care.

Call EMS.
Prepare the delivery area.
Wash hands with soap and water.
Do not restrain or delay delivery.
Do not place your hands in the vagina.

Wipe out the baby's mouth and nose.
Hold the baby firmly.
Dry the baby immediately, and keep it warm.
The baby should be crying; if not, snap or slap your fingers against the bottom of the baby's feet.

No — Did the baby start breathing within 30 seconds of birth? — **Yes**

Begin CPR.

Keep the baby level with the mother's vagina.
If in a remote location:
• Tie the umbilical cord tightly after it stops pulsating.
• Cut the cord between two ties.
• Save the placenta.
• Massage the mother's abdomen.

Seek medical care.

like any other victim, has the right to refuse first aid and transport to a hospital.

5. Even if the victim refuses aid, do not leave him or her alone. Try to have a trusted friend or relative stay with the victim. Protect the privacy of the victim. Emotional support is vital. Most large communities have rape crisis centers; furnishing the victim with the name and number of the nearest center (look in the telephone directory) is probably as important as treating any physical injuries. Trained volunteers can talk to the survivor and give you and the survivor information about what to do next.

6. Get the survivor medical care. The survivor could be in shock and unaware of the severity of her/his injuries. Strongly encourage a rape victim to receive medical care, even if the person does not show any signs of injury and does not want medical care. However, be aware that the medical exam following a rape is intrusive and includes a full gynecological exam. Survivors will need information about what is going to happen before receiving medical care.

FYI

Urinary Tract Infections
What Should Be Done About Urinary Tract Infections?

- Women, especially during pregnancy, are very susceptible to urinary tract infections. Often, when one infection clears, another replaces it.

- Seek advice from a doctor. Self-care measures to help relieve the burning pain include taking shallow, lukewarm sitz baths sprinkled with baking soda; urinating while standing in the shower; and practicing good personal hygiene. Wiping from front to back after going to the bathroom helps keep bacteria, including *Escherichia coli*, away from the urinary tract. Drinking more fluids helps prevent and treat urinary tract infections. Some experts report that drinking cranberry juice (tablets are also available with fewer calories) might help inhibit urinary tract infections.

- A urinary tract (bladder) infection can lead to the more serious kidney infection. Signs of a kidney infection include blood in the urine, pain in the lower back or flank, fever, and nausea or vomiting.

prep kit

▶ Ready for Review

- Miscarriages usually occur during the first trimester of pregnancy.
- If a woman experiences vaginal bleeding late in her pregnancy, it usually constitutes an emergency.
- Emergency childbirth occurs when a baby is born at an unplanned time or at an unplanned place.
- In most cases, childbirth is normal and natural. Sometimes complications can arise.
- Perhaps one of the most difficult emergency situations that a first aider might have to deal with is sexual assault.

▶ Vital Vocabulary

amniotic sac A thick, transparent sac that holds the fetus suspended in the amniotic fluid.

birth canal The vagina and the lower part of the uterus.

bloody show The bloody mucus plug that is discharged from the vagina when labor begins.

cervix The small opening at the lower end of the uterus through which the baby passes.

crowning The stage of birth when the presenting part of the baby is visible at the vaginal orifice.

labor The process or period of childbirth; especially, the muscular contraction of the uterus designed to expel the fetus from the mother.

miscarriage Delivery of the fetus before it is mature enough to survive outside the womb (about 20 weeks), from either natural (spontaneous abortion) or induced causes.

placenta The vascular organ attached to the uterine wall that supplies oxygen and nutrients to the fetus; also called afterbirth.

umbilical cord The flexible structure that connects the fetus to the placenta.

▶ Assessment in Action

It is a brisk autumn day and your very pregnant sister is visiting you at your weekend cabin to get a few days of relaxation before the arrival of her first child. You are sitting on the porch, enjoying a mug of tea when your sister puts her mug down and begins to rub her back. You are a little over than 45 minutes away from the nearest hospital.

Directions: Circle Yes if you agree with the statement, circle No if you disagree.

Yes   No   **1.** Since this is her first baby, the labor will probably be very short.

Yes   No   **2.** It is normal for the contractions to move from the back to the lower abdomen.

Yes   No   **3.** If the contractions are more than 5 minutes apart, you should have time to get her to the hospital.

Yes   No   **4.** If the amniotic sac ruptures, you should assume that delivery is imminent.

Yes   No   **5.** If there is time to transport your sister, place her on her left side.

Answers: **1.** No; **2.** Yes; **3.** Yes; **4.** No; **5.** Yes

▶ Check Your Knowledge

Directions: Circle Yes if you agree with the statement, circle No if you disagree.

Yes   No   **1.** An aching in the lower back is a sign of a miscarriage.

Yes   No   **2.** It is normal for a woman to experience vaginal bleeding in her last trimester.

Yes   No   **3.** Most babies in the United States are delivered at home.

Yes   No   **4.** Place a pregnant woman on her left side when transporting her to the hospital.

Yes   No   **5.** Labor is a four-stage process.

Yes   No   **6.** The second stage of labor lasts from 30 minutes to 2 hours.

Yes   No   **7.** New or clean shoelaces can be used to tie the umbilical cord.

Yes   No   **8.** A prolapsed umbilical cord is a normal occurrence.

Yes   No   **9.** The placenta is also called the afterbirth.

Yes   No **10.** Whether or not the woman has given birth before will usually affect the length of the labor.

Answers: **1.** Yes; **2.** No; **3.** No; **4.** Yes; **5.** No; **6.** Yes; **7.** Yes; **8.** No; **9.** Yes; **10.** Yes

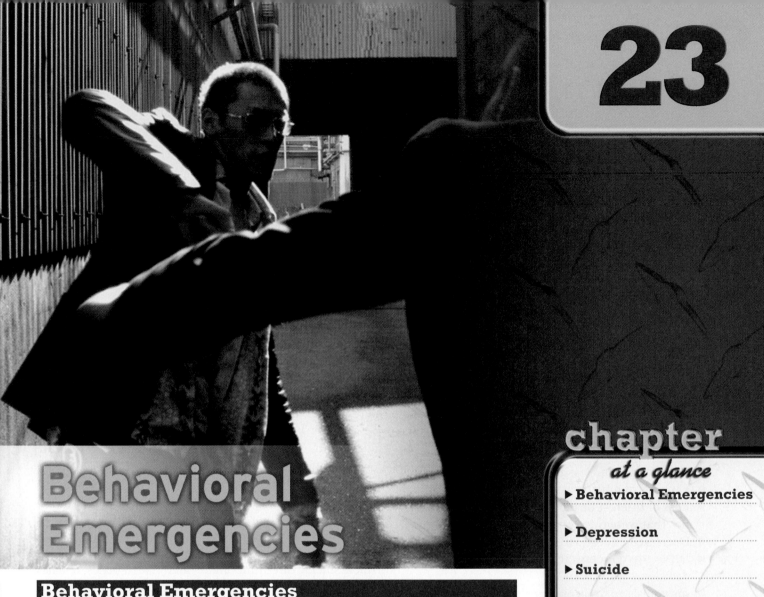

Behavioral Emergencies

Behavioral Emergencies

Behavior is how a person acts. Although each person acts or behaves differently, sometimes a person exhibits unacceptable or intolerable behavior. The abnormal behavior may be due to a psychological condition (such as a mental illness) or a physical condition. For example, a person with diabetes who has an uncorrected low blood sugar level can display aggressiveness, restlessness, or anxiety. Because the brain lacks energy in the form of blood sugar (glucose), altered mental status results. Likewise, lack of oxygen and inadequate blood flow to the brain also cause altered mental status, resulting in similar behavior. Behavior that leads to violence or other inappropriate activities is known as a <u>behavioral emergency</u>.

Several factors can change a person's behavior, including situational stresses, medical illnesses, psychiatric problems, alcohol, and drugs. The following are common reasons for behavioral changes:

- Low blood sugar level in a person with diabetes
- Lack of oxygen (known as *hypoxia*)
- Inadequate blood flow to the brain
- Head trauma
- Excessive cold
- Excessive heat
- Mind-altering substances, such as alcohol, depressants, stimulants, hallucinogens, and narcotics
- Psychogenic or psychiatric illness that leads to psychotic thinking, depression, or panic

▶ Depression

Depression is more than the sad feeling that everyone experiences at times. Depression is one of the most common and treatable of all mental illness. There are several types of depression: *reactive depression* (following tragic events), *major* or *clinical depression* (with no apparent cause, lasts more than 2 weeks, and prevents functioning in top form at work or socially), and *bipolar depression*, a type that includes episodes of euphoria. *Depression* is believed to be due to a chemical imbalance in the brain, which causes the nerves in the brain to not work properly. This is why it is often treated using medications that act on the brain. Depression can lead to suicide; in fact, untreated depression is the main cause of suicide.

Recognizing Depression

Not everyone who is depressed experiences every symptom. Some people experience a few symptoms, others many. Severity of symptoms varies with individuals and also varies over time.

- Persistent sad, anxious, or "empty" moods
- Feelings of hopelessness, pessimism
- Feelings of guilt, worthlessness, helplessness
- Loss of interest or pleasure in hobbies and activities that were once enjoyed, including sex
- Decreased energy, fatigue, feeling "slowed down"
- Difficulty concentrating, remembering, making decisions
- Insomnia, early-morning awakening, or oversleeping
- Appetite and/or weight loss or overeating and weight gain
- Thoughts or death or suicide; suicide attempts
- Restlessness, irritability
- Persistent physical symptoms that do not respond to treatment such as headaches, digestive disorders, and chronic pain

Care for Depression

Some depressed people do not feel like talking. In such cases, saying, "You look very sad," often allows the person to talk about the depressed feelings. The person might burst into tears. Do not discourage the crying. Maintain a sympathetic silence and let the person "cry it out."

A depressed person needs empathetic attention and reassurance and needs to know that the first aider is concerned. It is usually best to interview a depressed person in private because the presence of several people may make the person uncomfortable. Ask open-ended questions such as, "Tell me how you feel." Tell the depressed person that many people have periods of unhappiness, but they can be helped to feel better. Mention community resources where such help can be found.

▶ Suicide

Suicide is defined as any willful act that ends one's own life. Each year, about 30,000 Americans commit suicide; it is the eleventh reported leading cause of death in the United States. Many experts, however, believe that suicide is vastly underreported. Suicide in the United States is increasingly a problem of adolescents, college-age students, and the very old.

The male rate for suicides is more than three times that for females. It is most common in men who are single, widowed, or divorced. Slightly more than half of all suicides—both men and women—use firearms. The next most common method is hanging. Poisoning by solids or liquids is the most common method used by people who attempt but do not complete suicide. Jumping from high places, carbon monoxide poisoning by auto exhaust, drowning, and self-inflicted (non-firearm) wounds are less common methods.

The number of suicides peaks during spring months and is lowest in the winter. Suicide rates are lowest in the Northeast and highest in the mountain states.

Suicide attempts are eight times more common than completed suicides. In addition, although males complete suicide three times more often than females, females are reported to attempt suicide three times more often. It is not known if males are more reluctant to seek help and, thus, less likely to report their attempts. It also is not known if the lower rate of suicide among females results from their choice of less-lethal methods.

Despite its ranking as a major cause of death, suicide is rare. Except in the case of suicide clusters (three or more completed suicides closely related in time and place), no community is likely to experience many suicides.

Suicide is often attempted by people who are depressed or have alcoholism. About 60% of all suicide victims previously attempted suicide, and about 75% gave clear warning that they intended to kill themselves. Typically, a suicide attempt occurs when an individual's close emotional attachments are in danger or when he or she physically loses a significant family member or friend. Suicidal people often feel unable to manage their lives. Frequently, they lack self-esteem.

Many suicidal people make last-minute attempts to communicate their intentions. When a person phones to threaten suicide, try to keep the suicidal person on the line until EMS reaches the scene.

If you encounter a person who is attempting or threatening suicide, discreetly remove any dangerous articles. Talk quietly with the person and encourage the person to discuss the situation. Ask the following: Have you attempted suicide before? Have you made any concrete plans for a method of suicide? Has any family member committed suicide? People who have made a previous suicide attempt, who have detailed suicide plans, or who have a close relative who committed suicide are more likely to try to kill themselves Table 23-1 . They must be reassured and taken to medical help, usually at a hospital. Do not leave them alone under any circumstances.

When a person attempts suicide, first aid care has priority. Drug overdoses must be managed. Bleeding from slashed wrists must be controlled. As you give first aid, try to encourage the person to talk about the situation. If a drug overdose is involved, collect any medication containers, pills, or other drugs found on the scene and take the items to the hospital emergency department with the victim. In many cases, law enforcement authorities should be contacted.

Recognizing a Potential Suicide Victim

If you observe someone:

- Getting their affairs in order (paying off debts, making or changing a will)
- Giving away articles of either personal or monetary value
- Signs of planning a suicide such as obtaining a weapon or writing a suicide note

If someone says:

- Life isn't worth living.
- My family would be better off without me.
- Next time I'll take enough pills to do the job right.
- Take my (prized collection, valuables); I don't need this stuff anymore.
- I won't be around to deal with that.
- You'll be sorry when I'm gone.
- I won't be around much longer.
- I just can't deal with everything—life's too hard.
- Nobody understands me; nobody feels the way I do.
- There's nothing I can do to make it better.

Table 23-1 Suicide Risk Factors

The SAD PERSONS scale is a mnemonic list of known suicide high-risk characteristics. A score of nine or greater indicates the probable need for psychiatric consultation.

Mnemonic	Characteristics	Score
S Sex	Male	1
A Age	Younger than 19 or older than 45 years	1
D Depression or hopelessness	Admits to depression or decreased concentration, appetite, sleep, libido	2
P Previous attempts or psychiatric care	Previous impatient or outpatient psychiatric care	1
E Excessive alcohol or drug use	Chronic addiction or recent frequent drug use	1
R Rational thinking loss	Brain dysfunction (unknown or nonspecific cause) or psychosis	2
S Separated, widowed, or divorced		1
O Organized or serious attempt	Well-thought-out plan or life-threatening display	2
N No social support	No close family, friends, job, or active religious affiliation	1
S Stated future intent	Determined to repeat attempt	2

Determining whether high-risk factors are involved will help first aiders maintain objectivity. It is important to maintain a nonjudgmental approach. Using the SAD PERSONS mnemonic acknowledges the seriousness of the situation and reminds first aiders that ridiculing, making demeaning comments, or ignoring the person are not helpful or proper.

Take precautions by keeping the person under close observation, removing any potentially dangerous items (for example, glass, razors, and medicines) from the immediate area, and not allowing the person to go *anywhere*, even to the bathroom, unaccompanied.

Source: Hockberger RS, Rothstein RJ: Assessment of suicide potential by non-psychiatrists using the SAD PERSONS score. *J Emerg Med* 6(2):99-107.

- I'd be better off dead.
- I feel like there is no way out.

Care for a Potential Suicide Victim

If someone tells you they are thinking about suicide, you should take their distress seriously. Here are some ways to be helpful to someone who is threatening suicide:

- Be direct. Talk openly and matter-of-factly about suicide.
- Be willing to listen. Allow expressions of feelings. Accept the feelings.
- Be nonjudgmental. Don't debate whether suicide is right or wrong.
- Get involved. Become available. Show interest and support.
- Do not dare him or her to do it.

- Do not act shocked. This will put distance between the two of you.
- Do not be sworn to secrecy. Seek support.
- Offer hope that alternatives are available but do not offer glib reassurance.
- Take action. Remove means of suicide, such as guns or stockpiled pills.
- Get help from persons or agencies specializing in crisis intervention and suicide prevention.

CAUTION

DO NOT ignore a suicide threat. Every suicidal act or gesture should be taken seriously and the person referred to a professional counselor.

FYI

Fables and Facts About Suicide

Fable	Fact
People who talk about suicide do not commit suicide.	Of every 10 people who kill themselves, 8 have given definite warnings of their suicidal intentions. Suicide threats and attempts must be taken seriously.
Suicide happens without warning.	Studies reveal that the suicidal person gives many clues and warnings about suicidal intentions. Being alert to these cries for help may prevent suicidal behavior.
Suicidal people are fully intent on dying.	Most suicidal people are undecided about living or dying, and they gamble with death, leaving it to others to save them. Almost no one commits suicide without letting others know how he or she is feeling. Often this cry for help is given in code. Decoding these distress signals can save lives.
Once a person is suicidal, he or she is suicidal forever.	Fortunately, people who want to kill themselves are suicidal only for a limited time. If they are saved from self-destruction, they can lead useful lives.
Improvement following a suicidal crisis means that the suicidal risk is over.	Most suicides occur within 3 months after the beginning of improvement, when the individual has the energy to put morbid thoughts and feelings into effect. Relatives and physicians should be especially vigilant during this period.
Suicide strikes more often among the rich— or, conversely, it occurs more frequently among the poor.	Suicide is neither the rich man's disease nor the poor man's curse. Suicide is democratic and is represented proportionately at all levels of society.
Suicide is inherited or runs in a family (that is, is genetically determined).	Suicide does not run in families. It is an individual matter and can be prevented.
All suicidal people are mentally ill, and suicide is always the act of a psychotic person.	Studies of hundreds of genuine suicide notes indicate that although a suicidal person is extremely unhappy, he or she is not necessarily mentally ill. The overpowering unhappiness may result from a temporary emotional upset, a long and painful illness, or a complete loss of hope.

Source: US Department of Health and Human Resources.

► Emotional Injury

First aid for an emotional "injury" means being supportive of people with emotional injuries, whether the injuries are from physical injury or excessive or unbearable strain on the victim's emotions.

Emotional first aid often goes hand in hand with physical first aid because a physical injury and the circumstances surrounding it may actually cause emotional injury. On the other hand, emotional injury may occur when there is no physical injury. Emotional injuries usually are not as obvious as physical injuries, but both can be severe and require "first aid."

Although most emotional reactions are temporary, lasting only minutes, hours, or, at the most, a few days, they are seriously disabling and may upset others. It is important to know that first aid can be applied to emotional as well as to physical injuries.

Typical Reactions

With few exceptions, all people experience fear in the face of an emergency. Feeling shaky, perspiring profusely, and becoming nauseated are common. Such reactions are normal and no cause for concern. Most people are able to regain their composure reasonably quickly.

Extensive training is not needed to recognize severe, abnormal reactions. To determine whether a person needs help, find out whether he or she is doing something that makes sense and is able to take care of him- or herself. For the most part, emotional first aid measures are simple and easy to understand.

However, improvisation is often needed, just as it is in splinting a fracture. Whatever the situation, you will have your own emotional reactions toward the victim. These reactions are important; they can enhance or hinder your ability to help the person. Especially when you are tired or worried, you may easily become impatient with the victim who seems to be "making a mountain out of a molehill." You may feel resentful toward the victim for being a burden. Be on guard against becoming impatient, intolerant, or resentful. Victims who can see the first aider's calmness, confidence, and competence will be reassured.

On the other hand, do not be overly sympathetic or overly solicitous. Excessive sympathy for an incapacitated person can be as harmful as negative feelings. The victim needs solid help but does not need to be overwhelmed with pity.

Recognizing Aggressive, Hostile, and Violent Behavior

When you are faced with aggressive, hostile, or violent behavior, size up the situation before you do anything. It may be unsafe for you and for others. The person may be standing or sitting in a threatening position. For example, does the person have clenched fists? Is he or she holding a lethal object? Is the person yelling or verbally threatening harm to anyone? If the scene appears unsafe, do not enter. If necessary, contact law enforcement officers.

An angry, violent person is ready to fight with anyone who approaches and may be difficult to control. Remember that anger may be a response to illness or that aggressive behavior may be a person's way of coping with feelings of helplessness. Avoid responding with anger. Many angry or violent persons can be calmed by someone who is trained and who appears confident that the person will behave well. Encourage the person to speak directly about the cause of his or her anger. A statement like "I'm not sure I understand why you are angry" often brings results. Reassure the person that you are there to help.

A person who is violent and out of control presents a special problem. Notify the police if you are unable to communicate with a person who is dangerous to him- or herself or to others.

Care for Aggressive, Hostile, and Violent Behavior

Confronting a person who is experiencing a behavioral emergency can be a trying and frustrating experience. Use these guidelines if you must try to calm a person who is upset:

- Acknowledge that the person seems upset, and reiterate that you are there to help.
- Maintain a comfortable distance.
- Encourage the person to state what is troubling him or her.
- Do not make quick moves.
- Respond honestly to the person's questions.
- Do not threaten, challenge, or argue with a disturbed person.
- Tell the truth—do not lie.
- Do not "play along" with any of a disturbed person's visual or auditory disturbances.
- Involve trusted family members or friends.
- Be prepared to stay with the person for an extended period of time.
- Never leave the person alone.
- Avoid unnecessary physical contact.
- Maintain eye contact.

Table 23-2   Psychological First Aid for Reactions to Emergency Situations

Reaction	Symptoms	Do . . .	Do Not . . .
Normal	Trembling Muscle tension Perspiration Nausea Mild diarrhea Urinary frequency Pounding heart Rapid breathing Anxiety	Give reassurance. Provide group identification. Motivate. Talk with the person. Observe to see that the person is gaining composure, not losing it.	Show resentment. Overdo sympathy.
Individual panic (flight reaction)	Unreasoning attempt to flee Loss of judgment Uncontrolled weeping Wildly running about	Try kind firmness. Give the person something warm to eat or drink. Get help to isolate the person from others, if necessary. Be empathetic. Encourage the person to talk. Be aware of your own limitations.	Use brutal restraint. Strike the person physically. Douse the person with water. Give sedatives.
Depression (underactive reactions)	Stands or sits without moving or talking Vacant expression Lack of emotional display	Make contact gently. Secure a rapport. Get the person to tell you what happened. Be empathetic. Recognize feelings of resentment in the person and yourself. Give the person a simple, routine task to complete. Offer warm food or drink.	Tell the person to "snap out of it." Overdo the sympathy. Give sedatives. Argue with the person.
Overactive	Argumentative Talks rapidly Jokes inappropriately Makes endless suggestions Jumps from one activity to another	Let the person talk about the situation. Find them jobs that require physical effort. Offer warm food or drink. Supervision is necessary. Be aware of your own feelings.	Suggest that victim is acting abnormally. Give sedatives. Argue with victim.
Physical (conversion disorder)	Severe nausea and vomiting Cannot use some part of the body.	Show interest in the person. Find a small job for the person to distract and occupy his or her thoughts. Make them comfortable. Get medical help as soon as possible.	Tell the person that there's nothing wrong with him or her. Place blame. Ridicule the person. Ignore the disability.

Source: Modified from M51-400-603-1, Department of Nonresident Instruction, Medical Field Service School, Brooke Army Medical Center, Fort Sam Houston, Texas.

▶ Sexual Assault and Rape

The definitions of rape and sexual assault vary widely. *Rape* is generally defined as forcible sexual intercourse without the consent of one participant. Categories of rape include the following:

- *Acquaintance rape,* which involves people who knew each other before the rape; includes relatives, neighbors, or friends.
- *Date rape,* which takes place within a relationship but without the consent of one person and may involve harm or the threat of harm by the other person.
- *Marital rape,* which occurs when the victim and the offender are married to each other.
- *Stranger rape,* which occurs when the victim and the offender have no relation to each other.

The victim may hesitate to report a rape for various reasons, such as shame, guilt, fear of retaliation, or reluctance to deal with law enforcement officials or the judicial system. The victim may even begin to doubt whether a "real" rape occurred. Rape is a traumatic crisis that disrupts the physical, psychological, social, and sexual aspects of the victim's life. The most common physical injuries are bruises, black eyes, and cuts.

As a first aider, you must be tactful and sensitive with the victim. The victim may find it extremely difficult to discuss what happened and may feel fear or hostility toward a first aider of the opposite sex. Every effort should be made to understand the victim's feelings and to respond with kindness and reassurance. The emotional trauma of rape is usually more prolonged and severe than the physical trauma. The attitude shown toward the victim during the initial care can have a substantial influence—for good or ill—on future psychological and physical recovery. Convince the victim to seek counseling through community resources such as a rape crisis center and to report the crime to the police. Ask the victim not to change clothes or to bathe because doing so can alter legal evidence. For the same reason, suggest that the victim not urinate, douche, defecate, or wash before being examined by a physician. Care for any injuries incurred during the attack. For more information, see Chapter 22.

▶ Child Abuse and Neglect

Because child abuse and neglect usually occur in the privacy of the home, no one knows exactly how many children are affected. More than 2.5 million cases of child abuse and neglect cases are reported each year. Of these, 35% involve physical abuse, 15% involve sexual abuse,

and 50% involve neglect. Child abuse and neglect can cause permanent damage to a child's physical, emotional, and mental development. The physical effects can include damage to the brain, vital organs, eyes, ears, arms, and legs, which, in turn, can result in mental retardation, blindness, deafness, or loss of a limb. At its most serious, abuse or neglect can result in a child's death.

Child abuse and neglect are usually divided into four major categories: physical abuse, neglect, sexual abuse, and emotional maltreatment. Each has recognizable characteristics, and all may be encountered by a first aider.

The National Center on Child Abuse and Neglect has set forth physical and behavioral indicators of child abuse and neglect. The list is not intended to be exhaustive; many more indicators exist than can be included. The presence of a single indicator does not necessarily prove that child abuse or neglect has occurred Table 23-3.

However, the repeated occurrence of an indicator, the presence of several indicators in combination, or the appearance of serious injury should alert the first aider to the possibility of child abuse Figure 23-1.

Recognizing Child Abuse and Neglect

It is not always easy to recognize when a child has been abused. Children who have been mistreated are often afraid to tell anyone because they think they will be blamed or that no one will believe them. Other parents or teachers also tend to overlook symptoms because they do not want to face the truth. The longer a child continues to be abused or is left to deal with the situation on his or her own, the less likely he or she is to make a full recovery.

The best way to check for signs of abuse is to be alert to any unexplainable changes in a child's body or behavior.

- Physical abuse: any injury (bruise, burn, fracture, abdominal or head injury) that cannot be explained.
- Sexual abuse:
  - fearful behavior (nightmares, depression, unusual fears, attempts to run away)
  - abdominal pain, bedwetting, urinary tract infection, genital pain or bleeding, sexually transmitted disease
  - extreme sexual behavior that seems inappropriate for the child's age
- Emotional abuse:
  - sudden change in self-confidence
  - headaches or stomachaches with no medical cause
  - abnormal fears, increases nightmares
  - attempts to run away

Table 23-3 Physical and Behavioral Indicators of Child Abuse and Neglect

Type of Child Abuse or Neglect	Physical Indicators	Behavioral Indicators
Physical Abuse	Unexplained bruises and welts on face, lips, mouth, torso, back, buttocks, and/or thighs in various stages of healing Clustered injuries on several different surface areas; formed by regular patterns reflecting the shape of the articles used to inflict the injury (electric cord, belt buckle) Regularly appearing injuries after an absence, weekend, or vacation, especially about the trunk and buttocks Be particularly suspicious if there are old bruises in addition to fresh ones Unexplained burns (such as those from a cigar or cigarette) especially on soles, palms, back, or buttocks Immersion burns (socklike, glovelike, doughnut shaped on buttocks or genitalia) Pattern burns as from an electric burner or iron, for example Rope burns on arms, legs, neck, or torso Unexplained fractures (particularly if multiple) to skull, nose, and/or facial structures in various stages of healing Multiple or spiral fractures Unexplained lacerations or abrasions to mouth, lips, gums, eyes, and/or external genitalia	Wary of adult contacts Apprehensive when other children cry Behavioral extremes: aggressiveness or withdrawal Frightened of parents Afraid to go home Reports injury by parents Acts apathetic and does not cry despite injuries Has been seen by emergency personnel for related complaints Was injured several days before medical attention was sought
Physical Neglect	Consistent hunger, poor hygiene, inappropriate dress Consistent lack of supervision, especially in dangerous activities or for extended periods of time Unattended physical problems or medical needs Abandonment	Begs, steals food Extended stays at school (early arrival and late departure) Constant fatigue, listlessness, or falling asleep in class Alcohol or drug abuse Delinquency (for example, thefts) States there is no caretaker
Sexual Abuse	Difficulty walking or sitting Torn, stained, or bloody underclothing Pain or itching in genital area Bruises or bleeding in external genitalia or vaginal or anal areas Venereal disease, especially in preteens Pregnancy	Unwillingness to change for gym or participate in physical education class Withdrawal, fantasizing, or infantile behavior Bizarre, sophisticated, or unusual sexual behavior or knowledge Poor peer relationships Delinquency or truancy Reports sexual assault by caretaker
Emotional Maltreatment	Speech disorders Lags in physical development Failure to thrive	Habit disorders (for example, sucking, biting, rocking) Conduct disorders (for example, antisocial, destructive) Neurotic traits (sleep disorders, inhibition of play) Psychoneurotic reactions (hysteria, obsession, compulsion, phobias, hypochondria) Behavior extremes: compliant, passive-aggressive, demanding Overly adaptive behavior: inappropriately adult or inappropriately infantile Developmental lags (mental, emotional) Attempted suicide

Source: National Center on Child Abuse and Neglect.

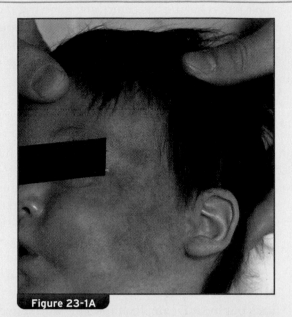

Figure 23-1A

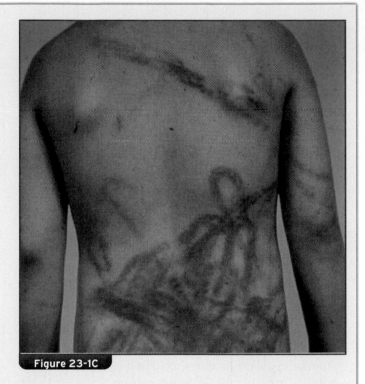

Figure 23-1C

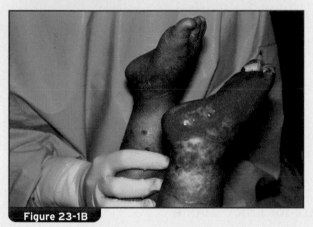

Figure 23-1B

A. The face is a common target for physical abuse.
B. Stocking-glove burns of the hands and feet are almost always inflicted injuries. **C.** Rope or cord bruises are a commonly inflicted injury.

- Emotional neglect:
  - failure to gain weight (especially in infants)
  - desperately affectionate behavior
  - large appetite and stealing of food

Care for Child Abuse and Neglect

The care of the neglected infant or child is extremely important.

- Give appropriate first aid for injuries.
- Do not accuse parents or caregivers, especially at the scene.
- Report any suspected abuse to the local welfare and social service agency responsible for investigating the problem. Report what you saw and heard, not what you think.

▶ Domestic Violence

Domestic violence, also known as *partner abuse, spouse abuse,* or *battering,* occurs when one person inflicts injury—either emotional or physical—upon another person who they had or have a relationship with. It occurs between spouses and partners, parents and children, children and grandparents, and brothers and sisters. Domestic violence may be the single most common source of serious injury to women.

Recognizing Domestic Violence

Physical domestic violence includes slapping, punching, kicking, and choking. Women also have been shot, stabbed, and bludgeoned. Injuries tend to be on the head, neck, chest, breast, abdomen, and perineum rather than the extremities. The injuries listed here should raise suspicion about potential domestic violence:

- Bruises or injuries on the head, neck, or chest
- Types or extent of an injury that is inconsistent with the victim's explanation
- Substantial delay between when the injury occurred and when the victim sought help
- Injuries during pregnancy
- Evidence of alcohol or drug abuse
- Needs medical care as a result of a suicide attempt or rape

---

FYI

Are You Being Abused?

Just one "yes" answer means you're involved in an abusive relationship. If so, you're not alone and you have choices. No one deserves to be abused.

- Threatens to hurt you or your children
- Says it is your fault if he or she hits you; then promises it will not happen again (but it does)
- Puts you down in public or keeps you from contacting family or friends
- Throws you down, pushes, hits, chokes, kicks, or slaps you
- Forces you to have sex when you do not want to

Source: American College of Obstetricians and Gynecologists, www.acog.org.

Care for Domestic Violence

- Talking with the suspected abuser about the problem is not likely to help.
- If you are not aware of immediate danger, but you suspect abuse, check with welfare and social service agencies. Most cities and counties, according to state law, will investigate and protect vulnerable adults. The problem cannot be remedied until it is reported.
- Call the police if a person is in imminent danger.
- First aid includes calling 9-1-1 and treating any injuries.

▶ Elder Abuse

Elder abuse ranges from passive neglect to active assault and includes emotional abuse. Some physically abused el-

derly people report having had something thrown at them; some are pushed, grabbed, or shoved; others are slapped, bitten, or kicked. Elder abuse occurs most often in women older than 75 years. Signs of abuse may be quite obvious or subtle. Burns are a common form of elder abuse.

Recognizing Elder Abuse

When concerned about an older adult who might be abused, look for these signs:

- Physical injury: Examples of questionable injuries include bruises, cuts, burn or rope marks, and broken bones that cannot be explained. Other signs of potential problems include sudden changes in behavior, comments about being battered, or the refusal of the caregiver to allow you to visit the older person alone.
- Lack of physical care: Examples include dehydration, malnourishment, weight loss, and poor hygiene. Bed sores, soiled bedding, unmet medical needs, and comments about being mistreated also may indicate a problem. Lack of physical care can happen to older adults living in their homes, as well as those in institutional care, such as a long-term care facility.
- Unusual behaviors: Examples include agitation, withdrawal, fear or anxiety, apathy, or reports of being treated improperly.

Care for Elder Abuse

- Talking with the suspected abuser about the problem is not likely to help.
- If you are not aware of immediate danger, but you suspect abuse, check with welfare and social service agencies. Most cities and counties, according to state law, will investigate and protect vulnerable adults. The problem cannot be remedied until it is reported.
- If you suspect elder abuse in an institutional setting, such as a nursing home, report your concerns to your state long-term care ombudsman. Each state has a long-term care ombudsman to investigate and address nursing home complaints.
- Call the police if a person is in imminent danger.
- First aid includes calling 9-1-1 when needed and treating any injuries.

▶ Ready for Review

- Behavior that leads to violence or other inappropriate activities is known as a behavioral emergency.
- Depression is one of the most common and treatable of all mental illness.
- Suicide in the United States is increasingly a problem of adolescents, college-age students, and older people.
- First aid for an emotional injury means being supportive of people with emotional injuries, whether the injuries are a result of physical injury or excessive or unbearable strain on the victim's emotions.
- Because child abuse and neglect usually occur in the privacy of the home, no one knows exactly how many children are affected.
- Domestic violence may be the single most common source of serious injury to women.
- The types of physical abuse of elders vary from passive neglect to active assault.

▶ Vital Vocabulary

behavioral emergency Situations in which a person exhibits abnormal behavior that is unacceptable or cannot be tolerated by the victims themselves, or by family, friends, or the community.

▶ Assessment in Action

Your roommate has not been acting like himself lately. He used to run every morning and led an active social life. Now he's given up running and he spends most of his free time alone in his room. He's also been gaining weight and complaining of headaches.

Directions: Circle Yes if you agree with the statement, circle No if you disagree.

Yes No 1. According to some of these symptoms, your roommate could be suffering from depression.

Yes No 2. The best thing to do is leave your roommate alone.

Yes No 3. You should confront your roommate and tell him to "snap out of it."

Yes No 4. You should provide empathy and attention to your roommate.

Yes No 5. Always discourage crying in a depressed person.

Answers: 1. Yes; 2. No; 3. No; 4. Yes; 5. No

▶ Check Your Knowledge

Directions: Circle Yes if you agree with the statement, circle No if you disagree.

Yes No 1. Abnormal behavior may be due to a psychological condition or a physical condition.

Yes No 2. Low blood sugar in a person with diabetes can affect behavior.

Yes No 3. Depression cannot be treated.

Yes No 4. The male rate for suicide is higher than the female rate.

Yes No 5. Most people who talk about suicide are not serious.

Yes No 6. The only way to react to an aggressive person is with anger.

Yes No 7. A failure to gain weight may be a sign of emotional neglect in an infant.

Yes No 8. Domestic violence rarely occurs to women.

Yes No 9. Burns are a common form of elder abuse.

Yes No 10. Feeling shaky during an emergency is not normal.

Answers: 1. Yes; 2. Yes; 3. No; 4. Yes; 5. No; 6. No; 7. Yes; 8. No; 9. Yes; 10. No

Wilderness First Aid

Wilderness First Aid

At some time, anyone living, working, traveling, or recreating in the wilderness will probably encounter dangers unfamiliar to most people. Regardless of precautions, injuries and illnesses happen.

Wilderness, as defined by the Wilderness Medical Society (WMS), is a remote geographical location more than 1 hour from definitive medical care. According to that definition, wilderness could describe a variety of situations, including the following:

- Recreation (for example, fishing, camping, hiking, hunting)
- Occupations in remote areas (such as farming, forestry, fishing)
- Urban areas with overwhelmed EMS after a natural or manmade disaster
- Residences in remote communities, such as farms, ranches, vacation homes
- Developing countries

The millions of people in these wildernesses should be as medically prepared as possible to manage a problem for others and for themselves. First aid with a wilderness focus seems indispensable in the following situations:

- Occurrence of injuries and illnesses in the outdoors where adverse environmental conditions such as heat, cold, altitude, rain, or snow may be a major concern
- Delay of definitive medical care for hours or days because of location, bad weather, lack of transportation, or lack of communication

- Occurrence of injuries and illnesses not commonly seen in urban or suburban areas (for example, altitude illness, frostbite, wild animal attacks)
- The need for advanced medical care (for example, reduction of some dislocations, wound cleansing)
- Limited first aid supplies and equipment
- Need to make difficult decisions (CPR, evacuation) in a remote setting

Most first aid books and training courses describe situations in which the EMS response is expected within 10 to 20 minutes. In these cases, the first aider usually helps for only a few minutes before an ambulance arrives. When the victim is transported, the first aider's job is finished.

Wilderness first aid is similar to that needed in urban situations, except that extra or extended skills are needed. Consideration must be given to time, distance, and availability of medical care. A first aider in the wilderness may have to remain many hours or days with a sick or injured person.

▶ Cardiac Arrest

Because heart activity must be restored within a short time (which requires defibrillation and medications) for a cardiac arrest victim to survive, CPR has limited use in a wilderness or remote setting, especially if severe trauma such as massive head or chest injury, severe blood loss, or a severed spinal cord accompanies the cardiac arrest. In addition, CPR is difficult to continue during a wilderness evacuation.

The WMS recommends *stopping* CPR if the:
- victim revives
- rescuers are exhausted
- rescuers are in danger
- victim is turned over to higher level trained personnel
- victim does not respond to prolonged (about 30 minutes) of resuscitation efforts

The State of Alaska Cold Injuries Guidelines, the WMS, and the NAEMSP says that CPR should *not be started* if the victim:
- Has been submerged in cold water for more than 1 hour
- Has a core temperature of less than 50° F
- Has obvious signs of death or fatal injuries (e.g., rigor mortis, decapitation, decomposition)
- Is frozen (e.g., ice formation in the airway)
- Has a chest wall that is so stiff that compressions are impossible
- Rescuers are exhausted or in danger

CPR for Hypothermia Victims

Avoid rough handling and seek medical care as soon as possible. The American Heart Association recommends that health care providers take 30 to 45 seconds to feel for a pulse in an unresponsive hypothermic victim. Determining the existence of a pulse is difficult in cold environments because the victim will have an extremely slow heart rate and the rescuer may have cold fingers. If the victim is not breathing, start CPR immediately. If there is any doubt about whether a pulse is present, begin CPR.

Lay rescuers should follow the procedures as for any cardiac arrest victims. Hypothermia is one of the cases in which CPR should be continued for more than 30 minutes. See Chapter 20 for additional information on cold emergencies.

CPR for Avalanche Victims

It is suffocation and/or blunt trauma that kills avalanche victims. For nonbreathing victims, stabilize the cervical spine and start CPR immediately; continue for more than 30 minutes if necessary.

CPR for Lightning-Strike Victims

Start CPR on nonbreathing victims immediately. In the case of multiple victims, treat the unresponsive ones first.

CPR for Submersed Victims

For a victim not breathing, start CPR as soon as possible. Be ready to roll the victim and clear the airway should water fill the airway or if the victim vomits. CPR can be stopped in 30 minutes if the victim has not recovered. If the victim has been submersed for more than 60 minutes, do not start CPR.

▶ Dislocations

In a wilderness situation, *reducing* (a technical term that means aligning) some dislocated joints is recommended. The WMS gives the following reasons for reducing a joint dislocation quickly after it happens:
- Reduction is easier immediately after the injury, before swelling develops.
- It is easier to transport a victim after reduction.
- Reduction dramatically relieves pain.
- The joint can be stabilized and better protected.
- Reduction lessens the possibility of jeopardizing circulation in the extremity. (If the blood supply is cut off, gangrene could develop, which could result in amputation.)

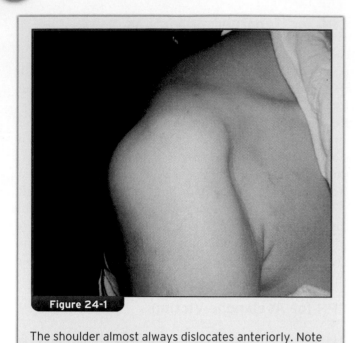

Figure 24-1

The shoulder almost always dislocates anteriorly. Note the absence of the normal rounded appearance of the shoulder.

- Several simple dislocations can be reduced by using simple and safe techniques.

A dislocation is considered simple if it involves the anterior (front) part of the shoulder, a finger, or the patella (the kneecap, not the knee itself). Do not attempt to reduce a dislocated elbow or hip. Elbow and hip dislocations resemble fractures; reduction techniques for those joints are painful and can cause further injury.

Shoulder Dislocation

Anterior (frontal) shoulder joint dislocations account for more than 90% of shoulder dislocations **Figure 24-1** .

Recognizing a Shoulder Dislocation

- The victim is in extreme pain.
- Because the problem often recurs, the victim can identify the dislocation if it has happened before.
- The upper arm is held away from the body in various positions and cannot be brought next to the body into a sling-type position.
- The victim is unable to touch the uninjured shoulder with the hand of the injured extremity.
- Compare the injured shoulder with the uninjured one. The shoulder joint will appear squared off or flattened and a prominence may be seen or felt in the front of the shoulder.

Care for a Shoulder Dislocation

There are two methods for reducing a shoulder dislocation. With either method, stop if pain increases or resistance is met. Do not try pulling on the victim's arm with your foot in the victim's armpit. Check the circulation, sensation, and movement of the hand before and after splinting.

Care for a Shoulder Dislocation: Traction and External Rotation

Traction and external rotation is the easiest and most effective method for reducing an anterior shoulder dislocation **Figure 24-2** .

1. Gently but steadily pull the arm out to the side while another rescuer provides countertraction against the chest wall, just below the armpit, using straps, a sleeping bag, clothing, or a flotation vest.
2. Tell the victim to relax. Massage may help.
3. As you pull, gently and slowly rotate the arm into a baseball-throwing position (take 5 to 15 minutes). Keep the arm in that position; the muscles will fatigue within 15 minutes, allowing the joint to slip back into place.
4. After successful reduction, stabilize the arm with a sling and swathe (binder).

If there is only one rescuer, countertraction can be applied by the rescuer's padded or bare feet against the victim's chest (not armpits).

Care for a Shoulder Dislocation: Simple Hanging Traction

Using the simple hanging traction method:

1. Lay the victim face down on a surface high enough so the injured arm can hang over the side. Place some cushioning (a folded towel or clothing) under the armpit, between the arm and the surface **Figure 24-3** .
2. Attach a 10- to 15-lb weight to the victim's lower arm, between the elbow and the wrist. Cushion and strap the weight, being careful not to impede circulation. Keep the victim's palm facing inward.
3. It may take up to 60 minutes to stretch and tire the muscles, allowing the joint to pop back in.
4. After successful reduction, stabilize the arm with a sling and swathe.

If available, place a small pillow, folded towels, or some type of pad under the person's armpit. Secure a sling and swathe (binder) using the method shown in Chapter 16.

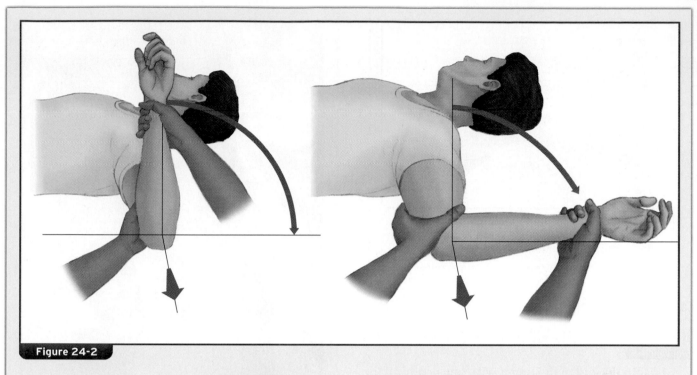

Figure 24-2

Applying traction (left) and external rotation (right) to anterior shoulder dislocation.

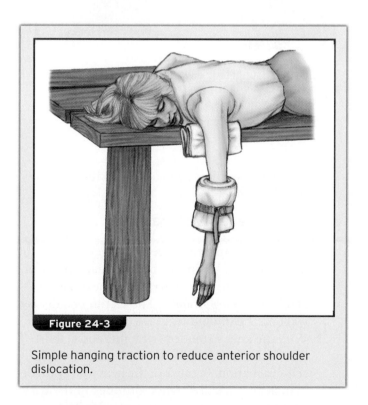

Figure 24-3

Simple hanging traction to reduce anterior shoulder dislocation.

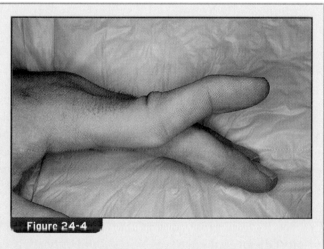

Figure 24-4

Dislocation of the finger joint. Do not be tempted to try to "pop" the joint back into place.

Finger Dislocation

The fingers are injured easily, and even a minor injury may cause a dislocation **Figure 24-4**.

Recognizing a Finger Dislocation

- Deformity and inability to use or bend the finger
- Pain and swelling
- An abnormal position of the two adjoining bones; looks like a lump at the joint

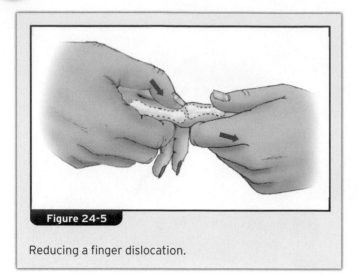

Figure 24-5

Reducing a finger dislocation.

Care for a Finger Dislocation

To reduce a finger dislocation, use one of two methods
Figure 24-5 :

1. Hold the end of the finger with one hand and the rest of the finger in the other.
2. Gently hyperextend the dislocated joint (bend it backwards).
3. Pull gentle traction.
4. Push the dislocated bone into place.
5. Unbend the finger.
6. Buddy-tape it to the next finger.
7. Splint the finger in a functional position.

Often, persons with this injury can reduce the finger dislocation themselves. In a remote location, you should try to reduce a finger dislocation only once. Stabilize and protect the finger by the *buddy-taping method*—using adhesive tape to secure the injured finger to an adjacent uninjured finger.

Kneecap Dislocation

For most dislocated kneecaps, you should only apply an ice pack and use a splint to stabilize the leg in place as you found it. For remote locations, however, always consider reducing a dislocated kneecap by using the following method. All dislocations, whether successfully reduced in the field or not, should be seen by a physician.

Recognizing a Kneecap Dislocation

Some victims have recurrent dislocations of the patella and can tell you what is wrong.

- The patella has moved to the outside of the knee joint (large bulge under the skin) with the leg bent **Figure 24-6** .
- The victim is in pain.

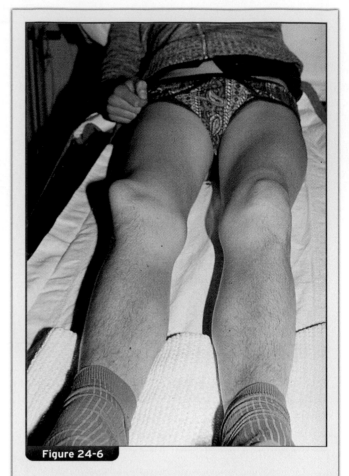

Figure 24-6

A dislocated patella typically will appear with the patella displaced lateral to the knee and with the knee moderately flexed.

- Compare the injured portion with the patella on the other leg.

Care for a Kneecap Dislocation

1. Slowly straighten the knee as you gently push the kneecap back into its normal position. Straightening alone may replace the kneecap.
2. Stabilize the leg straight. The victim usually can walk on the injured leg.
3. With the knee extended (straight) and stabilized, the victim may be able to walk well enough for self-evacuation. Because of the heavy physical demands and usually higher altitudes in the backcountry, carrying a victim can take 8 to 16 rescuers rotating the task. In the wilderness, a ski pole or a tree branch makes a good walking aid. Helicopter evacuation usually is not justified for a kneecap dislocation.

▶ Spinal Injury

The necessity of stabilizing the spine after trauma is well known. An unconscious victim with a cervical spinal injury who is moved without stabilization may become quadriplegic or die. In urban settings, spine stabilization is almost always automatically applied for survivors of violent accidents, such as automobile crashes or falls from a height.

In the wilderness, full-spine stabilization may not always be necessary—such a procedure can be difficult, impractical, impossible, or even dangerous during prolonged evacuation in severe environments. For example, an injured climber far above the timberline could wait for hours or days, depending on the distance someone has to go for help. The injured climber would have to wait in a hostile environment and risk death from avalanche, rockfall, or hypothermia. If the victim were cleared of a spinal injury, he or she could self-evacuate.

Spinal fractures can be difficult to determine, even by physicians reading radiographs. One study found that all of the spinal fracture cases reviewed had at least one of the following findings: midline neck tenderness, altered mental status, evidence of intoxication, or a separate painful injury away from the neck.

FYI

Spinal Injury

Question: Should a suspected spinal injury be stabilized as found or moved to an in-line position?

Answer: The National Emergency Medical Technician curriculum says that the head can be placed in an in-line position unless the victim complains of pain or the head is not easily moved into that position. The anatomic (normal) position is the most stable position for all bony structures, including the spine, and movement toward that position from the position found generally is considered safe. Therefore, in wilderness settings, it is best to reposition patients with suspected spinal injuries into the normal, anatomic ("eyes forward") position. If movement causes increased pain or if there is resistance to movement, it is best to splint the spine in the position found.

Recognizing a Possible Spinal Injury Victim

Assessing a spinal injury can be done through a process of elimination. First, ask these questions:

- Is the victim alert and oriented? Has the victim been drinking alcohol or using drugs?
- Does the victim have any major painful injury? Distracting injuries include fractures, deep lacerations, severe contusions, and large burns.

- Is the victim complaining of neck pain?
- Does the victim have tingling, numbness, or weakness in the extremities?

Next, perform these physical exams:

- Check for neck tenderness by pressing firmly on the bony part of the spine. This is a safe procedure, and there is little chance of injuring the spinal cord by feeling the bony spinal column as long as movement of the spine is prevented.
- Determine whether the victim has sensation in the hands or feet and whether he or she can move the fingers and toes.

Here is a simple protocol for clearing a spinal injury in the wilderness: The victim does not need to be stabilized in one position if he or she is completely alert, not intoxicated, has no distracting injuries, does not complain of neck pain, can feel normal touch, and can move the fingers and toes.

Follow these guidelines to assess a suspected spinal injury:

- The victim is responsive:
  - Determine whether the mechanism of injury was a violent-impact force capable of damaging the bony spinal column. Examples include a fall from a height, a gunshot wound near the spine, and a high-velocity vehicle crash.
  - Ask questions: Does your neck or back hurt? What happened? Can you move your hands and feet? Can you feel me touching your fingers and toes?
  - Look and feel for D-O-T-S (deformity, open wounds, tenderness, swelling) along the bony spinal column.
  - Assess the equality of strength of the extremities: Have the victim grip your hands; have the victim push his or her feet against your hand.
- The victim is unresponsive:
  - Determine the mechanism of injury.
  - Look for deformity, open wounds, and swelling along the spinal bones.
  - Feel for deformity and swelling along the spinal bones.
  - Obtain information from others at the scene to determine information relevant to mechanism of injury and victim's mental status before your arrival.

Care for a Spinal Injury

Providing effective spine stabilization in the wilderness often requires you to improvise methods. Initially, you can use your hands or knees to hold the victim's head in place. While kneeling at the victim's head, use your hands or knees to stabilize the victim's neck in relation to the long axis of the spine.

Improvised cervical collars such as a blanket, or a SAM splint alone are inadequate. Improvise supports by placing dirt or sand in garbage bags, stuff sacks, or roll up extra articles of clothing. Place them on both sides of the victim's head, and secure them in place.

Leave the victim on the ground, and avoid moving him or her. If necessary to prevent heat loss, log roll the victim, keeping the spine straight, and place insulating materials underneath. For spinal injury procedures when EMS response time is less than 1 hour, see Chapter 12.

▶ Splinting Femur Fractures

Victims with a femur fracture can easily lose 2 quarts of blood in the thigh and develop massive swelling. Because EMS personnel have the training, experience, and equipment, it is best to let them apply traction splints, if possible. However, first aiders can use the methods on page 224 to stabilize a femur fracture.

FYI

Femur Fracture

Question: Do improvised traction splints work?

Answer: Although the advantages of stabilizing a broken femur by applying a traction splint are cited in various manuals, there are dissenting opinions about the effectiveness of improvised traction splints. For example, the Outward Bound organization says, "Improvised traction splints for field use employing ski poles, canoe paddles, and other pieces of equipment are usually more architecturally interesting than medically useful. The simplest, safest, and most universal splint is firm immobilization on a long board or litter without traction." The WMS suggests stabilizing the fractured extremity to the uninjured leg with adequate padding, and to place padding behind the knee to create a slight bend which is more comfortable than being straight.

▶ Avalanche Burial

Avalanches are falling masses of snow that may also contain rocks, soil, or ice. Since the early 1970s, the number of deaths caused by avalanches has increased rapidly as a result of the tremendous growth in backcountry win-

ter mountain travel (skiing, mountaineering, snowmobiling). Recent statistics show that the average annual number of deaths is about 20 per year in the United States and 10 in Canada.

Snow sets up solid after an avalanche. It is almost impossible for victims to dig themselves out, even if they are buried under less than a foot of snow. The pressure of several feet of snow sometimes is so great that victims are unable to expand their chests to breathe.

Most avalanche victims die of suffocation, therefore, in the absence of fatal injuries, speed of extrication from the avalanche and existence of an air pocket are the main factors that determine survival of a buried victim. There are no documented reports of anyone surviving a burial of 7 feet or more.

FYI

Avalanche Rescue

If you survive an avalanche, follow these steps to find other victims:

1. With a piece of equipment, clothing, or tree branch, mark the spot where a victim was last seen.
2. Search the area below the last-seen point for any clues of the victim. Make probes into likely burial spots with a ski, ski pole, or tree limb.
3. If beacons were being used, all survivors must immediately switch their units to the receive mode and listen for a beeping sound from buried beacons.
4. If a second avalanche is possible, place one person in a safe location to shout a warning so rescuers can flee to safety.
5. Send a person to notify the ski patrol immediately if you are near a ski area and there are several rescuers. If you are the only rescuer, do a fast surface search for clues before leaving to notify the ski patrol. In remote backcountry, all survivors should remain and search until they cannot or should not continue.

Rescue transceivers or beacons are an efficient way of locating victims. Organized probe lines have found more victims than any other method, but because of the time involved, most of the victims were dead. Trained search dogs can locate buried victims quickly, but they often are brought to the scene only after long periods of burial. One trained dog can search more effectively than 30 searchers.

Recognizing an Avalanche Victim

Avalanches kill and injure in two ways. The first is from the serious injury the victim acquires while tumbling down an avalanche path. Trees, rocks, cliffs, and the wrenching action of snow are hazards. About one third of all deaths are related to trauma, especially trauma to the head and neck. The second way is snow burial, which causes suffocation in the other two thirds of avalanche deaths. Inhaled snow clogs the mouth and nose, and victims can suffocate quickly if they are buried with the airway already blocked.

Care for an Avalanche Victim

A completely buried victim has a poor chance of survival. During the first 15 minutes, more people are found alive than dead. Between 16 and 30 minutes after an avalanche, an equal number are found dead and alive (50% chance of survival). After 30 minutes, more are found dead than alive.

After you have first checked for further avalanche danger and then found a victim, follow these steps:

1. Quickly free the victim's head, chest, and stomach.
2. Send for help.
3. Clear the victim's airway and check breathing.
4. If not breathing, begin CPR.
5. Check for severe bleeding.
6. Examine for and stabilize a spinal injury.
7. Treat for hypothermia.

▶ Altitude Illness

If you live in or visit mountainous regions, you need to know about altitude illness. Altitude illness is not simply an exotic affliction of mountaineers but is a common environmental risk to which millions of people are exposed, often without adequate knowledge.

Altitude illnesses actually are a spectrum of a single problem, <u>hypoxia</u>. *Hypoxia* occurs when the body's tissues do not have enough oxygen. Altitude illnesses include *acute mountain sickness (AMS)*, *high-altitude pulmonary edema (HAPE)*, and *high-altitude cerebral edema (HACE)* Table 24-1 .

The least serious altitude illness is acute mountain sickness and affects about one in four people from lower elevations who visit areas 6,000 to 12,000 feet above sea level. Such elevations are common at ski resorts and on mountain hiking trails.

The actual incidence of altitude illness varies with rate of ascent and altitude attained. About 67% of climbers on Mt Rainier in Washington have at least mild AMS because of rapid ascent to a moderately high altitude. The incidence of AMS in a study of Colorado skiers at lower altitudes (usually 1 day's ascent from Denver or lower) was only 15% to 40%.

Table 24-1 Characteristics of Altitude Illnesses

	AMS	HAPE	HACE
Elevation	Above 8,000 ft	Usually above 10,000 ft	Above 12,000 ft
Time after ascent	1-2 days	3-4 days, possibly later	4-7 days, possibly later
Cause and symptoms	Symptoms of hypoxia: headache, sleep disturbance, fatigue, shortness of breath, dizziness, loss of appetite, vomiting	Symptoms of fluid in the lungs: shortness of breath, dry cough, mild chest pain, weakness, insomnia, rapid pulse, cyanosis, *rales* (crackles), or gurgling sounds	Symptoms of increased fluid and pressure on brain: severe headache (unrelieved), vomiting, Cheyne-Stokes breathing (irregular breathing pattern that includes periods of apnea [no breathing]), ataxia (irregular gait or lack of coordination), unconsciousness
First aid	Stop ascending or return to a lower altitude. Drink fluids. Rest. Take aspirin or ibuprofen. Take acetazolamide.	Descend at least 2,000 ft. Seek medical attention *immediately.*	Descend 4,000 ft. Seek medical attention *immediately.*

HAPE and HACE occur when reduced oxygen causes capillary leakage and swelling of body tissues. Both conditions are life threatening.

Although anyone can get altitude illness, certain factors increase the risk. Under similar conditions, different people sometimes respond quite differently to altitude. For most people, at least four factors determine whether they will be sick or well at a higher altitude: (1) the speed of ascent (the slower the climb, the fewer the symptoms); (2) the altitude reached (the higher one goes, the more likely one will have problems); (3) health at the time (malnutrition, dehydration, fatigue, and any of several illnesses increase the risk); and (4) individual differences and genetic influences.

Altitude illness occurs because oxygen levels decrease as elevation increases, and it takes a few days to adapt to the "thinner" air. At 11,500 feet, the amount of oxygen in the air is about 65% the amount at sea level, so the body struggles to maintain normal levels of oxygen. As the person breaths more deeply he or she "blows off" more carbon dioxide than normal, creating a more alkaline (less acidic) condition in the body, which in turn causes altitude illnesses.

Recognizing Altitude Illness

Altitude illness typically strikes during the first 12 hours, and a headache is the most common symptom. Other symptoms include loss of appetite, nausea, insomnia, fatigue, and shortness of breath with exertion. Three fourths of all people who travel from sea level to above 8,000 feet have at least one symptom (usually a headache), and the rest have two or more symptoms. Many people mistake the symptoms for a cold, the flu, or a hangover and wonder why it had to happen on their long-awaited mountain vacation.

Care for Altitude Illness

It is important to recognize the symptoms of altitude illness and take steps to treat it. In a small number of people, acute altitude illness can progress to pulmonary edema (HAPE), in which fluid builds up in the lungs, or cerebral edema (HACE), in which fluid collects in the brain. Although they are uncommon, both conditions can be fatal in less than 12 hours. Seek medical help if any of the following, more serious symptoms appear: persistent cough, shortness of breath while resting, noisy breathing, loss of balance, confusion, or vomiting.

Most people who have altitude illness get better with rest as the body acclimatizes. However, anyone who has recently ascended to above 6,000 feet, is feeling ill, and whose condition does not improve in 1 to 2 days should see a physician. If that is not possible, the victim should descend 2,000 to 3,000 feet, rest, and drink plenty of fluids. Aspirin or a similar pain reliever can be taken for a mild headache. If rest and over-the-counter (OTC) medications do not provide relief, a physician should be consulted and might administer oxygen or prescribe medication.

FYI

Preventing Altitude Illness

You can take several measures to lower your risk of getting altitude sickness. Start slowly, and avoid overexerting yourself. If possible, gain altitude slowly to allow your body to adjust. By going easy, you allow your body to acclimatize; that is, adjust to different conditions. Simply put, your body becomes more efficient at using oxygen. Unfortunately, the effects of acclimatization last after you return to your normal altitude. You must repeat the process whenever you return to higher elevations.

If you cannot or will not take the time, protective medications are available by prescription. Acetazolamide (Diamox) has been effectively used to prevent AMS for more than 30 years. Acetazolamide also seems to prevent HAPE and HACE, although that is almost impossible to prove because HAPE and HACE are rare.

Side effects of acetazolamide include increased urination and tingling or numbness in the fingers and toes. If you are allergic to sulfa drugs, you may be allergic to acetazolamide. Also, you should wear a sunscreen with a sun protection factor (also called SPF) of at least 15 while taking the drug, since it may increase the risk of sunburn.

Acetazolamide is effective for most lowlanders going to moderate altitudes and perhaps for high-altitude residents returning after a short stay at low altitude. It has been called an *artificial acclimatizer*. Just how much acetazolamide to take and when to take it are debated. Follow the prescribed dosage; for adults it is 125 mg twice a day starting the day of ascent.

Because dehydration can be a factor at high altitudes, drink plenty of fluids such as water and juice. Mountain air is drier than air at lower elevations. You are drinking enough fluid when your urine is clear. Tea, coffee, and alcohol cause more frequent urination and may lead to dehydration. Eat lightly for a few days.

Avoid taking sleeping pills because they tend to cause shallow breathing while you sleep, which can make it difficult for your body to get enough oxygen. Likewise, do not smoke because it increases carbon monoxide levels in the blood, which diminishes the body's ability to use oxygen.

The condition of people with acute altitude illness usually improves, even at higher elevations, after a few days of rest, and they can continue with their plans. As long as the condition does not worsen and the victim can be carefully watched, a day or two of rest at a lower altitude may be sufficient.

All forms of altitude illness will improve when the victim simply descends a few thousand feet. If HACE or HAPE is suspected, early descent is wise, because these conditions are serious. The next best step after descent is to breathe additional oxygen so that the inspired oxygen pressure equals that at sea level. This will also relieve the headache and make breathing easier.

At 18,000 feet, humans reach their ceiling and cannot stay for more than a few weeks. Any sea-level person taken quickly to 20,000 feet will be almost incapacitated in less than half an hour, and death will occur soon thereafter.

Other Altitude-Related Illnesses

- *Pharyngitis* and *bronchitis*. Because of dry air, a sore throat and coughing may develop. Care involves drinking fluids, applying an OTC antibiotic ointment in the nostrils, and sucking on hard candy or throat lozenges.
- *Peripheral edema.* The hands, ankles, and/or face (around the eyes) may swell at high altitude. If possible, raise the affected arms and/or legs. After descending or with acclimatization to higher altitudes, the swelling diminishes. Descend if signs of the more serious altitude illness appear.

FYI

Altitude Increases Sunburn Risk

Skiers, hikers, and others who enjoy outdoor activities in the mountains have long believed that it took less time to sunburn in the mountains than at lower levels. Research confirms that the higher the altitude, the quicker a person will develop sunburn. UV (ultraviolet) light energy readings were taken at solar noon in direct sunlight on cloudless days at Vail, Colorado; Orlando, Florida; and New York, New York. The high-altitude regions in the United States include areas with some of the fastest population growth, and it is vital that people living or visiting these regions recognize the increase in UV exposure at higher altitudes and take precautions to prevent sunburn.

Source: Rigel DS, Rigel EG, Rigel AC: Effects of altitude and latitude on ambient UVB radiation. *J Am Acad Dermatol* 40:114-116.

▶ Lightning

Lightning is awesome and frightening **Figure 24-7**. About 30% of lightning strikes to humans result in death. Lightning strikes claim more lives in the United States than any other natural disaster, including earthquakes, blizzards, tornadoes, floods, and hurricanes.

In the past, farmers, sailors, and other outdoor workers in isolated areas tended to be the most frequently injured. Today, a larger proportion of victims are hikers, campers, golfers, and others who are outdoors for recreational purposes.

Almost 70% of lightning deaths involve just one person; 15% involve groups of two; and groups of three or more account for another 15%. Lightning deaths occur more often during daytime hours when people are active and outdoors. Most occur during the months of June through September, when thunderstorms are most frequent. There are more thunderstorm days in the South

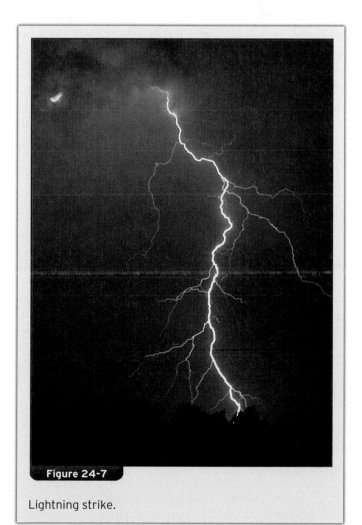

Figure 24-7

Lightning strike.

than in any other region of the United States. Thunderstorms occur frequently over high mountains. People are better protected in urban areas where high buildings have metal frames and lightning devices.

How Lightning Injures

Lightning injures in five ways. A *direct strike* is actually being struck by lightning. Lightning is most likely to hit a person in the open who has been unable to find shelter. Any conductor of electricity that the victim carries, especially if it is metal and carried above the shoulder level (for example, an open umbrella or a bag of golf clubs slung over the shoulder) increases the chances of a direct hit.

A more frequent cause of injury is a *splash*, which occurs when lightning strikes a tree or a building and "splashes" onto a victim seeking shelter nearby. The electrical current seeks the path of least resistance and may jump to the person because bodies have less resistance than trees or other objects. Frequently, a splash can kill groups of animals as they stand near a fence or seek shelter under trees. *Contact injury* occurs when a person is holding an object that is directly hit or splashed by lightning.

Ground current is produced when lightning hits the ground or a nearby object. The current spreads like a wave in a pond. Although ground current is less likely to produce fatalities than direct hits or splashes, it often creates multiple victims and injuries. Large groups have been injured on baseball fields and hiking paths and during military maneuvers.

Finally, people can be injured by the explosive force of the *shock wave* produced as lightning strikes nearby. Victims actually can be thrown by this blast effect.

Differences Between Generated High-Voltage Electricity Injuries and Lightning Injuries

Lightning contact with the body is instantaneous, leading to flashover, where the current flashes over the body.

The current flashes over the body as well as going through it. With flashover there are seldom burns of any magnitude. Lightning injuries disrupt electrical activity in the heart and nervous system. Exposure to

FYI

Flash-to-Bang: How Close

Be aware of how close lightening is occurring. The flash-to-bang method is the easiest and most convenient way to estimate how far away lightning is occurring. Thunder always accompanies lightning even though its audible range can be diminished due to background noise in the immediate environment and its distance from you. To use the flash-to-bang method, count the seconds from the time the lightning is sighted to when the clap of the thunder is heard. Divide this number by five to obtain how far away (in miles) the lightning is occurring. For example, if you count 15 seconds between seeing the flash and hearing the bang, 15 divided by 5 equals 3. Therefore the lightning flash is about 3 miles away.

FYI

30/30 Rule: When to Find Shelter

The 30/30 rule states that people should seek shelter if the flash-to-bang delay (length of time in seconds between a lightning flash and its subsequent thunder) is 30 seconds or less, and that they remain under cover until 30 minutes after the final clap of thunder.

A 30-second lead time is necessary prior to a storm's arrival because of the possibility of distant strikes. A 30-minute wait after the last thunder clap is heard is necessary because the trailing storm clouds still carry a lingering charge. This charge can—and does—occasionally produce lightning on the back edge of a storm, several minutes after the rain has ended.

Studies have shown most people struck by lightning are struck not at the height of a thunderstorm, but before and after the storm has peaked. DO NOT wait for the rain to start before seeking shelter, and do not leave shelter just because the rain has ended. Half of all lightning deaths occur after a storm passes.

FYI

Avoid Lightning Injury

- Be alert about weather conditions and predictions before going outdoors.
- Do not stand under a natural lightning rod such as a tall, isolated tree in an open area.
- Avoid projecting above the surrounding landscape, as you would do if you were standing on a hilltop, in an open field, on the beach, or fishing from a boat on the open water.
- Get out of and away from open water.
- Get away from tractors and other metal farm equipment.
- Get off of and away from motorcycles, scooters, golf carts, and bicycles. Lay down golf clubs.
- Stay away from wire fences, clotheslines, metal pipes, rails, and other metallic paths that could carry lightning to you from some distance away.
- Avoid standing in small, isolated sheds or other small structures in open areas.
- In a forest, seek shelter in a low area under a thick growth of small trees.
- In open areas, go to a low place such as a ravine or valley.
- If you are hopelessly isolated in a level field or prairie and you feel tingling or your hair stand on end—indicating lightning is about to strike—drop to a baseball catcher's crouching position or stance and put your hands over both ears to help avoid an eardrum rupture. Do not lie flat on the ground. You want as small an area of your body as possible touching the ground to minimize the possibility of your body acting as a conductor.
- If you are indoors during a thunderstorm, avoid open doors and windows, fireplaces, and metal objects such as pipes, sinks, and plug-in electrical appliances. Avoid using the telephone.
- If you are in an automobile (without a cloth top), stay in it. The vehicle will diffuse the current around you to the ground. It is a myth that the rubber tires will provide insulation but it is true that the metal body affords protection.
- If a group of people is exposed, they should spread out and stay several yards apart. That way, should a strike hit, the smallest number will be seriously injured.

household electricity tends to be much more prolonged, because the victim freezes to the circuit. The electrical energy surges through the tissues with little resistance to flow, causing thermal injury with severe tissue damage that can result in amputation. Electric current can also disrupt the body's electrical activity as does lightning.

Recognizing a Lightning Injury

- Breathing may be absent.
- Seizures, paralysis, and loss of responsiveness can result if the central nervous system is damaged.
- Minor burns. Most people believe that a lightning-strike victim will be severely burned. However, owing to the flashover effect, most victims have

only minor burns. The entrance and exit burn points common with electrical current burns are rare with lightning. The types of burns seen with lightning strikes are *punctate burns* (small, circular injuries resembling cigarette burns), *feathering* or *ferning burns, linear burns,* and burns from ignited clothing and heated metal. On rare occasions, clothing is ignited by lightning. A victim wearing metal, such as a necklace or a belt buckle, or carrying coins in a pocket may be burned as the objects heat.

Care for a Lightning Injury

1. If more than one victim has been struck by lightning at the same time, go to the quiet and motionless victim first, check for breathing, and treat accordingly.
2. If the victim is not breathing, start CPR. Persistent care is crucial for such victims.
3. If the victim is unresponsive but breathing, place the victim on his or her side.
4. Because spinal injuries can occur with lightning strikes, precautions should be taken to stabilize the spine.
5. Check for injuries.
6. Evacuate to medical care even if responsive.

▶ Wild Animal Attacks

Despite the fact that few large wild animals (bears, bison, cougars, and alligators) remain in the United States, attacks on humans still occur **Figure 24-8**. Wild animal attacks outside the United States are more common.

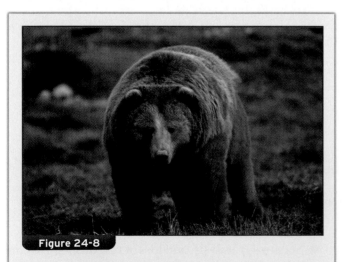

Figure 24-8

Large animals do not always retreat from humans and may attack rescuers.

Attacks, especially involving death, are often reported and sensationalized in the media.

The incidence of injuries from wild animal attacks is not known. Reporting is not mandatory, and many attacks are not recorded. Perhaps one or two deaths occur each year in the United States. Outside the United States, animal attacks by hippopotami, crocodiles, elephants, cape buffalo, lions, and tigers are a much greater cause of injury and death.

Wild animal attacks occur most often in rural or wilderness settings, a long distance from medical care. Preventing wild animal attacks is largely common sense and awareness. An increasing number of parks and wilderness areas are posting warning signs. Recreationalists should be aware of and knowledgeable about the animal habitats through which they travel and take precautions in food handling so as not to attract animals.

Generally, if you encounter a large wild animal, try to remove yourself from the scene quietly and slowly. Running will elicit a predatory response. Never get between an adult animal and its offspring. In most cases, a general rule is to fight back if you are attacked. Vigorous physical resistance, including striking the attacking animal with fists, a weapon, or any other object, has been effective in repelling attacks by cougars, lions, tigers, brown and black bears, and even crocodiles. Exceptions to this recommendation are the grizzly bear and a mother black bear with cubs. In these cases, you should lie down and play dead.

Recognizing Wild Animal Attacks

Not all injuries are bites. Severe injuries result from victims being thrown in the air, gored by an antler, butted, or trampled on the ground. Injuries include puncture wounds, bites, lacerations, bruises, fractures, rupture of internal organs, and evisceration.

Care for Wild Animal Attacks

See Chapters 8, 9, and 10 for what to do. Depending upon the severity of the injury, either evacuate the victim to medical care or contact local authorities for evacuation.

▶ Wilderness Evacuation

Determining the best way to evacuate a victim (helicopter evacuation versus walking the victim out versus carrying the victim on a litter) must be based on several factors. The following list is adapted from the WMS Practice Guidelines and suggests factors for determining the level of evacuation:

- Severity of the illness or injury
- Rescue and medical skills of the rescuers

- Physical and psychological condition of the rescuers and the victims
- Availability of equipment and aid for the rescue
- The time it would take to evacuate the victim by other means as determined by distance, terrain, weather, and other conditions
- Cost

When requesting outside assistance, you must consider the safety of incoming rescuers, their time commitment, and the cost of the rescue.

As a general rule, you should delay travel plans or start evacuating a victim from the wilderness for any of the following reasons:

- The victim's condition is not improving.
- The victim is experiencing debilitating pain.
- The victim is unable to travel at a reasonable pace owing to a medical problem.
- The victim is passing blood via the mouth or rectum (not from an obviously minor source).
- The victim has signs and symptoms of serious altitude illness.
- Infections are not improving.
- Chest pain is not caused by a rib cage injury.
- Wounds are severe enough to require medical care.
- The victim's dysfunctional psychological status is impairing the safety of others.

When to Evacuate

Use these guidelines to decide whether a victim should be evacuated.

Immediate Evacuations

Rapidly evacuate the following injuries, where medical care is needed in 30 to 60 minutes or less:

- Open fractures
- Extremity injuries with deformity
- Extremity injuries in which circulation is absent
- Spinal injuries with no sensation in the fingers or toes or inability of the victim to move fingers or toes
- Severe altitude illness (signs of HACE or HAPE)
- Decreased level of consciousness
- Signs of shock
- Severe bleeding

In the wilderness, all bleeding should be controlled. Wounds should be cleaned and irrigated under pressure. The standard rule is not to remove blood-soaked dressings, locate the bleeding vessels, and reapply pressure directly over the bleeding vessels. Never attempt to clamp or tie a vessel—more damage can result. Do not close a wound with adhesive strips, butterfly bandages, staples, or sutures.

Delayed Evacuations

Medical care should be obtained within 6 to 24 hours of injury:

- Limb injuries with deformity, severe pain, or inability to walk
- Severe frostbite
- Open wounds: Evacuate a wounded victim so that a physician can suture a wound within 6 hours for hand or foot injuries and within 24 hours for head or trunk injuries. (If necessary, closure can be done by a physician up to about the fourth day).
- Hypothermia: It is not necessary to evacuate a victim of mild hypothermia if the victim has normal mental status and is shivering. Evacuate victims who have severe hypothermia (shivering has stopped but the victim is still cold, altered mental status). It is impossible to rewarm a severely hypothermic victim in a wilderness or remote location. See Chapter 20 for more information on cold-related emergencies.

Guidelines for Ground Evacuation

If the victim is walking out, at least two people should accompany the victim. If the victim is being carried out, one or two people should be sent to notify authorities that assistance is needed and to give them specifics about the problem.

During a litter evacuation, there should be at least four, and preferably six, litter bearers at all times. Over rough terrain, eight carriers (six over smooth trail) should carry the litter 100 yards and then rest or rotate with eight other carriers. It is very demanding to carry a loaded litter for more than 15 minutes without a break.

Guidelines for Helicopter Evacuation

Helicopters can reduce the time the victim has to wait to receive medical care. Evacuate by helicopter only if the following conditions apply **Figure 24-9** :

- The victim's life will be saved or the victim will have a significantly better chance for full recovery.
- The pilot believes conditions are safe enough for helicopter evacuation.
- Ground evacuation would be unusually dangerous or excessively prolonged or not enough rescuers are available for ground evacuation.
- In general, helicopters are not beneficial if ground transport can get the victim to the hospital within 30 to 60 minutes.

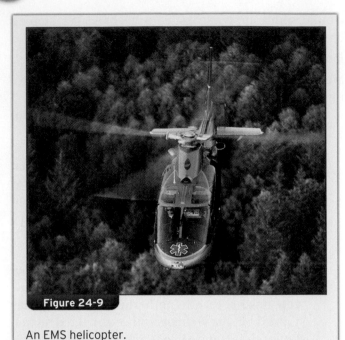

Figure 24-9

An EMS helicopter.

CAUTION

DO NOT approach a helicopter until one of the aircraft personnel signals it is safe for you to approach.

DO NOT approach a helicopter from the rear, where the fast-spinning tail rotor is invisible and dangerous. Many people walk into spinning rotors each year.

DO NOT forget to protect against wind chill from the rotor blades in the winter or to protect the eyes against flying dirt and debris.

DO NOT approach from the uphill side. The rotor is closer to the ground on the uphill side **Figure 24-10**.

DO NOT stand up when approaching a helicopter. Keep as low as possible in a crouched position. Because the blade is flexible, it may dip as low as 4 feet off the ground.

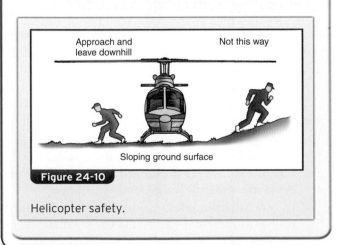

Approach and leave downhill   Not this way

Sloping ground surface

Figure 24-10

Helicopter safety.

FYI

Hiking: How to Protect One's Health on the Trail
The popularity of backpacking and day hiking has greatly increased, but so have related injuries. A survey of 224 backpackers who hiked the entire 2,100-mile mountainous Appalachian Trail showed that 82% had injuries (mostly muscle sprains, strains, and stress fractures) and illnesses (mostly diarrhea, skin irritations, foot blisters, and colds). Medical help was needed in 25% of the incidents. Hikers lost an average of 5 days of hiking because of these problems. Because these problems are common, hikers should carry supplies such as water-purification equipment, pain medicine, antibiotic ointment, and bandages.
Source: Crouse BJ, Josephs D: Health care needs of Appalachian Trail hikers. *J Fam Pract* 36:521-525.

FYI

Preparedness of Wilderness Hikers
A study of 301 hikers in Yosemite National Park showed they were healthy people but that injuries and illnesses requiring first aid attention were common. The hikers were not adequately prepared for the medical problems commonly encountered, such as acute mountain sickness, hypothermia, bee stings, minor cuts, blisters, and sunburns. Although the hikers demonstrated considerable knowledge about most first aid topics, they lacked knowledge about common injuries and injuries with high morbidity (likely to cause permanent disability) and mortality (likely to cause death).
Source: Kogut KT, Rodewald LE: A field survey of the emergency preparedness of wilderness hikers. *J Wilderness Med* 5:171-178.

▶ Signaling for Help

Many emergency conditions require a search for people in distress. Under such circumstances, it is always better if the people being sought know how to make their presence and their location conspicuous.

Signaling Aircraft

When creating a ground signal that people in an aircraft can see, remember that there are few straight lines or right angles in nature and that things are a lot smaller when viewed from the air. Bigger is almost always better. For ground signals, make a large "V" for immediate assistance or an "X" if medical assistance is needed. Make the lines of these signals as large as you can. Construct your signal so that each line is six times as long as it is wide, such as a "V" with each side 12 feet long and 2 feet wide. Contrast is another key to ground signals. Examples of materials to use include toilet paper, strips of plastic tarp, strips of tent material, tree branches, logs, and light-colored rocks. In snow and on open ground or sandy shores, signals may be tramped or dug into the surface using shadows to make the signals stand out.

Other Signals

A series of three of almost anything indicates "Help." Examples include three shouts, three shots, three blasts from a whistle, or three flashes from a light. Use smoke by day and bright flame by night if other signaling devices are not available. Add engine oil, rags soaked in oil, or pieces of rubber to your fire to make black smoke (best against a light background). Keep plenty of spare fuel on hand. If you are tending a fire as you wait for help, keep fuel handy and throw it on the fire when you hear an aircraft; do not wait, because it takes time for smoke to form and rise. Make sure to start the fire away from combustibles such as grass or trees.

A mirror is an effective means of sending a distress signal. On hazy days, aircraft pilots can see the flash of a mirror before survivors can see the aircraft, so it is wise to flash the mirror in the direction of a plane when you hear it, even when you cannot see it. Mirror flashes have been spotted by rescue aircraft more than 20 miles away.

To use a mirror, follow this procedure:

1. Hold the mirror up to the sun with one hand, and stretch your other hand out in front of you. Use

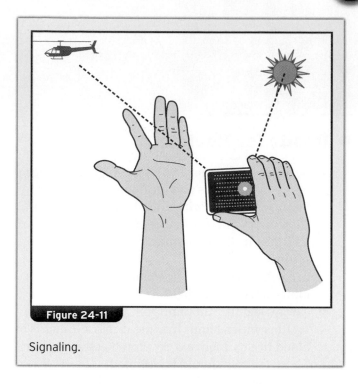

Figure 24-11

Signaling.

your finger or thumb to block your view of your target.

2. Hit your extended finger or thumb with a reflection of the sun from the mirror.

3. Repeatedly flick the spot of light from the mirror across the finger or thumb and the target.

4. Try to hit the aircraft or rescuers with a flash as much as possible. Do not attempt to do series of three flashes—it is too difficult **Figure 24-11**.

FYI

Survival Kit: The Bare Essentials

Minimal items	Purpose
One or two large plastic trash bags or an emergency blanket ("space blanket") made of Mylar	Protects against weather (wind, rain, snow). Wear one trash bag by cutting a hole in the bottom of the bag for your head; use the second bag to cover your legs.
Whistle (Mini Fox 40 or Windstorm)	Signal for help.
Signal mirror	Signal for help.
Metal match with striker (magnesium)	Start a fire.
Waterproof match case containing windproof and waterproof matches	Start a fire.
Waterproof match case or empty film canister containing several cotton balls smeared with petroleum jelly (such as Vaseline) or commercial tinder tabs	Petroleum jelly is flammable. Make tinder using cotton balls smeared with petroleum jelly. When using, open a cotton ball up to catch sparks from metal match.
Knife (multitool) and/or wire blade survival saw	Cutting
Food (such as energy bars and MREs [US military surplus meals-ready-to-eat])	Provides calories and a psychological boost

prep kit

▶ Ready for Review

- Be as medically prepared as possible to manage a problem for others and for themselves.
- Because heart activity must be restored within a short time for a cardiac arrest victim to survive, CPR has limited use in a wilderness or remote setting.
- In a wilderness situation, reducing some dislocated joints is recommended.
- Always stabilize an unresponsive victim.
- Victims with a femur fracture can lose 2 quarts of blood in the thigh and develop massive swelling. These injuries should be splinted.
- Since the early 1970s, the number of deaths caused by avalanches has increased rapidly.
- Altitude illnesses actually are a spectrum of a single problem: hypoxia.
- Determining the best way to evacuate a victim must be based on several factors.
- Many emergency conditions require a search for people in distress.

▶ Vital Vocabulary

hypoxia A low oxygen content in the blood; lack of oxygen in inspired air.

▶ Assessment in Action

You and your friend decide to spend the day hiking in a park about 3 hours away from your town. This park is known for its natural beauty and seclusion, and you are looking forward to a day of peace and quiet. Being experienced hikers, you and your friend properly pack your day sacs and bring along a first aid kit.

The day goes by quickly. A little after noon, you reach the top of a summit and enjoy a light lunch. As you are climbing down, your friend slips and stops his slide with his left shoulder. As you rush to help him, you find him groaning and holding his arm in a weird way.

Directions: Circle Yes if you agree with the statement, circle No if you disagree.

Yes   No   **1.** Should you believe your friend when he says, "I think I dislocated my shoulder"?

Yes   No   **2.** If your friend cannot touch his uninjured shoulder with the hand from his injured shoulder, than the shoulder is fine.

Yes   No   **3.** The shoulder is probably dislocated because the joint is squared off.

Yes   No   **4.** You should leave the shoulder alone.

Yes   No   **5.** You should call for a medical evacuation immediately.

Answers: **1.** Yes; **2.** No; **3.** Yes; **4.** Yes; **5.** No

▶ Check Your Knowledge

Directions: Circle Yes if you agree with the statement, circle No if you disagree.

Yes   No   **1.** Injuries in the wilderness rarely happen.

Yes   No   **2.** CPR in the wilderness should be stopped if the victim does not respond after 30 minutes.

Yes   No   **3.** Reduction of a dislocation dramatically relieves pain.

Yes   No   **4.** When it comes to spinal stabilization, never improvise!

Yes   No   **5.** After an avalanche, it is easy for victims to dig themselves out.

Yes   No   **6.** Speed of ascent can affect altitude illness.

Yes   No   **7.** Headache is a common symptom of altitude illness.

Yes   No   **8.** A victim of altitude illness should keep moving.

Yes   No   **9.** Most lightning deaths occur during the night.

Yes   No   **10.** Most lightning victims will have only minor burns.

Answers: **1.** No; **2.** Yes; **3.** Yes; **4.** No; **5.** No; **6.** Yes; **7.** Yes; **8.** No; **9.** No; **10.** Yes

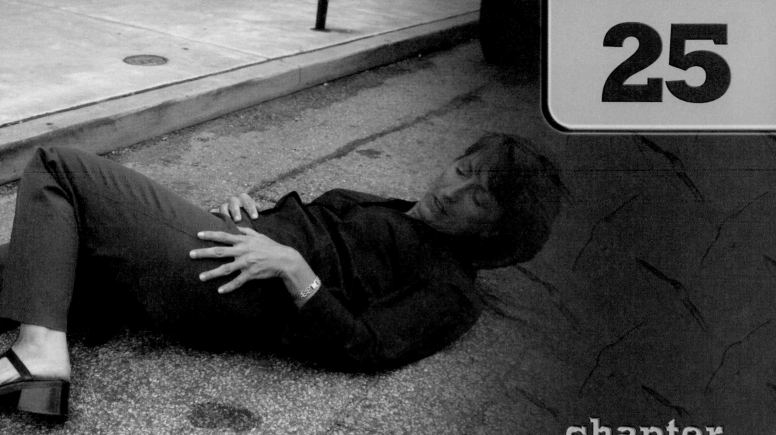

25

chapter
at a glance

▶ Victim Rescue

▶ Triage: What to Do
with Multiple Victims

▶ Moving Victims

Rescuing and Moving Victims

Victim Rescue

▶ Water Rescue

Reach-throw-row-go identifies the sequence for attempting a water rescue. The first and simplest rescue technique is to reach for the victim. Reaching requires a lightweight pole, ladder, long stick, or any object that can be extended to the victim. Once you have your "reacher," secure your footing, and have a bystander grab your belt or pants for stability. Secure yourself before reaching for the victim.

You can throw anything that floats—an empty picnic jug, an empty fuel or paint can, a life jacket, a floating cushion, a piece of wood, or an inflated spare tire—whatever is available Table 25-1. If there is a rope handy, tie it to the object to be thrown so you can pull the victim in, or, if you miss, you can retrieve the object and throw it again. The average untrained rescuer has a throwing range of about 50 feet.

If the victim is out of throwing range and there is a rowboat, canoe, motor boat, or boogie board nearby, you can try to row to the victim. Maneuvering these craft requires skill learned through practice. Wear a personal flotation device for your own safety. To avoid capsizing, never pull the victim in over the side of a boat; instead, pull the victim in over the stern (rear end) or tow the victim to safety.

If reach, throw, and row are impossible and you are a capable swimmer trained in water lifesaving procedures, you can go to the drowning victim by swimming.

Table 25-1	Effect of Flotation Devices on Survival Times	
Situation (50° F water)	**Predicted Survival Time (hours)**
No Flotation Device	
Drownproofing	1.5
Treading water	2.0
With Flotation Device	
Swimming	2.0
Holding still	2.7
HELP (heat escape lessening position)	4.0
Huddle position	4.0

Entering even calm water makes a swimming rescue difficult and hazardous. All too often a would-be rescuer becomes a victim as well.

Near-Drowning

In the United States, there are about 4,000 deaths each year due to drowning. In addition to the drownings, there are many cases of extreme, permanent disability that result from near-drowning.

Drowning means suffocation by immersion in water or other liquid. *Near-drowning* occurs when a victim survives an immersion incident. About two thirds of drowning victims are younger than 30 years. Most are males.

Usually, the initial reaction to drowning is panic. Then violent struggling occurs. Frequently, as victims become short of breath, they swallow water during attempts to breathe, and the water is often vomited. Further attempts to breathe may then result in aspiration of water, vomitus, or foreign bodies into the lungs. Sometimes the vocal cords (larynx) close and will not allow any water to enter the lungs. A seizure may occur, followed by death.

Drownings are classified into three basic types. In *dry drownings* (10% to 15%), no water passes the vocal cords. Presumably, in these cases, the cords shut tightly (*laryngospasm*) when water touches them. Other things being equal, a near-drowning without aspiration is easier to resuscitate because water has not entered the airway.

In *wet drownings* (85% of near-drownings), water, vomitus, or foreign bodies are aspirated into the lungs. Fresh water in the lungs enters the bloodstream and has a profoundly destructive effect on blood cells (which swell and burst) and leads to cardiac arrest (ventricular fibrillation). In saltwater drownings, water is taken from the bloodstream and enters the lungs. As much as 25% of the total blood volume can be lost as fluids move into the lungs. The victims drown in their own fluids as much as in the saltwater itself.

A *secondary drowning* is one in which a victim who was resuscitated dies within 96 hours. Aspiration pneumonia (due to inhalation of vomitus) is a late complication of near-drowning and occurs 48 to 72 hours after the episode. Near-drowning victims should be hospitalized or closely monitored.

CAUTION

DO NOT swim to and grasp a drowning person unless you are trained in lifesaving.

FYI

Typical Drowning Situations
Immediate-Disappearance Syndrome
- Victim enters water but does not return to the surface
- Little chance of rescue
- Caused by:
  1. Diving from height and striking the head
  2. Hyperventilation before underwater swimming
  3. Cold-induced heart attack

Distressed Nonswimmer
- Struggles 20 to 60 seconds before sinking
- Signs of distress: flailing arms, head tilted back, no vocalizing, appears to be playing

Sudden-Disappearance Syndrome
- Victim fully clothed
- Victim apparently able to swim but is fatigued, a poor swimmer, and/or cold
- Victim disappears after 5 to 10 minutes on surface (after clothing loses entrapped air)

Hypothermia-Induced Drowning
- Victim seriously affected after about 15 minutes of cold-water exposure
- Rule of 50s: Average unaware, unpracticed, and unprotected 50-year-old man would approach the 50-50 life-or-death point after 50 minutes of exposure to 50° F water.

Source: Adapted from David S. Smith.

Care for Drowning

1. Survey the scene (see Chapter 2), then carry out a water rescue 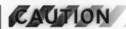.
2. If the victim was diving (or it is unknown whether he or she was diving), suspect a possible spinal injury. Keep the victim in-line floating on the wa-

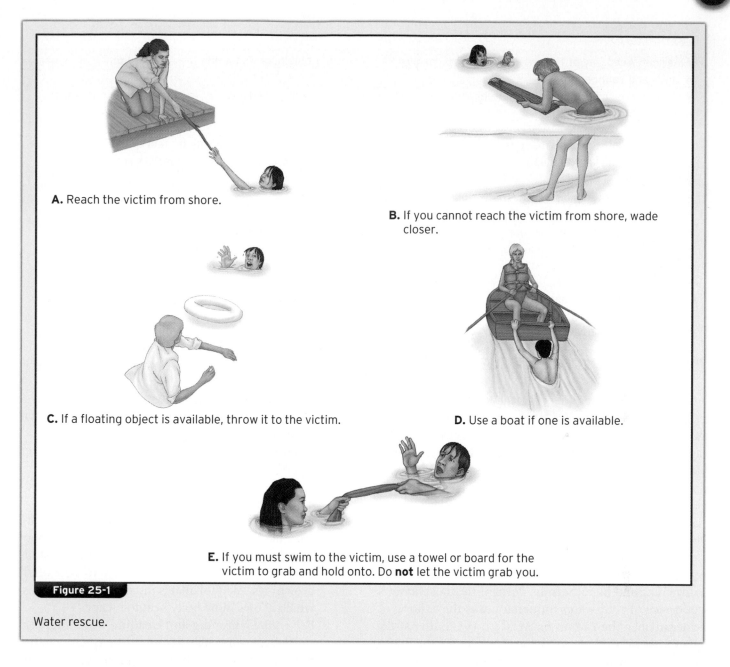

A. Reach the victim from shore.

B. If you cannot reach the victim from shore, wade closer.

C. If a floating object is available, throw it to the victim.

D. Use a boat if one is available.

E. If you must swim to the victim, use a towel or board for the victim to grab and hold onto. Do **not** let the victim grab you.

Figure 25-1

Water rescue.

ter surface until properly trained rescuers arrive with a backboard.

3. Check breathing and treat accordingly. Any non-breathing victim who has been submerged in cold water should be resuscitated unless submerged for more than 60 minutes.

4. If no spinal injury is suspected, place the victim on his or her side to allow fluids to drain from the airway.

Cold-Water Immersion

Immersion in cold water is a potential hazard for anyone who participates in activities in the oceans, lakes, and streams of all but the tropical regions of the world. The US Coast Guard defines *cold water* as water with a tem-

perature less than 70° F. However, water does not need to be that cold for a person to become hypothermic. A person can become hypothermic in water that is 77° F. Most North American lakes, rivers, and coasts are colder than that year-round. The risk of immersion hypothermia in North America is nearly universal most of the year. A person immersed in cold water loses heat about 25 times faster than someone exposed to cold air.

The US Coast Guard and other rescue organizations recommend that survivors get as much of their bodies out of the water as possible to minimize cooling rate and maximize survival time. A widespread misunderstanding of the concept of wind chill often causes people to conclude that survivors have higher heat losses if they are exposed to wind, especially if they are wet, than

FYI

American Academy of Pediatrics Recommendations for Preventing Childhood Drowning (by Age Group)

4 years and younger
- Never leave children alone in bathtubs, spas, or wading pools or near nearly filled buckets, toilets, irrigation ditches, or other standing water.
- Recognize that swimming lessons do not "drownproof" children.
- Fence the entire pool so that it is separated from the house. Pool covers are not a substitute for fences.
- Learn CPR and keep a telephone and emergency equipment—such as life preservers and a shepherd's crook—poolside.

5 to 12 years
- Provide with swimming lessons that include safety rules.
- Never let the children swim alone or without adult supervision.
- Make sure the children wear approved flotation devices when playing in or near a body of water.
- Teach the children the dangers of jumping or diving into water and of being on thin ice.

13 to 19 years
- In addition to relaying the preceding safety tips, counsel about the dangers of substance abuse combined with swimming, diving, or boating.
- Teach adolescents how to perform CPR.

Source: Pediatrics 112(2):437-439.

if they are immersed in water. During recreational activities at beaches, lakes, and swimming pools, most people have experienced feeling colder after leaving the water than they do while swimming. That reinforces the misunderstanding, which has sometimes led accident victims to abandon a safe position atop a capsized vessel and reenter the water, usually with tragic results.

Cold-water immersion is associated with two potential medical emergencies: drowning and hypothermia. Numerous case histories and statistical evidence document the prominence of cold-water immersion as a cause of drowning and hypothermia. Perhaps the most famous occurrence of cold-water immersion was the sinking of the ocean liner, the *Titanic*, on April 14, 1912. After striking an iceberg, the ship sank in calm seas. Of the 2,201 people on board, only 712 were rescued, all from the ship's lifeboats. The remaining 1,489 people died in the water, despite the arrival of a rescue vehicle within 2 hours. Nearly all of those victims were wearing life preservers, yet the cause of death was officially listed as drowning. More likely, the cause of death was immersion hypothermia.

The speed at which a person cools depends on several factors:

- *Body fat.* The more body fat a person has, the slower cooling occurs. More fat increases survival chances.
- *Body type.* Bigger people cool more slowly than smaller people. Children cool faster than adults. Women have more fat but are usually smaller, so they cool at the same rate as men.
- *Physical fitness.* Cardiovascular fitness can help meet the stress of cold-water immersion, but physically fit people usually have less subcutaneous fat for insulation.
- *Water temperature.* The colder the water, the faster a person cools.
- *Clothing.* Clothing can insulate, and some types of fabric, such as wool, are better than others.
- *Alcohol.* People who have been drinking alcohol are more likely to get into dangerous situations. Alcohol impairs judgment and coordination. Research studies have implicated alcohol in 10% to 50% of all drownings. Alcohol dilates the skin's blood vessels, which allows more body heat to escape.
- *Behavior.* Swimming and treading water increase the flow of warm blood from the body's core to the muscles, increasing the cooling rate. Thus, swimmers often die first because they are more likely to try to tread water or swim rather than float. Likewise, so-called *drownproofing,* a technique of bobbing in the water (like a jellyfish), markedly increases heat loss as water circulates around the head.

A *heat escape lessening position (HELP)* has been devised, in which the victim draws the knees up close to the chest, presses the arms to the sides, and remains as quiet as possible **Figure 25-2**. For two or more people, huddling quietly and closely together (huddle position) will decrease heat loss from the groin and the front of the body. Both of these positions require personal flotation devices (life jackets).

Surviving long periods of submersion has been explained by the diving reflex found in mammals. Some say

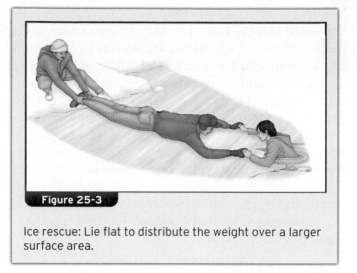

Figure 25-3

Ice rescue: Lie flat to distribute the weight over a larger surface area.

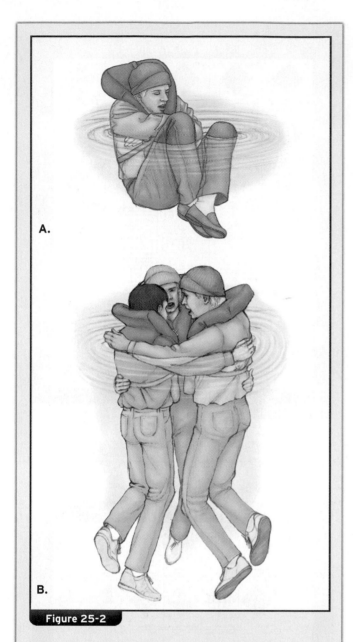

Figure 25-2

HELP or huddle. **A.** A person wearing a flotation device can minimize heat loss and increase chances of survival by assuming the heat escape lessening position (HELP) in which the knees are pulled up to the chest and the arms crossed. **B.** Groups of three or more can conserve heat by wrapping their arms around one another and pulling into a tight circle or huddle.

that the diving reflex slows the heart rate, shunts blood to the brain, and closes the airway. Recent research, however, suggests that the diving reflex is present in marine mammals such as seals, porpoises, whales, and walruses but not in humans. If the diving reflex is discounted, the most likely explanation for prolonged submersion survival is that cold water produces hypothermia, which reduces the body's demand for oxygen and protects the brain.

► Ice Rescue

If a person has fallen through the ice near the shore, extend a pole or throw a line with a floatable object attached to it. When the person has hold of the object, pull him or her toward the shore or the edge of the ice.

If the person has fallen through the ice away from the shore and you cannot reach him or her with a pole or a throwing line, lie flat and push a ladder, plank, or similar object ahead of you **Figure 25-3**. You can also tie a rope to a spare tire and the other end to an anchor point on the shore, lie flat, and push the tire ahead of you. Pull the person ashore or to the edge of the ice.

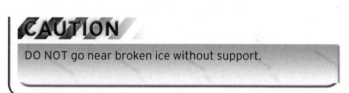

CAUTION

DO NOT go near broken ice without support.

► Electrical Emergency Rescue

Electrical injuries can be devastating. Just a mild shock can cause serious internal injuries. A current of 1,000 V or more is considered high voltage, but even the 110 V of household current can be deadly.

When a person receives an electrical shock, electricity enters the body at the point of contact and travels along the path of least resistance (nerves and blood vessels). The current travels rapidly, generating heat and causing destruction.

Most indoor electrocutions are caused by faulty electrical equipment or the careless use of electrical appliances. Before you touch the victim, turn off the electricity at the circuit breaker, fuse box, or outside switch box or unplug the appliance if the plug is undamaged.

If the electrocution involves high-voltage power lines, the power must be turned off before anyone approaches the victim. If you approach a victim and feel a tingling sensation in your legs and lower body, stop. You are on energized ground, and an electric current is entering one foot, passing through your lower body, and leaving through the other foot. You should raise one foot off the ground, turn around, and hop to a safe place. Wait for trained personnel with the proper equipment to cut the wires or disconnect them. If a power line falls over a car, tell the driver and passengers to stay in the car. A victim should try to jump out of the car only if an explosion or fire threatens and then without making contact with the car or the wire.

CAUTION

DO NOT touch an appliance or the victim until the current is off.

DO NOT try to move downed wires.

DO NOT use any object, even dry wood (broomstick, tools, chair, stool) to separate the victim from the electrical source.

▶ Hazardous Materials Incidents

Almost any highway crash scene involves the potential danger of hazardous chemicals. Clues that indicate the presence of hazardous materials include the following:

- Look for warning signs on the vehicle (for example, "explosive," "flammable," "corrosive"). If you are unable to read the placard or labels, do not move closer and risk exposure. If you are able to read the placard with the naked eye, you may be too close and should consider moving farther away. **Figure 25-4** shows a chart illustrating the hazardous materials warning placards, and **Figure 25-5** shows a chart illustrating the warning labels.
- Watch for a leak or spill from a tank, container, truck, or railroad car with or without hazardous material placards or labels.
- A strong, noxious odor can denote a hazardous material.
- A cloud or strange-looking smoke from the escaping substance "says" stay away.

Stay well away and upwind from the area. Only people who are specially trained in handling hazardous materials and who have the proper equipment should be in the area.

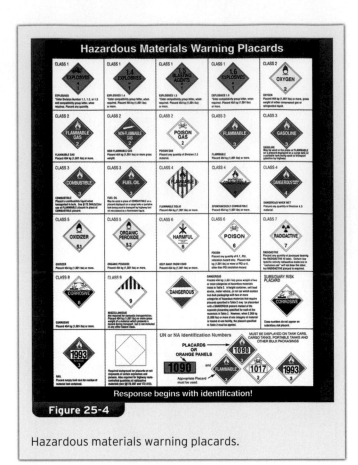

Figure 25-4

Hazardous materials warning placards.

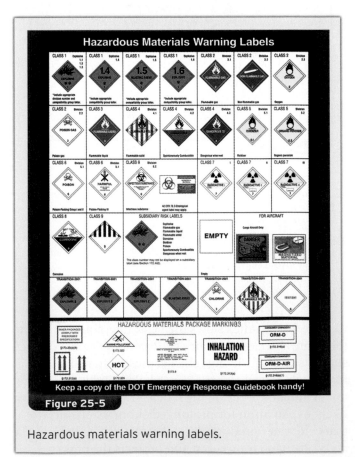

Figure 25-5

Hazardous materials warning labels.

▶ Motor Vehicle Crashes

In most states, you are legally obligated to stop and give help when you are involved in a motor vehicle crash. If you arrive at a crash shortly after it happens, the law does not require you to stop, although it might be argued that you have a moral responsibility to provide any aid that you can.

1. Stop and park your vehicle well off the highway or road and out of active traffic lanes. Park at least five car lengths from the crash. If the police have taken charge, do not stop unless you are asked to do so. If the police or other emergency vehicles have not arrived, call or send someone to call 9-1-1 or the local emergency number as soon as possible. Ways to call include the following:
   - Finding a pay phone or roadside emergency phone
   - Using a cellular phone or CB (citizen's band) radio
   - Using a phone at a nearby house or business

2. Turn on your vehicle's emergency hazard flashers. Raise the hood of your vehicle to draw more attention to the scene.

3. Make sure everyone on the scene is safe.
   - Ask the driver to turn off the ignition or turn it off yourself.
   - Ask bystanders to stand well off the roadway.
   - Place flares or reflectors 250 to 500 feet behind the crash scene to warn oncoming drivers of the crash. Do not ignite flares around leaking gasoline or diesel fuel.

4. If the driver or passenger is unresponsive or might have spinal injuries, use your hands to stabilize the person's head and neck.

5. Check and keep monitoring the victim's breathing. Treat any life-threatening injuries.

6. Whenever possible, wait for EMS personnel to extricate the victims from vehicles because they have training and the proper equipment. In most cases,

CAUTION

DO NOT rush to get the victims out of a car that has been in a crash. Contrary to opinion, most vehicle crashes do not involve fire, and most vehicles stay in an upright position.

DO NOT move or allow victims to move unless there is an immediate danger such as fire or oncoming traffic.

DO NOT transport victims in your car or any other bystander's vehicle.

keep the victims' conditions stabilized inside the vehicle.

7. Allow the EMS ambulance to take victims to the hospital.

▶ Fires

Should you encounter a fire, you should:
1. Get all the people out of the vehicles and area quickly.
2. Call the emergency telephone number (usually 9-1-1).

Then—and *only* then—if the fire is small and if your own escape route is clear, should you fight the fire yourself with a fire extinguisher. You may be able to put out the fire or at least hold damage to a minimum. Because a fire can spread quickly, efforts to contain it within the first 5 minutes of a blaze can make a substantial difference in the eventual outcome.

To use a fire extinguisher, aim directly at whatever is burning and sweep across it. Extinguishers expel their contents quickly; it takes just 8 to 25 seconds for most home models containing dry chemicals to empty.

If clothing catches fire, tear the article off, in a motion away from the face. Keep the victim from running, because running fans the flames. Wrap a rug or a woolen blanket around the victim's neck to keep the fire from the face or throw a blanket on the victim. In some cases, you may be able to smother the flames by throwing the victim to the floor and rolling him or her in a rug.

CAUTION

DO NOT let victims run if their clothing is on fire.

DO NOT become trapped while fighting a fire. Always keep a door behind you so you can exit if the fire gets too big.

▶ Threatening Dogs

When you enter any emergency scene, look for signs of a dog and proceed with caution if the animal is not threatening. Ask the owner to control a threatening dog. If you cannot be delayed, consider using a fire extinguisher, water hose, or pepper spray. For a vicious dog, call the police for assistance.

▶ Farm Animals

Emergencies involving farm animals can be dangerous to rescuers. Horses kick and bite. Cattle kick, bite, gore, or squeeze people against a pen or barn. Pigs can deliver severe bites.

- Approach a situation involving animals with caution.
- Do not frighten an animal. Speak quietly to reassure it.
- If food is available, use it to lure the animal away from the victim.

▶ Confined Spaces

A *confined space* is any area not intended for human occupancy that may have or develop a dangerous atmosphere. There are three types of confined spaces: below ground, ground level, and above ground. Below-ground confined spaces include manholes, below-ground utility vaults and storage tanks, old mines, cisterns, and wells. Ground-level confined spaces include industrial tanks and farm storage silos. Above-ground confined spaces include water towers and legged storage tanks.

An accident in a confined space demands immediate action. If someone enters a confined space and signals for help or becomes unresponsive, follow these steps:

1. Call 9-1-1 for immediate assistance.
2. Do not rush in to help.
3. When help arrives, try to rescue the victim without entering the space.
4. If rescue from the outside cannot be done, allow trained and properly equipped (respiratory protection plus safety harnesses or lifelines) rescuers to enter the space and remove the victim.
5. Give first aid or CPR if necessary.

Triage: What to Do With Multiple Victims

You may encounter emergency situations in which there are two or more victims. This often occurs in multiple-car accidents or disasters. After making a quick scene survey, decide who must be cared for and transported first. This process of prioritizing or classifying injured victims is called *triage*. Triage comes from the French word *trier*, to sort. The goal is to do the greatest good for the greatest number of victims. Triage may require unpleasant decisions to withhold care from victims who are unlikely to survive so that lifesaving care can be given to those more likely to survive.

▶ Finding Life-Threatened Victims

A variety of systems are used to identify care and transportation priorities. To find the people needing immediate care for life-threatening conditions, first tell all victims who can get up and walk to move to a specific area. Victims who can get up and walk rarely have life-threatening injuries. These victims (*walking wounded*) are classified as needing delayed care (see the following definitions). Do not force a victim to move if he or she complains of pain.

Find the life-threatened victims by performing only an initial check on all remaining victims. Assess motionless victims first. You must move rapidly (spend less than 60 seconds with each victim) from one victim to the next until all have been assessed. Classify victims according to the following care and transportation priorities:

1. Immediate care: Victim needs immediate care and transport to medical care as soon as possible.
   - Breathing difficulties
   - Severe bleeding
   - Severe burns
   - Signs of shock
   - Unresponsiveness
2. Delayed care: Care and transport can be delayed up to 1 hour.
   - Burns without airway problems
   - Major or multiple bone or joint injuries
   - Back injuries with or without suspected spinal cord damage
3. Walking wounded: Care and transportation can be delayed up to 3 hours.
   - Minor fractures
   - Minor wounds
4. Dead: Victim is obviously dead or unlikely to survive because of the type and extent of the injuries. This includes most cases of cardiac arrest due to injury.

Do not become involved in treating the victims at this point, but ask knowledgeable bystanders to provide care for immediate life-threatening problems (that is, rescue breathing, bleeding control).

Reassess victims regularly for changes in their condition. Only after victims with immediate life-threatening conditions receive care should people with less-serious conditions be given care.

You may have to care for multiple victims without adequate help until more highly trained emergency personnel arrive. You will usually be relieved when more highly trained emergency personnel arrive on the scene. You may then be asked to provide first aid, to help move

FYI

Principles of Lifting

- Know your capabilities. Do not try to handle a load that is too heavy or awkward; seek help.
- Use a safe grip. Use as much of your palms as possible.
- Keep your back straight. Tighten the muscles of your buttocks and abdomen.
- Bend your knees to use the strong muscles of the thighs and buttocks.
- Keep your arms close to your body and your elbows flexed.
- Position your feet shoulder width apart for balance, one in front of the other.
- When lifting, keep and lift the victim close to your body.
- While lifting, do not twist your back; pivot with your feet.
- Lift and carry slowly, smoothly, and in unison with the other lifters.
- Before you move a victim, explain to him or her what you are doing.

CAUTION

DO NOT move a victim unless absolutely necessary, such as if the victim is in immediate danger or must be moved to shelter while waiting for EMS personnel to arrive.

DO NOT make the injury worse by moving the victim.

DO NOT move a victim who could have a spinal injury unless absolutely necessary due to other threats to life such as fire.

DO NOT move a victim without stabilizing the injured part.

DO NOT move a victim unless you know where you are going.

DO NOT leave an unconscious victim alone except for taking a short time to call EMS.

DO NOT move a victim when you can send someone for help. Wait with the victim.

DO NOT try to move a victim by yourself if other people are available to help.

victims, or to help with ambulance or helicopter transportation.

Moving Victims

A victim should not be moved until he or she is ready for transportation to a hospital, if required. All necessary first aid should be provided before moving a victim. A victim should be moved only if there is an immediate danger, such as the following:

- There is a fire or danger of a fire.
- Explosives or other hazardous materials are involved.
- It is impossible to protect the scene from hazards.
- It is impossible to gain access to other victims in the situation who need lifesaving care (such as in a vehicle crash).

A cardiac arrest victim is usually moved unless he or she is already on the ground or floor because CPR must be performed on a firm, level surface.

▶ Emergency Moves

The major danger in moving a victim quickly is the possibility of aggravating a spinal injury. In an emergency, every effort should be made to pull the victim in the direction of the long axis of the body to provide as much

protection to the spinal cord as possible. If the victims are on the floor or ground, you can drag them away from the scene by using the various techniques shown in **Figure 25-6** to **Figure 25-19** .

▶ Nonemergency Moves

All injured parts should be stabilized before and during moving. If rapid transportation is not needed, it is helpful to practice on another person about the same size as the injured victim.

Stretcher or Litter

The safest way to carry an injured victim is on some type of stretcher or litter, which can be improvised. Before using it, test an improvised stretcher by lifting a rescuer about the same size as the victim.

- *Blanket-and-pole improvised stretcher.* If the blanket is properly wrapped, the victim's weight will keep it from unwinding **Figure 25-20** .
- *Blanket with no poles.* The blanket is rolled inward toward the victim and grasped for carrying by four or more rescuers.
- *Board-improvised stretcher.* These are sturdier than a blanket-and-pole stretcher but heavier and less comfortable. Tie the victim on to prevent him or her from rolling off **Figure 25-21** .
- *Commercial stretchers and litters.* These usually are not available except through the EMS.

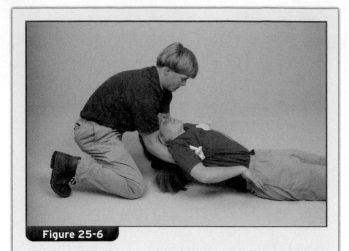

Figure 25-6

Shoulder drag. Use for short distances over a rough surface; stabilize the victim's head with your forearms.

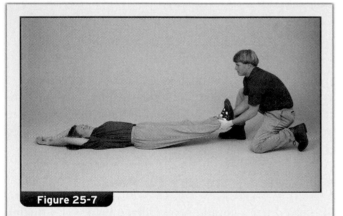

Figure 25-7

Ankle drag. This is the fastest method for a short distance on a smooth surface.

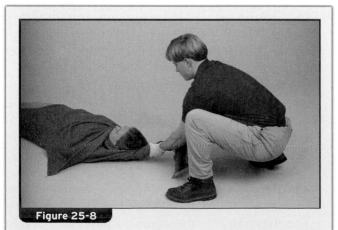

Figure 25-8

Blanket pull. Roll the victim onto a blanket, and pull from behind the victim's head.

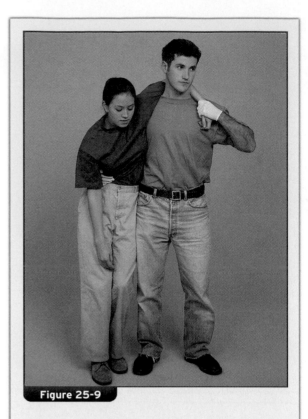

Figure 25-9

Human crutch (one person helps victim to walk). If one leg is injured, help the victim to walk on the good leg while you support the injured side.

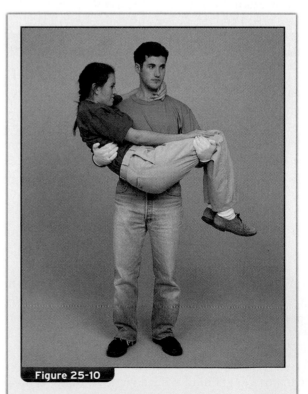

Figure 25-10

Cradle carry. Use this method for children and lightweight adults who cannot walk.

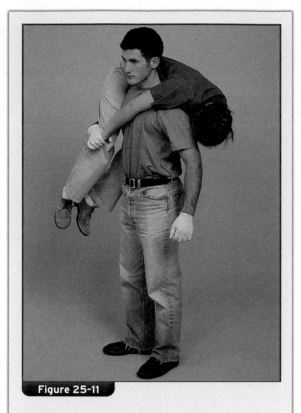

Figure 25-11

Firefighter's carry. If the victim's injuries permit, you can travel longer distances if you carry the victim over your shoulder.

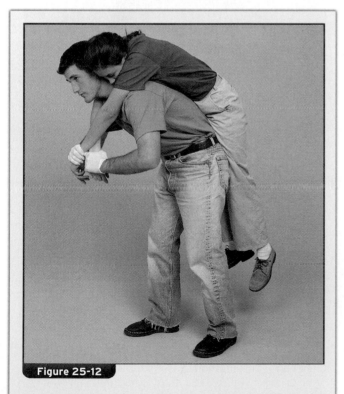

Figure 25-12

Pack-strap carry. When injuries make the firefighter's carry unsafe, this method is better for longer distances.

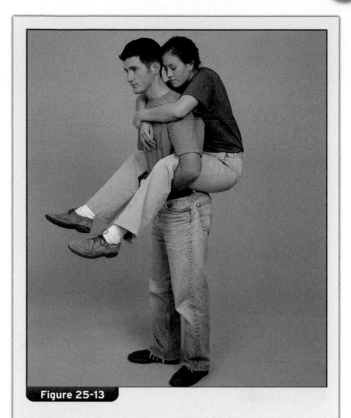

Figure 25-13

Piggyback carry. Use this method when the victim cannot walk but can use the arms to hang onto the rescuer.

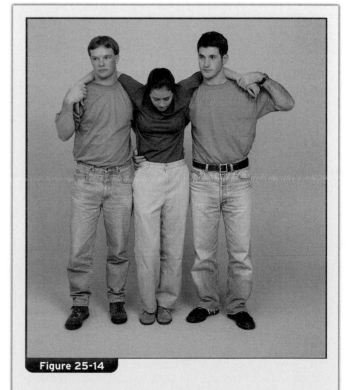

Figure 25-14

Two-person assist. This method is similar to the human crutch.

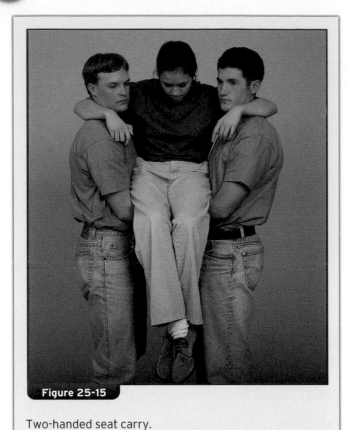

Figure 25-15

Two-handed seat carry.

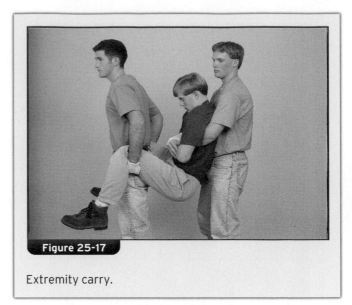

Figure 25-17

Extremity carry.

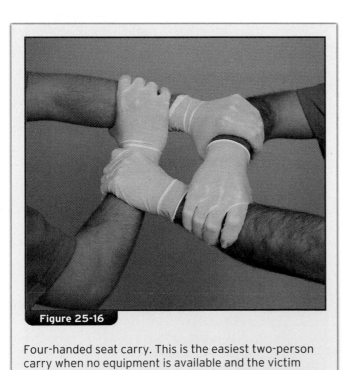

Figure 25-16

Four-handed seat carry. This is the easiest two-person carry when no equipment is available and the victim cannot walk but can use the arms to hang onto the two rescuers.

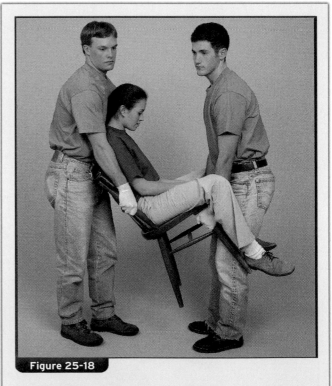

Figure 25-18

Chair carry. This method is useful for a narrow passage or up or down stairs. Use a sturdy chair that can take the victim's weight.

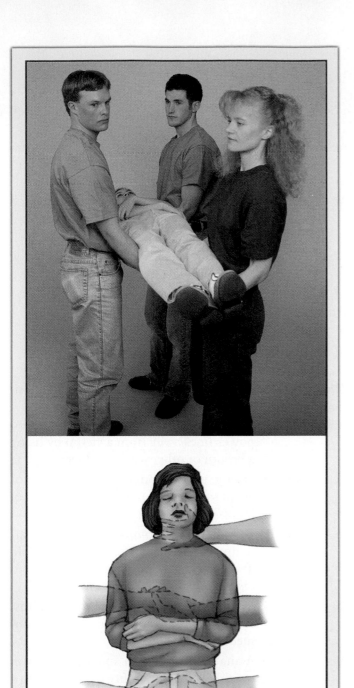

Figure 25-19

Hammock carry. Three to six people stand on alternate sides of the injured person and link hands beneath the victim.

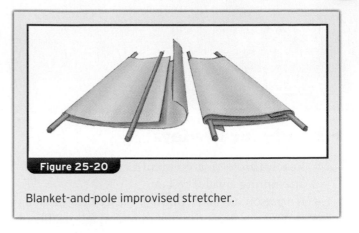

Figure 25-20

Blanket-and-pole improvised stretcher.

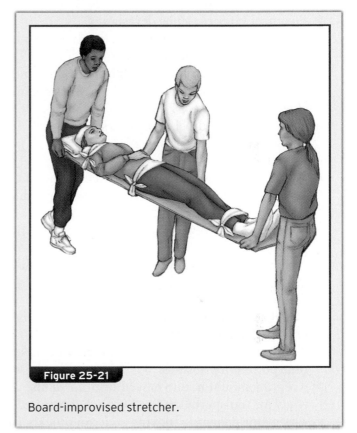

Figure 25-21

Board-improvised stretcher.

prep kit

▶ Ready for Review

- Reach-throw-row-go identifies the sequence for attempting a water rescue.
- If a person has fallen through the ice near the shore, extend a pole or throw a line with a floatable object attached to it.
- Electrical injuries can be devastating.
- Almost any highway crash scene involves the potential danger of hazardous chemicals.
- In most states, you are legally obligated to stop and give help when you are involved in a motor vehicle crash.
- Should you encounter a fire, you should:
  - Get all people out fast.
  - Call 9-1-1.
- When you enter any emergency scene, look for signs of an animal and proceed with caution if the animal is not threatening.
- Emergencies involving farm animals can be dangerous to rescuers.
- A confined space is any area not intended for human occupancy that may have or develop a dangerous atmosphere.
- The goal of triage is to do the greatest good for the greatest number of victims.
- A variety of systems are used to identify care and transportation priorities.
- A victim should not be moved until he or she is ready for transportation to a hospital, if required.
- The major danger in moving a victim quickly is the possibility of aggravating a spinal injury.
- All injured parts should be stabilized before and during moving.

▶ Vital Vocabulary

triage A system used for sorting victims to determine the order in which they will receive medical attention.

▶ Assessment in Action

You see a single car leave the highway and crash into an electrical power line pole, knocking down some of the high-voltage power lines. One victim is ejected from the car, and another remains in the car yelling for help.
Directions: Circle Yes if you agree with the statement, circle No if you disagree.

Yes No 1. You should go first to the victim in the car because he or she is pleading for help.
Yes No 2. If one of the victims is in contact with the high-voltage power line, a dry tree branch could be used to move the electrical line.
Yes No 3. Most state laws require a driver of another car witnessing a car crash to stop and render care.
Yes No 4. For the quiet, motionless victim ejected from the car, you should stabilize the head and neck against movement.
Yes No 5. You could consider moving either of the victims if their lives are threatened by a fire.

Answers: 1. No; 2. No; 3. No; 4. Yes; 5. Yes

▶ Check Your Knowledge

Directions: Circle Yes if you agree with the statement, circle No if you disagree.
Yes No 1. You should attempt to move downed power lines away from a victim by using a broom or other wooden object.
Yes No 2. Strong, unusual odors or clouds of vapor are possible indications of the presence of hazardous materials.
Yes No 3. To keep from becoming trapped while attempting to extinguish a fire, you should always keep a door behind you for rapid exit.
Yes No 4. In a situation involving several victims, those with breathing difficulties need immediate attention.
Yes No 5. A major concern in moving a victim quickly is the possibility of aggravating a spine injury.
Yes No 6. "Row-throw-reach-go" represents the safe order for executing a water rescue.
Yes No 7. In most states, you are legally obligated to stop and give help when you are involved in a motor vehicle crash.
Yes No 8. The first thing to do in case of a fire is to use a fire extinguisher and try to put out the fire.
Yes No 9. When using a fire extinguisher, aim it at the base of the flames.
Yes No 10. When several people are injured, those crying or screaming should receive your attention first.

Answers: 1. No; 2. Yes; 3. Yes; 4. Yes; 5. Yes; 6. No; 7. Yes; 8. No; 9. Yes; 10. No

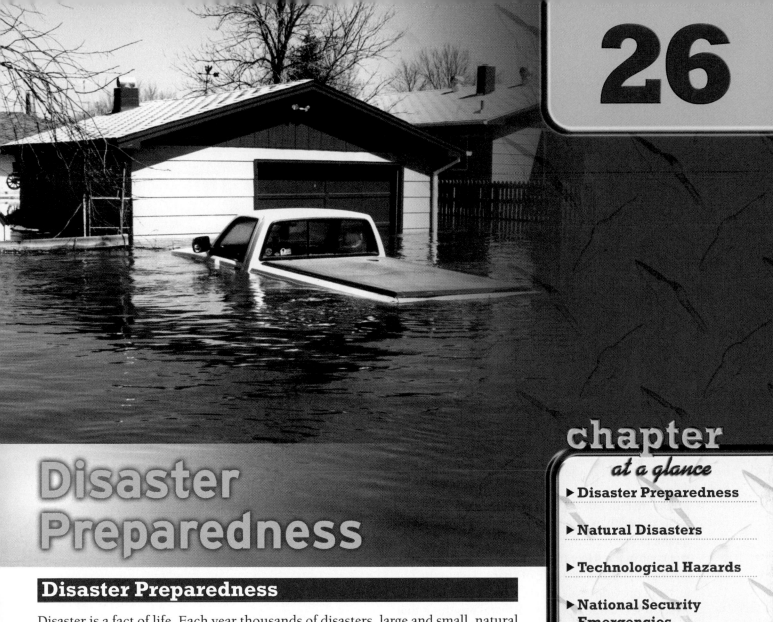

Disaster Preparedness

Disaster Preparedness

Disaster is a fact of life. Each year thousands of disasters, large and small, natural and caused by humans, strike somewhere in the world. Many people have survived disasters, thanks to good luck and willpower, but that is not enough. Training about disasters needs to be modified from "nice to know" to "must know."

Valuable information about disasters is discussed in this chapter. This information is adapted from US government documents provided by the Federal Emergency Management Agency (FEMA), the US Department of Homeland Security, the National Weather Service, and the US Geological Survey.

▶ Natural Disasters

Natural disasters such as earthquakes, floods, hurricanes, and tornados claim many lives each year. Becoming informed about the dangers of natural disasters and the steps you can take to protect yourself and others can help minimize injuries and deaths.

Earthquake

An earthquake is a sudden, rapid shaking of the earth caused by the breaking and shifting of rock deep beneath the earth's surface. This shaking can cause buildings and bridges to collapse; disrupt gas, electric, and phone service; and sometimes trigger landslides, avalanches, flash floods, fires, and huge, destructive ocean

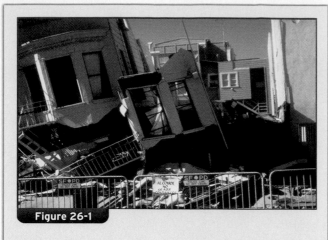

Figure 26-1

Devastation resulting from the California earthquake that crippled San Francisco in 1989.

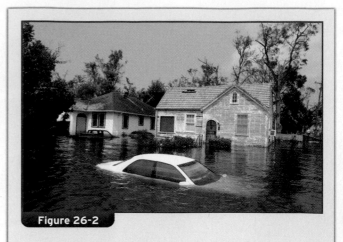

Figure 26-2

Hurricane Katrina caused massive floods in New Orleans.

waves known as *tsunamis*. Earthquakes can occur at any time of the year **Figure 26-1**.

What to Do During an Earthquake

Follow these safety guidelines if you experience an earthquake:

- If you are indoors, take cover under a sturdy desk, table, or bench or against an inside wall. If the earthquake is severe, crouch next to a large, sturdy object such as a refrigerator or file cabinet. Should the ceiling collapse, a triangle of space next to the object will provide a safe place. Stay away from glass, windows, outside doors, walls, and anything that could fall. If there is not a table or desk nearby, cover your face and head with your arms and crouch down, a door frame may offer some protection. Stay inside until the shaking has stopped and you are sure exiting is safe. It is dangerous to try to leave a building during an earthquake because objects can fall on you. Beware of aftershocks, and follow the same precautions as for an earthquake.
- If you are in bed, stay there, and protect your head with a pillow, unless you are under a heavy light or fan fixture that could fall. If the earthquake is severe, get on the floor next to but not under the bed. This will also provide a safe space if the ceiling collapses.
- If you are in a high-rise building, expect the fire alarms and sprinklers to go off during an earthquake. Do not use the elevators; use the stairs.
- If you are outdoors, find a clear spot away from buildings, trees, streetlights, and power lines. Drop to the ground and stay there until the shaking stops.

- If you are in a vehicle, pull over and stay there with your seatbelt fastened until the shaking has stopped. If the earthquake is severe and you are under a highway overpass, exit your car and lie next to, but not underneath your vehicle. The falling debris may crush the roof of the car, but beside the car will be a safe place for you to stay until help arrives.
- If you are trapped in debris, do not panic. Move carefully.
  - Do not use a flame for light due to gas leaks.
  - Do not move about or kick up dust.
  - Cover your mouth with a handkerchief or clothing.
  - Tap on a pipe or wall so rescuers can locate you.
- Learn how to turn off your gas supply where it enters the house. Turn off the gas if you smell gas or have to evacuate.
  - If you smell gas, do not use light switches or any other devices that can spark.

Flood

With the exception of fire, floods are the most common and widespread of all natural disasters. Most communities have experienced some type of flooding after heavy storms, or winter snow thaws **Figure 26-2**. Pay attention to flash flood warnings even if skies are clear in your location, because run-off can occur from storms miles away. Be especially aware of storms in hills above you. Flash floods occur when heavy rain causes run-off into channels and low-lying areas. The flood can be very fast and can occur miles from the rain, often catching people off-guard.

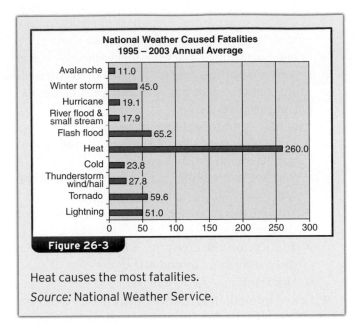

**National Weather Caused Fatalities
1995 – 2003 Annual Average**

Avalanche	11.0
Winter storm	45.0
Hurricane	19.1
River flood & small stream	17.9
Flash flood	65.2
Heat	260.0
Cold	23.8
Thunderstorm wind/hail	27.8
Tornado	59.6
Lightning	51.0

Figure 26-3

Heat causes the most fatalities.

Source: National Weather Service.

most vehicles, including sport utility vehicles and pickups.

- If flood water rises around your car and you cannot drive out, abandon the car and move to higher ground, but only if you can do so safely.

Heat Wave

In extreme heat and high humidity, cooling of the body by evaporation is slowed and it is difficult for the body to maintain normal temperature **Figure 26-3**. People living in urban areas may be at greater risk from the effects of a prolonged heat wave than those living in rural areas. Asphalt and concrete store heat longer and gradually release heat at night. A devastating heat wave struck Europe in 2003, resulting in thousands of injuries and deaths.

What to Do During a Heat Wave

Follow these safety guidelines if you experience a heat wave emergency:

- Stay in the coolest available location. Stay indoors as much as possible. If air-conditioning is not available, stay on the lowest floor out of the sunshine. Circulate the air with a fan, and use cool, wet cloths to help keep your body temperature down.
- Drink plenty of water regularly, even if you do not feel thirsty.
- Avoid drinking alcoholic beverages because they cause further body dehydration.
- Never leave children or pets alone in vehicles.
- Dress in loose-fitting clothes. Lightweight, light-colored clothing reflects heat and sunlight and helps maintain normal body temperature.
- Protect your face and head outdoors by wearing a wide-brimmed hat.
- Avoid too much sunshine. Sunburn slows the skin's ability to cool itself.
- Avoid strenuous work during the warmest part of the day (usually 10 AM to 3 PM).
- Spend at least 2 hours of the day in an air-conditioned place. If your home is not air-conditioned, consider spending the warmest part of the day in public buildings (for example, libraries, movie theaters, and shopping malls).
- Check on family, friends, and neighbors who do not have air-conditioning and who spend much of their time alone. Refer to Chapter 19 for first aid procedures for heat-related emergencies (for example, heat stroke, heat exhaustion, and heat cramps).

What to Do During a Flood

Follow these safety guidelines if conditions exist that could cause a flood:

- Be aware of the likelihood of flooding in your area. If there is any possibility of a flood or flash flood, move immediately to higher ground. Be aware of streams, drainage channels, canyons, and other areas prone to flooding quickly and suddenly.
- Listen to the radio or television stations for local information.
- If local authorities issue a flood watch, prepare to evacuate.
  - Secure your home, if you have time. Move essential items to upper floors.
  - If instructed, turn off utilities at the main switches or valves. Disconnect electrical appliances. Do not touch electrical equipment if you are wet or standing in water.
  - If you are not evacuating, you still need to prepare for the worst. If you do not have access to adequate bottled water, you can fill the bathtub with water in case water becomes contaminated or services are cut off. Before filling the tub, sterilize it with a diluted bleach solution (1 part bleach to 10 parts water).
- Do not walk through moving water. Six inches of moving water can knock you off your feet. Use a stick or pole to check the firmness of the ground and water depth in front of you.
- Do not drive into flooded areas. A foot of water can float a vehicle. Two feet of water can carry away

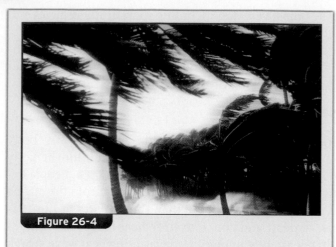

Figure 26-4

Hurricanes are among the most costly and dangerous disasters.

Hurricane

A hurricane is a tropical storm with winds that have reached a constant speed of at least 74 miles per hour. As a hurricane nears land, it can bring torrential rains, high winds, and flooding from the ocean, called storm surges. All Atlantic and Gulf of Mexico coastal areas are subject to hurricanes or tropical storms. August and September are the peak months of hurricane activity during the storm season, which lasts from June to November **Figure 26-4**. In the Pacific Ocean these storms are called typhoons.

What to Do During a Hurricane

Follow these safety guidelines if you experience the threat of a hurricane:

- Listen to the radio or television stations for local information. If a hurricane *watch* is issued, you usually have 24 to 36 hours before the hurricane hits land.
- Secure your home. Close any storm shutters. Secure outdoor objects or bring them indoors. Attach boards to window frames or tape windows to prevent or reduce the risk of broken glass. Park cars remaining at home along the side of the house. Make sure that all vehicles have a full tank of gas.
- If you are not evacuating, you need to prepare for the worst. Gather several days' supply of water and food for each household member. If you do not have access to adequate bottled water, fill the bathtub with water in case water becomes contaminated or services are cut off. Before filling the tub, sterilize it with a diluted bleach solution (1 part bleach to 10 parts water).

- If you are evacuating, prepare backpacks to take your disaster supplies with you to the shelter.
- When preparing to evacuate, fuel your vehicle and review evacuation routes. If instructed, turn off utilities at the main valves or switches before departing your residence.
- Evacuate to an inland location early if:
  - Local authorities announce an evacuation and you live in an evacuation zone.
  - You live in a mobile home near the path of the hurricane.
  - You live in a high-rise building near the path of the hurricane.
  - You live on the coast, on a flood plain near a river, or near an inland waterway.
  - You think you are in danger.
- Leave immediately if local authorities order an evacuation. Follow evacuation routes, stay away from coastal areas, riverbanks and streams, and tell others where you are going.
- If you are not required to evacuate or are unable to evacuate, stay indoors during the hurricane and away from windows and glass doors.
- To protect yourself against the strong wind:
  - Take refuge in a small interior room, closet, or hallway.
  - Close all interior doors; secure and brace exterior doors.
  - In a multiple-story building, go to the first or second floor and stay in interior rooms away from the windows.
  - Lie on the floor under a table or other sturdy object if a hurricane or any associated tornado approaches.
- Phone lines are likely to be busy with emergency traffic. Avoid using the phone except for serious emergencies.

Landslides

Landslides occur in almost every US state when masses of rock, earth, or debris move down a slope. They may be small or large and can move at slow or high speeds. They are usually associated with periods of heavy rainfall or rapid snowmelt.

What to Do During a Landslide

Follow these safety guidelines if conditions exist that could cause a landslide:

- Stay alert. Many landslides occur when people are sleeping.

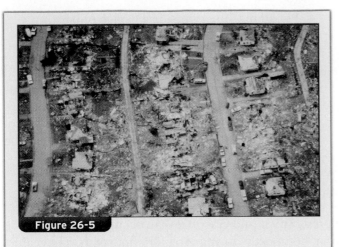

Figure 26-5

The tornado in Wichita Falls, Texas, in 1979 was one of the worst tornadoes in US history.

- If you are in an area susceptible to landslides, consider evacuating if it is safe to do so.
- Listen for unusual sounds that might indicate moving debris, such as trees cracking, boulders knocking together, or rumbling.
- If you are near a stream or channel, be alert for any sudden increase or decrease in water flow and for a change from clear to muddy water. Such changes may indicate landslide activity upstream, so be prepared to move quickly.
- Be alert when driving. Embankments along roadsides are susceptible to landslides. Watch the road for collapsed pavement, mud, fallen rocks, and other indications of possible debris flow.
- If you remain at home, move to a second level if possible to distance yourself from the direct path of landslide debris.

Tornado

A tornado is a violent windstorm characterized by a twisting, funnel-shaped cloud. It is spawned by a thunderstorm (or sometimes as a result of a hurricane). Tornado season is generally March through August, although tornadoes can occur at any time of the year. Every state is at some risk from this hazard, but tornados are most frequently reported east of the Rocky Mountains **Figure 26-5**.

What to Do During a Tornado

Follow these safety guidelines if you experience a tornado. If you are at home:

- Go immediately to a windowless interior room, storm cellar, basement, or the lowest level of the building. If there is no basement, go to an inner hallway or a smaller inner room without windows, such as a bathroom or closet.
- Get under a piece of sturdy furniture (such as a heavy table or desk) and hold on to it.

If you are outdoors:

- If possible, get inside a building.
- If shelter is not available or there is no time to get indoors, lie in a ditch or low-lying area or crouch near a strong building.

If you are at work or school:

- Avoid places with wide-span roofs such as auditoriums, cafeterias, large hallways, and shopping malls.
- Go to a predetermined shelter area (signs are usually posted)
- Get under a piece of sturdy furniture (such as a heavy table, desk, or workbench).

If you are in a vehicle:

- Do not try to outdrive a tornado.
- Get out of the vehicle immediately and take shelter in a nearby building. If there is no time to get indoors, get out of the car and lie in a ditch or low-lying area away from the vehicle.

Tsunami

A **tsunami** (pronounced soo-nahm'ee) is a series of waves generated by an undersea disturbance (for example, an earthquake). From the area of disturbance, the waves travel outward in all directions, much like the ripples caused by throwing a rock into a pond. Tsunamis reaching heights of more than 100 feet have been recorded near coastlines, although most waves are less than 18 feet high. Areas of greatest risk are less than 50 feet above sea level and within 1 mile of the shoreline. Drowning is the most common cause of death due to a tsunami.

What to Do During a Tsunami

Follow these safety guidelines if conditions exist that could cause a tsunami:

- Listen to the radio or television stations for the latest local emergency information. If you are advised to evacuate, do so immediately.
- Stay away from the area until local authorities say it is safe to return.
- Do not go to the shoreline to watch for a tsunami. If you can see the wave, you are too close to escape it. Because a tsunami is a series of waves, do not assume that one wave means the danger is over.

Volcano Eruption

A volcano is a mountain that opens downward to a reservoir of molten rock below the earth's surface. When the pressure from gases and molten rock become strong enough to cause an explosion, eruptions occur. Gases and rock shoot up through the opening and spill over the mountainsides and/or spew into the air. Most injuries and deaths are due to ash, falling rocks, landslides, and floods, rather than hot flowing lava.

What to Do During a Volcano Eruption

Follow these safety guidelines if a volcano erupts:
- Follow the evacuation order issued by local authorities. Avoid areas downwind from the volcano.

If caught indoors:
- Close all windows, doors, and chimney and stove dampers.

If caught outdoors:
- Seek shelter indoors.
- Avoid low-lying areas where poisonous gases can collect and flash floods and lava- and mudflows can be dangerous.

- Put all machinery inside a garage or barn.

Protect yourself:
- Wear long-sleeved shirts and pants.
- Use goggles to protect your eyes.
- Use a dust mask or hold a damp cloth over your face to keep from breathing in the hot ash or gases.
- Stay out of the area around the erupting volcano. Trying to watch an erupting volcano can be deadly.

Wildfire

Forest, brush, and grass fires can occur at any time of the year, but mostly during long, dry hot spells. The majority of these fires are caused by human carelessness or ignorance **Figure 26-6** .

What to Do During a Wildfire

Follow these safety guidelines if a wildfire occurs:
- Listen to local radio or television stations for the latest emergency information.
- If advised to evacuate, do so immediately. Choose a route away from the fire hazard. Watch for changes in the speed and direction of fire and smoke. Do not block firefighting entrance routes.

Winter Storm

Heavy snowfall and extreme cold can immobilize an entire region. Even areas that usually experience mild winters can be hit with a major snowstorm or extreme cold **Figure 26-7** .

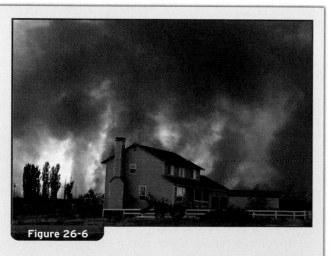

Figure 26-6

Wildfires can move quickly, threatening lives and homes.

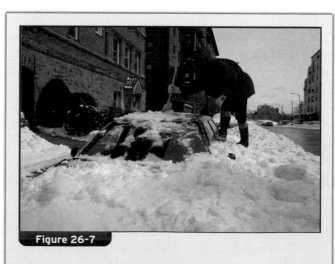

Figure 26-7

Major winter snowstorms can tie up a city.

What to Do During a Winter Storm

Follow these safety guidelines if a winter storm occurs. If indoors:

- Listen to the local radio or television stations or NOAA (National Oceanic and Atmospheric Administration) weather radio for weather reports and emergency information.
- Conserve fuel by lowering the thermostat to 65° F during the day and 55° F at night. Close off unused rooms.
- Eat regularly and drink ample fluids, but avoid caffeine and alcohol.
- If using kerosene heaters, maintain ventilation, refuel the heater outside, and keep heaters at least 3 feet from flammable objects.
- Never use heat sources designed for outside use in a closed space.

If outdoors:

- Dress warmly (that is, several layers of loose fitting clothing, a hat, and a scarf to cover your mouth and protect your lungs).
- Avoid overexertion (for example, shoveling snow or pushing a car), which can bring on a heart attack.
- Be aware of signs of frostbite and hypothermia.
- Keep dry by changing wet clothing, which does not insulate well.

If trapped in a vehicle during a winter storm:

- Pull off of the highway. Turn on the vehicle's hazard lights. Hang a distress flag from the window or radio antenna.
- Stay inside the vehicle. Rescuers are more likely to find you. Do not set out on foot unless you can see a building close by where you know you can take shelter.
- Run the engine and heater about 10 minutes each hour to keep warm. When the engine is running, open a window slightly for ventilation, and clear snow from the exhaust pipe to prevent carbon monoxide poisoning.
- Exercise (for example, clap your hands and move your arms and legs occasionally) to maintain body heat, but avoid overexertion.
- In extreme cold, use floor mats, seat covers, road maps, newspapers, and other available resources for insulation. Huddle with other passengers.
- Take turns sleeping. One person should be awake at all times to look for rescue crews.
- Drink fluids to avoid dehydration.
- Watch for signs of frostbite and hypothermia.
- Be careful not to waste battery power.

FYI

Winter Travel Supplies

When traveling during the winter, carry disaster supplies in the vehicle. The kit should include the following:

- Shovel
- Windshield scraper
- Flashlight
- Extra batteries
- Battery-powered radio
- Water
- Snack food
- Gloves and mittens
- Hat
- Blanket
- Tow chain or rope
- Tire chains
- Bag of road salt and sand
- Fluorescent distress flag
- Jumper or booster cables
- Road maps
- Emergency flares
- Cellular telephone
- Emergency heating candles and container

- At night, turn on the inside light so work crews or rescuers can see you.
- Once the winter storm passes, you may need to leave the car and proceed on foot.

▶ Technological Hazards

Hazardous Materials Incidents

Chemicals are found everywhere. They can become hazardous during their production, storage, transportation, and disposal. It is not always possible to identify a situation as one involving hazardous materials, but clues such as a leaking cargo trailer, color-coded placards (signs) on abandoned drums, and unusual odors can be good indicators **Figure 26-8** .

What to Do During a Hazardous Materials Incident

Follow these safety guidelines if a hazardous materials incident occurs:

- If you witness an incident that you believe to be a hazardous materials incident, call 9-1-1 or your local emergency telephone number.

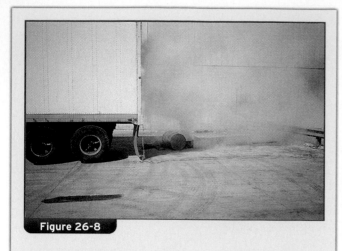

Figure 26-8

Fumes leaking from a cargo truck could be an indication of a hazardous materials incident.

- Stay away from the incident site.
- If caught outside, remember that gases and mists are usually heavier than air. Try to stay upstream, uphill, and upwind. Try to go at least one-half mile from the danger area.
- If in a vehicle, stop and seek shelter in a permanent building if possible. If you must remain in the vehicle, keep the windows and vents closed and shut off the air-conditioner and heater.
- If asked to evacuate your home, do so immediately.
- If requested to stay indoors rather than evacuate:
  - Follow all instructions, and close all exterior doors, windows, vents, and fireplace dampers.
  - Turn off air-conditioners and ventilation systems.
  - Go into an above-ground room with the fewest openings to the outside; close the doors and windows; tape around the sides, bottom, and top of the door; and cover each window and vent in the room with a single piece of plastic sheeting.
  - Listen to local emergency broadcasts.
  - When advised to leave your shelter, open all doors and windows and turn on air-conditioning and ventilation systems to flush out any chemicals that infiltrated the building.

Nuclear Power Plants

Nuclear power plants operate in most states and produce about 20% of the nation's power. Nearly 3 million Americans live within 10 miles of an operating nuclear power plant. Although these plants are closely monitored and regulated, unintentional radiation exposures are possible. Local and state governments, federal agencies, and electric utility companies have emergency response plans for nuclear power plant incidents.

What to Do During a Nuclear Power Plant Emergency

Follow these safety guidelines in a nuclear power plant emergency:
- Stay tuned to local radio and television stations. Local authorities will provide specific information and instructions.
- Evacuate if you are advised to do so.
- If told not to evacuate, remain indoors. Close the doors and windows, and turn off the air-conditioner, ventilation fans, furnace, and other air intakes. Go to a basement or other underground area if possible. Keep a battery-powered radio with you at all times.
- Do not use the telephone unless absolutely necessary. Lines will be needed for emergency calls.
- If you suspect exposure, take a thorough shower. Change clothes and shoes. Put all exposed clothing in a plastic bag. Seal the bag and place it out of the way.
- Seek medical treatment for any symptoms, such as nausea, which may be related to radiation exposure.

▶ National Security Emergencies

Terrorism

<u>Terrorism</u> is the use of force or violence against persons or property in violation of the criminal laws of the United States for purposes of intimidation, coercion, or ransom. Acts of terrorism range from threats of terrorism, assassinations, kidnappings, hijackings, bomb scares and bombings, and cyber attacks (computer based) to the use of chemical, biologic, and nuclear weapons **Figure 26-9**.

The Homeland Security Advisory System is designed to provide quick, comprehensive information about the potential threat of terrorist attacks or threat levels. Threat conditions can apply nationally, regionally, by industry, or by specific target. You should be aware of the current Homeland Security threat level at all times **Table 26-1**.

Chemical and Biologic Agents

<u>Chemical warfare agents</u> are poisonous vapors, aerosols, liquids, or solids that have toxic effects on people, animals, or plants. They can be released by bombs; sprayed from aircraft, boats, or vehicles; or used in liquid form to create a hazard to people and the environment. Some chemical agents may be odorless and tasteless. They can

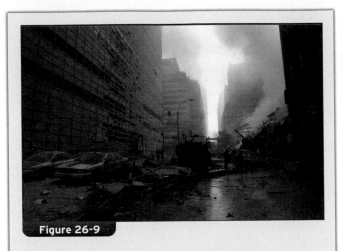

Figure 26-9

The September 11, 2001, terrorist attacks on the World Trade Center in New York City.

Table 26-1	Homeland Security Advisory System
Threat Level	**Protective Measures You Should Take**
Severe	Avoid high-risk areas such as public gatherings. Listen attentively to news for advisories and instructions. Contact employers to determine work status.
High	Review evacuation and sheltering measures for different types of attacks (chemical, biologic, or radiologic).
Elevated	Watch and report any suspicious activity. Contact school(s) to determine their emergency procedures.
Guarded	Review home disaster plan and update supplies. Meet with your family to discuss what to do, where to go, and how to communicate if an attack occurs.
Low	Develop a home disaster plan and disaster supply kit.

have an immediate effect (a few seconds to a few minutes) or a delayed effect (several hours to several days). Although potentially lethal, chemical agents are difficult to deliver in lethal concentrations. Outdoors, the agents often dissipate rapidly.

Biologic agents are organisms or toxins that can kill or incapacitate people, livestock, and crops. The three ba-

sic groups of biologic agents likely to be used as weapons are bacteria, viruses, and toxins.

What to Do During a Chemical or Biologic Attack

If a chemical or biologic weapon attack occurs near you, authorities will instruct you on the best course of action, which may be to evacuate the area immediately, seek shelter at a designated location, or take immediate shelter where you are and seal the premises. The best way to protect yourself is to take emergency preparedness measures ahead of time and get medical attention as soon as possible, if needed.

Follow these additional safety guidelines if a chemical or biologic attack occurs:

- Listen to the local radio or television stations for instructions from authorities, such as whether to remain inside or to evacuate.
- If instructed to remain in your home, office building, or other shelter during a chemical or biologic attack:
  - Turn off all ventilation, including furnaces, air-conditioners, vents, and fans.
  - Seek shelter in an internal room, preferably one without windows. Seal the room with duct tape and plastic sheeting.
  - Avoid the furnace or utility room.
  - Do not use any major appliances (for example, the furnace, oven or range, clothes dryer, or washing machine).
- Remain in protected areas where toxic vapors are reduced or eliminated, and take a battery-operated radio with you.
- If caught in an unprotected area, try to get upwind of the contaminated area, try to find shelter inside a building as quickly as possible, and listen to the radio for official instructions.

Nuclear and Radiologic Weapons

Nuclear explosions can cause deadly effects such as blinding light, intense heat (thermal radiation), initial nuclear radiation, blast fires started by the heat pulse, and secondary fires caused by the destruction. Surface level explosions also produce radioactive particles called *fallout* that can be carried by wind for hundreds of miles.

Terrorist use of a radiologic dispersion device—often called a dirty bomb—is considered far more likely than use of a nuclear device. These radiologic weapons are a combination of conventional explosives and radioactive material designed to scatter dangerous and sublethal amounts of radioactive material over a general area. There is no way of knowing how much warning time there would be before an attack by a terrorist using a nuclear or radiologic weapon.

What to Do During a Nuclear or Radiologic Attack

Follow these safety guidelines if a nuclear or radiologic attack occurs:

- Avoid looking at the flash or fireball; it can blind you.
- If you hear an attack warning:
  - Take cover as quickly as you can, below ground if possible, and stay there until instructed to do otherwise.
  - If caught outside and unable to get inside immediately, take cover behind anything that might offer protection. Lie flat on the ground and cover your head.
  - If the explosion is some distance away, it could take 30 seconds or more for the blast wave to hit. Be aware of a second, returning blast wave.
  - Protect yourself from radioactive fallout by taking shelter, even if you are many miles from the source of the explosion.
  - Keep a battery-powered radio with you, and listen for official information. Follow the instructions given. Local instructions should always take precedence; officials in your area know the local situation best.

▶ Summary

"The farther you are from the last disaster, the closer you are to the next one" is an oft-quoted statement made by emergency preparedness specialists. This is an age of catastrophe. Every American will likely be an unfortunate victim or witness to at least one disaster during his or her lifetime. The tragedy is that each citizen can be better prepared than he or she is now for that disaster. When a disaster strikes, you must be ready to act.

FYI

Disaster Preparedness

The US Department of Homeland Security offers these general guidelines for food and water needs for survival during emergency situations.

Water

- One gallon of water per person per day, for drinking and sanitation.
- Keep at least a 3-day supply of water per person.
- Children, nursing mothers, and people who are ill may need more water.
- If you live in a warm weather climate, more water may be necessary.

Food

- Store at least a 3-day supply of nonperishable food.
- Select foods that require no refrigeration, preparation, or cooking and little or no water.
- Pack a manual can opener and eating utensils.
- Choose foods your family will eat:
  - Ready-to-eat canned meats, fruits, and vegetables
  - Protein or fruit bars
  - Dry cereal or granola
  - Peanut butter
  - Dried fruit
  - Nuts
  - Crackers
  - Canned juices
  - Nonperishable pasteurized milk
  - High-energy foods
  - Vitamins
  - Food for infants
  - Comfort foods

First Aid Kit

- See Appendix A for suggestions for your first aid kit.

prep kit

▶ Ready for Review

- Disaster is a fact of life and you need to be prepared.
- Natural disasters such as earthquakes, floods, hurricanes, and tornados claim many lives each year.
- Chemicals are found everywhere; they can be hazardous during their production, storage, transportation, and disposal.
- Terrorism is the use of force or violence against persons or property in violation of the criminal laws of the United States for purposes of intimidation, coercion, or ransom.
- When disaster strikes, you must be ready to act.

▶ Vital Vocabulary

<u>biologic agents</u> Organisms or toxins that can kill or incapacitate people, livestock, and crops.

<u>chemical warfare agents</u> Poisonous vapors, aerosols, liquids, or solids that have toxic effects.

<u>terrorism</u> Use of force or violence against persons or property in violation of criminal laws for purposes of intimidation, coercion, or ransom.

<u>tsunami</u> A series of waves generated by an undersea disturbance.

▶ Assessment in Action

You are visiting with your grandfather at his ocean-front home on the Gulf Coast. It is late August and although the weather has been great all week, today it's not looking good. Because you are on vacation and your grandfather does not have a TV, you have not been paying attention to the weather, but you hear from your grandfather's neighbors that there's been talk of a possible hurricane. You turn on the local radio station and learn that a hurricane watch has been declared.

Directions: Circle Yes if you agree with the statement, circle No if you disagree.

Yes   No   1. No time to pack! You should grab your grandfather and get in the car to safety immediately.

Yes   No   2. You should board up the windows to prevent the risk of broken glass.

Yes   No   3. No need to worry that you only have half a tank of gas; there are plenty of gas stations along the highway.

Yes   No   4. You should include any medications that you or your grandfather are taking in your disaster supplies.

Yes   No   5. Review all possible evacuation routes before driving.

Answers: **1.** No; **2.** Yes; **3.** No; **4.** Yes; **5.** Yes

▶ Check Your Knowledge

Directions: Circle Yes if you agree with the statement, circle No if you disagree.

Yes   No   1. Earthquakes most often occur in the winter.

Yes   No   2. Never walk through moving water.

Yes   No   3. People in urban areas may be at greater risk from the effects of a prolonged heat wave than those in rural areas.

Yes   No   4. Hurricane season is from April until August.

Yes   No   5. Hide in a room with open windows if you are in the path of a tornado.

Yes   No   6. Never go near the shoreline to watch for a tsunami.

Yes   No   7. If you are trapped inside your car during a winter storm, run the engine and heater 10 minutes each hour to keep warm.

Yes   No   8. If you witness a hazardous materials incident, get up close to find out the name of the hazardous material before calling 9-1-1.

Yes   No   9. You should be aware of the Homeland Security threat level at all times.

Yes   No   10. All chemical agents have a smell or taste.

Answers: **1.** No; **2.** Yes; **3.** Yes; **4.** No; **5.** No; **6.** Yes; **7.** Yes; **8.** No; **9.** Yes; **10.** No

appendix A

First Aid Supplies

▶ First Aid Supplies

Many injuries and sudden illnesses can be cared for without medical attention. For these situations and for situations requiring medical attention later, it is a good idea to have useful supplies on hand for emergencies.

Supplies in a first aid kit should be customized to include those items likely to be used on a regular basis. For example, a kit for the home will be different from one at a workplace or one found on a boat.

The list here includes nonprescription (over-the-counter) medications. Some drug products lose their potency over time, especially after they have been opened. Therefore, buying a large, family size of a product that you use infrequently may not be economical. Note the expiration date on every medication.

Keep all medicines out of the reach of children. Read and follow all directions for properly using medications. Keep your first aid supplies in either a fishing tackle box or a tool box.

First Aid Kits

The following recommended items should be stocked inside a first aid kit in the workplace, at home, and for travel. First aid kits should be:

- impact resistant and made of durable material to protect against moisture, dust, and contamination.
- portable and easily carried by a handle.
- of sufficient size to store the equipment listed.
- clearly marked as being a first aid kit by words and/or symbols.
- regularly inspected and updated for completeness and content condition.

Workplace First Aid Kit

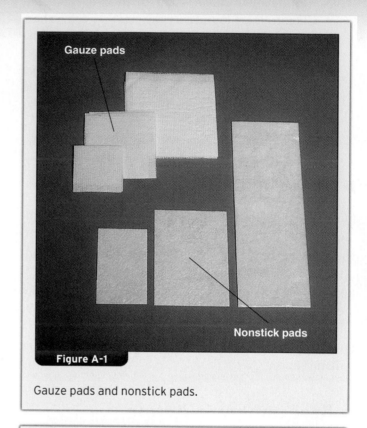

Figure A-1

Gauze pads and nonstick pads.

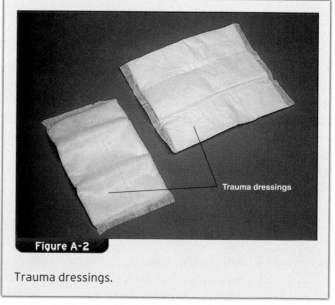

Figure A-2

Trauma dressings.

Equipment	Minimum Quantity
1. Adhesive strip bandages (1″ × 3″)	20
2. Triangular bandages (muslin, 36″–40″, 52″–56″)	4
3. Sterile eye pads (2⅛ × 2 ⅝″)	2
4. Sterile gauze pads (4″ × 4″) **Figure A-1**	6
5. Sterile nonstick pads (3″ × 4″) **Figure A-1**	6
6. Sterile trauma pads (5″ × 9″) **Figure A-2**	2
7. Sterile trauma pads (8″ × 10″) **Figure A-2**	1
8. Sterile conforming roller gauze (2″ width) **Figure A-3**	3 rolls

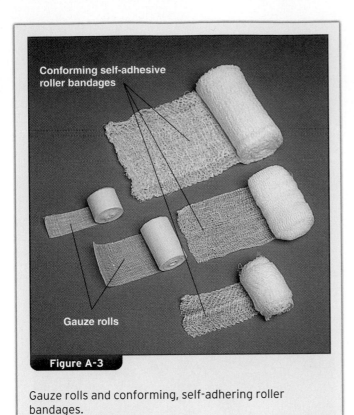

Figure A-3

Gauze rolls and conforming, self-adhering roller bandages.

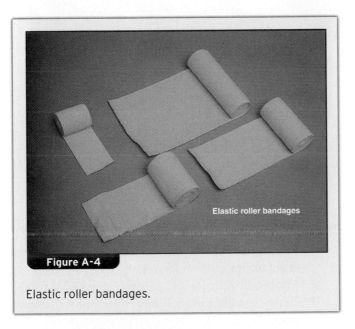

Figure A-4

Elastic roller bandages.

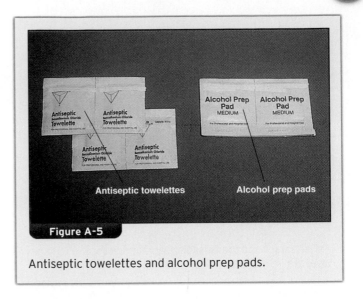

Figure A-5

Antiseptic towelettes and alcohol prep pads.

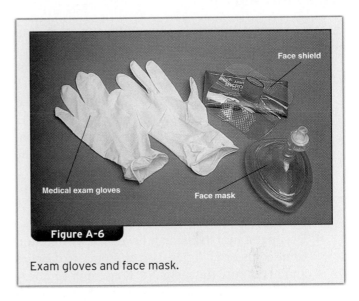

Figure A-6

Exam gloves and face mask.

9. Sterile conforming roller gauze (4½″ width) **Figure A-3** — 3 rolls
10. Waterproof tape (1″ × 5 yards) — 1 roll
11. Porous adhesive tape (2″ × 5 yards) — 1 roll
12. Elastic roller bandages (4″ and 6″) **Figure A-4** — 1 each
13. Antiseptic skin wipes, individually wrapped **Figure A-5** — 10

14. Medical-grade exam gloves (medium, large, extra large), conforming to FDA requirements **Figure A-6** — 2 pairs per size
15. Mouth-to-barrier device, either a face mask with a one-way valve or a disposable face shield **Figure A-6** — 1
16. Disposable instant-activating cold packs — 2
17. Resealable plastic bags (quart size) — 2
18. Padded malleable splint (4″ × 36″) — 1
19. Emergency blanket, Mylar — 1
20. Paramedic shears (with one serrated edge) **Figure A-7** — 1
21. Splinter tweezers (about 3″ long) — 1
22. Biohazard waste bag (3½ gallon capacity) — 2
23. First aid and CPR manual and list of local emergency telephone numbers — 1

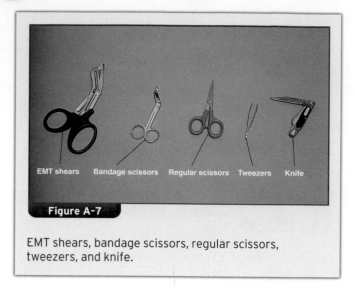

Figure A-7

EMT shears, bandage scissors, regular scissors, tweezers, and knife.

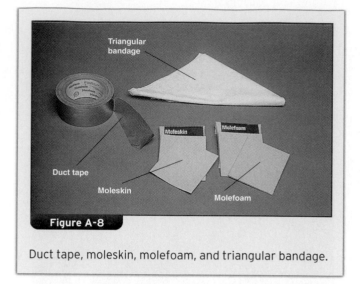

Figure A-8

Duct tape, moleskin, molefoam, and triangular bandage.

Home First Aid Kit

The American College of Emergency Physicians recommends that a home first aid kit include the following:

1. Acetaminophen, ibuprofen, and aspirin tablets: for headaches, pain, fever, and simple sprains or strains of the body. (Aspirin should not be used for relief of flu symptoms or given to children.)
2. Antihistamine: to relieve allergies and inflammation. Use appropriate dosages and make sure the medicine is age appropriate.
3. Cough suppressant: to relieve coughing. Use appropriate dosages and make sure the medicine is age appropriate.
4. Decongestant tablets: to relieve nasal congestion from colds or allergies. Use appropriate dosages and make sure the medicine is age appropriate.
5. Antiseptic wipes: to disinfect wounds or clean hands.
6. Thermometer: to take temperature. For babies under age 1, use a rectal thermometer.
7. Calamine lotion: to relieve itching and irritation from insect bites and stings and poison ivy.
8. Hydrocortisone ointment: to relieve irritation from rashes.
9. Activated charcoal: for treatment after ingestion of certain poisons. (Use only on the advice of a poison control center or the emergency department.)
10. Elastic wraps: for wrapping wrist, ankle, knee, and elbow injuries.
11. Triangular bandage: for wrapping injuries and making arm slings **Figure A-8**.
12. Scissors with rounded tips.
13. Adhesive tape **Figure A-9** and 2″ gauze: for dressing wounds.

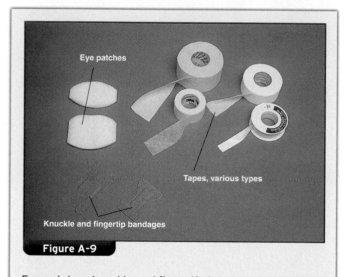

Figure A-9

Eye patches, knuckle and fingertip bandages, and tape.

14. Disposable, instant-activating ice bags: for icing injuries and treating high fevers.
15. Bandages of assorted sizes **Figure A-10**: for covering minor cuts and scrapes.
16. Antibiotic ointment: for burns, cuts, and scrapes.
17. Gauze in rolls and in 2″ and 4″ pads: for dressing wounds.
18. Bandage closures, ¼″ and 1″: for taping cut edges together.
19. Tweezers: to remove small splinters and ticks.
20. Safety pins: to fasten splints and bandages.
21. Medical-grade exam gloves to protect your hands and reduce the risk of infection when treating open wounds.
22. First aid manual.
23. List of emergency phone numbers.

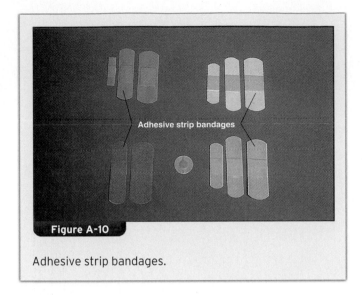

Figure A-10

Adhesive strip bandages.

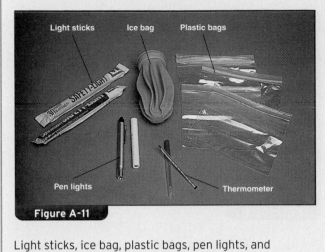

Figure A-11

Light sticks, ice bag, plastic bags, pen lights, and thermometer.

Travel First Aid Kit

The American College of Emergency Physicians recommends that a travel first aid kit include the following:

1. Aspirin, acetaminophen, or ibuprofen: for headaches, pain, fever, and simple sprains or strains of the body. (Aspirin should not be used for relief of flu symptoms or given to children.)
2. Antiseptic wipes: to disinfect wounds or clean hands, tweezers, scissors, and thermometer.
3. Calamine lotion: to relieve itching and irritation from insect bites and stings and poison ivy.
4. Gauze in rolls and 2-inch and 4-inch pads: to dress larger cuts and scrapes.
5. Antihistamine/decongestant cough medicine.
6. Antinausea/motion sickness medication.
7. Bandages of assorted sizes, including adhesive bandages.
8. Adhesive tape and 2″ gauze: for dressing wounds.
9. Elastic wraps: for wrapping wrist, ankle, knee, and elbow injuries.
10. Triangular bandage: for wrapping injuries and making arm slings.
11. Scissors with rounded tips.
12. Medical-grade exam gloves: to reduce the risk of infection.
13. Disposable, instant-activating ice bags: for icing injuries and treating high fevers.
14. Antifungal cream (tolnaftate 1% or clotrimazole 1%): good for athlete's foot or ringworm.
15. Antibiotic ointment: for burns, cuts, and scrapes.
16. Thermometer with case **Figure A-11** .
17. Sunscreen: SPF 15 or higher **Figure A-12** .

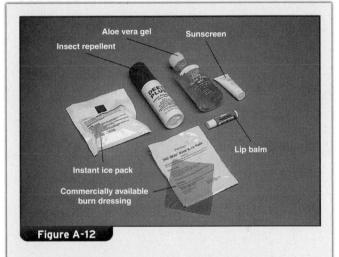

Figure A-12

Insect repellent, aloe vera gel, sunscreen, instant ice pack, commercially available burn dressing, and lip balm.

18. Insect repellent: those that contain 35%–55% DEET with stabilizer.
19. Antidiarrheal medications, tablets or liquid; follow directions carefully.
20. Antimalaria medications (if indicated).
21. Water-purifying pills or liquid (tincture of iodine or halazone tablets) or mechanical filtration devices.
22. Corcicosteroid cream, such as hydrocortisone cream: for insect bites.
23. Tweezers: to remove small splinters and ticks.
24. Safety pins: to fasten splints and bandages **Figure A-13** .

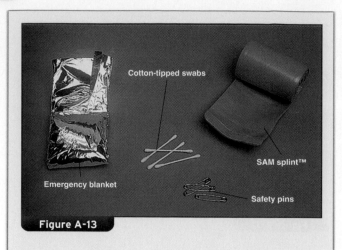

Figure A-13

Emergency blanket, cotton-tipped swabs, safety pins, and SAM splint.

Medication Information

As a first aider, you might be in a situation that requires you to give a victim certain medications (or to assist a victim in taking his or her own medication). A knowledgeable first aider should be familiar with the following medications:

Over-the-counter pain relievers:
- acetaminophen
- aspirin
- ibuprofen
- naproxen

Physician-prescribed medications:
- metered-dose inhaler
- nitroglycerin
- epinephrine

Over-the-counter medications carried in a first aid kit or available from the victim:
- oral glucose
- activated charcoal

▶ Pros and Cons of Popular Pain Relievers

Acetaminophen

Brand names: Tylenol, Datril
Advantages: Relieves pain and fever, does not irritate stomach
Disadvantages: Heavy or prolonged use can damage liver and kidneys

Aspirin

Brand names: Bufferin, Anacin
Advantages: Relieves pain, fever, inflammation; prevents heart attacks
Disadvantages: Interferes with blood clotting; might trigger stomach bleeding; can cause Reye's syndrome in children with viral infections

Ibuprofen

Brand names: Advil, Nuprin
Advantages: Relieves pain, fever, and inflammation
Disadvantages: Interferes with clotting; can cause stomach bleeding, ulcers, irritation; heavy or prolonged use can damage liver and kidneys

Naproxen

Brand name: Aleve
Advantages: Relieves pain, fever, and inflammation; one dose lasts 8 to 12 hours
Disadvantages: Can cause stomach bleeding, ulcers, irritation; prolonged use can harm kidneys

▶ Nitroglycerin

Give a victim nitroglycerin (trade name Nitrostat) if the following conditions exist:
- The victim is an adult.
- The victim has chest pain.
- The victim has physician-prescribed sublingual tablets or spray.

Do *not* give a victim nitroglycerin if any of the following conditions applies:
- The victim has a head injury.
- The victim is an infant or a child.
- The victim has already taken three doses.

Medication forms: tablet (about one tenth the size of an aspirin), sublingual spray, and patch.
Dosage: One dose, repeated in three to five minutes. If no relief, repeat again (maximum of three doses).

Procedure

Once you've decided to administer nitroglycerin, follow these steps:
1. Check the expiration date of nitroglycerin.
2. Ask the victim about the last dose taken.
3. Ask the victim to lift his or her tongue. Place the tablet or spray dose under the tongue or have the victim do so. Do not touch the tablet—wear gloves because your skin will absorb nitroglycerin and it will affect your heart rate.
4. Have the victim keep his or her mouth closed with the tablet under the tongue (without swallowing) until the tablet dissolves and is absorbed.

Actions

Nitroglycerin takes the following actions:
- relaxes (dilates) blood vessels
- reduces the workload of the heart

Side Effects

Side effects of nitroglycerin include the following:
- lowers blood pressure (victim should sit or lie down)
- headache
- heart rate changes

▶ Epinephrine Auto-Injector

Give a victim epinephrine (trade name Adrenaline) if both of the following conditions exist:
- The victim exhibits signs of a severe allergic reaction (includes breathing distress or shock).

The victim has physician-prescribed medication.
Medication form: liquid from automatic needle-and-syringe injection system.

Dosage

- Adult: One adult auto-injector (0.3 mg) **Figure B-1**
- Child/infant: One infant/child auto-injector (0.15 mg)

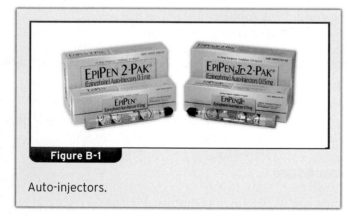

Figure B-1

Auto-injectors.

Procedure

Use these steps when administering epinephrine:
1. Obtain the victim's physician-prescribed auto-injector.
2. Remove the safety cap.
3. Place the tip of the auto-injector against the victim's thigh.
4. Push the injector firmly against the thigh to inject medication.
5. Hold the injector in place for 10 seconds.

Actions

Epinephrine takes the following actions:
- dilates the bronchioles (small tubes in lungs)
- constricts blood vessels

Side Effects

Epinephrine has the following side effects:
- increased heart rate
- dizziness
- headache
- chest pain
- nausea
- vomiting
- anxiety

Reassessment: Monitor breathing. If the victim worsens, give an additional dose; treat for shock.

Health Care Provider Basic Life Support

A health care provider is a person who provides health care as part of his or her job responsibilities. Examples include physicians, nurses, paramedics, and athletic trainers. Health care providers work in a variety of settings such as emergency medical services, hospitals, medical clinics, and athletic facilities. These professionals perform basic life support techniques differently than lay persons. Lifeguards are often taught two-rescuer CPR procedures.

▶ One-Rescuer Adult Rescue Breathing and CPR

If you see a motionless person, do the following:

1. *Check for response* **Figure C-1** .
   - Check the scene for hazards.
   - Tap the victim's shoulder.
   - Shout, "Are you OK?"
2. *If no response, call 9-1-1 and get an AED.*
   - If you are alone with the victim, shout for help.
   - If someone responds, send him or her to call 9-1-1 and get an AED.
   - If no one responds, call 9-1-1 and get an AED if available.

3. *Open an airway* **Figure C-2** .
   - Use the head tilt-chin lift method.
      - Place your hand that is nearest victim's head on his forehead and apply backward pressure to tilt his head back.
      - Place the fingers (not thumb) of your other hand under the body part of the jaw near the chin and lift. Avoid pressing on soft tissues under the jaw.
      - Tilt the head backward without closing victim's mouth.
   - If you suspect a neck injury, use the jaw thrust method without tilting the victim's head **Figure C-3** . If an airway does not open, use the head tilt–chin lift method.
4. *Check breathing for 5 to 10 seconds* **Figure C-4** .
   - Place your ear over the victim's mouth and nose while keeping the airway open.
   - Look at the victim's chest for rise and fall; listen and feel for breathing for 5 to 10 seconds.
   - If the victim is breathing, place him or her on his or her side (known as the recovery position).
   - If the victim is not breathing, go to Step 5.

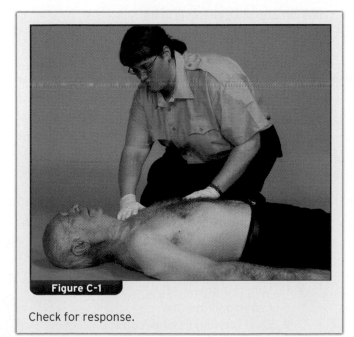

Figure C-1

Check for response.

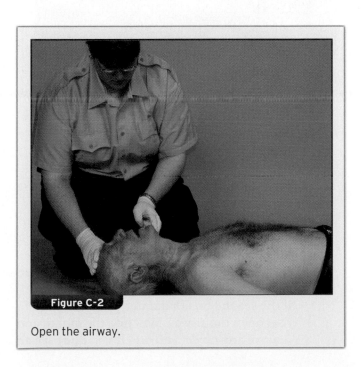

Figure C-2

Open the airway.

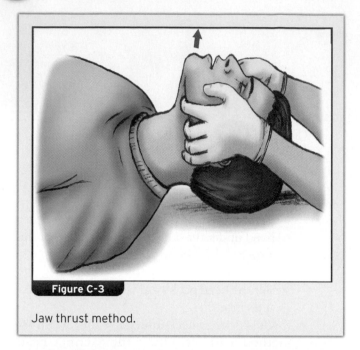

Figure C-3

Jaw thrust method.

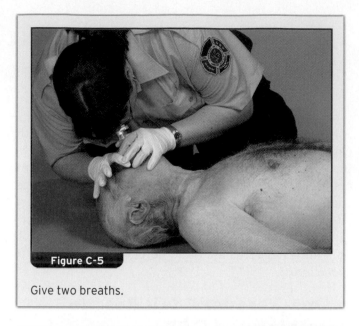

Figure C-5

Give two breaths.

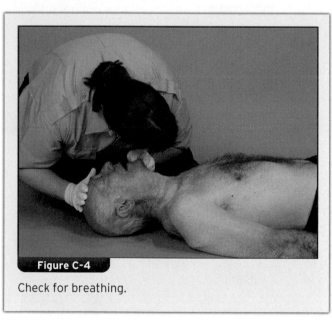

Figure C-4

Check for breathing.

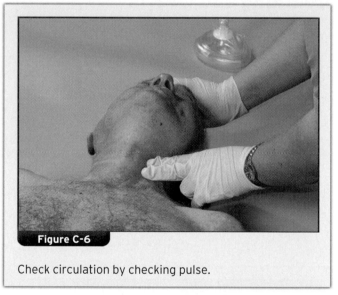

Figure C-6

Check circulation by checking pulse.

5. *Give two breaths* **Figure C-5**.
   - Use a barrier device, if available.
   - Each breath lasts 1 second.
   - Each breath is a normal breath and should cause the chest to rise.
   - If both breaths caused the victim's chest to rise, go to Step 6.
   - If the first breath did not cause the chest to rise, retilt the head and give the victim a second breath.
   - If the second breath did not cause the chest to rise, open the airway, look into the mouth and remove any object you see. If you don't see an

object, go to Step 7. While giving CPR, before giving breaths, open the victim's mouth, look for an object, and remove any you see.

6. *Check circulation by checking pulse* **Figure C-6**.
   - Keep the victim's head tilted with your hand that is nearest the head.
   - Using your hand nearest the victim's feet, locate the Adam's apple (trachea) with two or three fingers.
   - Slide your fingers down into the groove of the neck on the side closest to you (do not use your thumb because you might feel your own pulse).
   - Feel for carotid pulse for 5 to 10 seconds.
   - If there is a pulse:
   - Give normal breaths:
     - Each breath lasts 1 second.

- Repeat every 5 to 6 seconds (10 to 12 breaths per minute).
- Use the head tilt–chin lift method.
- After every 2 minutes (about 20 breaths), stop and check for a pulse.
- Continue until:
    - the victim is revived.
    - you are relieved by trained rescuers.
    - you are completely exhausted.
    - the victim needs CPR, which replaces rescue breaths.

If there is no pulse or you are not sure, go to Step 7.

7. *Perform CPR. The victim should be face up on a hard, level surface before you start CPR.*

Find hand position by:
- Placing the heel of one hand on center of chest between the nipples. Place your other hand on top of the first one and interlace, hold, or extend your fingers up off the chest.

Give chest compressions by **Figure C-7** :
- Placing your shoulders directly over your hands on the chest.
- Keeping your arms straight and your elbows locked.
- Pushing straight down 1.5 to 2 inches.
- Giving 30 compressions at a rate of about 100 per minute. Count as you push down: "one, two, three, four . . . 30." Push hard; push fast.
- Allowing chest to recoil completely after each compression.
- Keeping your fingers pointing across the victim's chest, away from you.

Open the airway, and give two normal breaths (1 second each).
- Give five cycles (2 minutes) of CPR. Recheck the pulse. If there is no pulse, repeat CPR. Continue CPR until:
    - the victim moves.
    - an AED becomes available.
    - you are relieved by trained rescuers.
    - you are completely exhausted.

8. *When an AED is available:*
- Turn the AED on.
- Attach adhesive pads to bare skin on the victim's chest and then attach the cable to the AED (use child pads for children, if available).
- The AED analyzes the victim's heart rhythm (no one should be touching victim).
- If shock is indicated by the AED (no one should be touching the victim), press the shock button.
- Start CPR with chest compressions.
- After five cycles of CPR, analyze rhythm with AED.

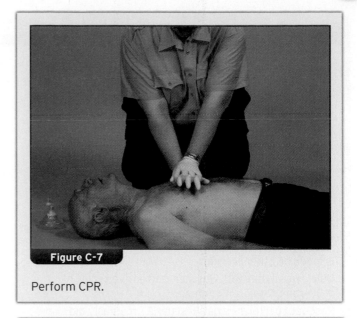

Figure C-7

Perform CPR.

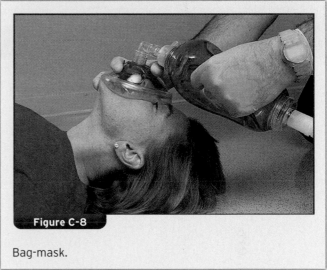

Figure C-8

Bag-mask.

- If shock is not indicated by the AED:
    - Start CPR with chest compressions.
    - After five cycles of CPR, analyze rhythm with AED.

▶ Two-Rescuer CPR for Adults and Children

Having two or more rescuers has two advantages:
- One rescuer can call 9-1-1 and obtain an AED, if available.
- It is less exhausting for the rescuers.

If a mask is available, a mouth-to-mask or bag-to-mask method should be used **Figure C-8** . The rescuer providing breaths should be at the victim's head while the other rescuer, who is giving chest compressions, should be at the victim's side. Ideally, the rescuers should be on opposite sides of the victim to enable a quicker switch.

Table C-1   Health Care Provider Basic Life Support

The rescuer performs an initial check.

- Is the victim responsive?
- Call 9-1-1.
- Position victim face up.
- A—Airway open? (Utilize head tilt-chin lift.)
- B—Breathing? If not, give two normal 1-second breaths.
- C—Circulation? (Check pulse.)

Rescuer 1	**Rescuer 2**
Gives 30 chest compressions (15 compressions for a child age 1 to puberty [12 to 14]) while counting out loud.	Keeps airway open during compressions.
Pauses after 30 compressions for two breaths to be given by other rescuer.	Gives two normal breaths during pause.
Quickly switches with Rescuer 2 after five cycles of 30 compressions (2 minutes).	Quickly switches with Rescuer 1 after five cycles of 30 compressions (2 minutes).
Rescuer 1 performs what Rescuer 2 previously did.	Rescuer 2 performs what Rescuer 1 previously did.

- D—Defibrillate when an AED arrives.

▶ Health Care Provider Procedural Differences Between Adult and Child (1 year of Age to Puberty)

Procedures are the same for *all* victims age 1 and over except:

If child (age 1 to puberty [12 to 14]) . . .	*Then* . . .
Is unresponsive.	• Call 9-1-1 after five cycles (2 minutes) of resuscitation (in adults, call 9-1-1 immediately after determining unresponsiveness). • A lone rescuer should use the adult procedures; call 9-1-1; and get an AED, if available, first.
Is not breathing, but has a pulse.	• Give enough breath to make chest rise, which will usually be less than that for larger children or adults. • Give one breath every 3 to 5 seconds (in adults give one breath every 5 to 6 seconds). • Rescuers might need to try several times to give two breaths to make the chest rise.
Does not have a pulse.	• Use one or two hands for giving chest compressions (depends upon the size of the child and the rescuer—adults require two hands). • Compress chest one third to half the depth of the chest (adults require 1½ to 2 inches).
Has a pulse less than 60 beats per minute (count pulse for 10 seconds and multiply by 6 for rate).	• Perform CPR.
Needs CPR and there are two rescuers.	• Use 15:2 compressions to breaths (30:2 is for one-rescuer CPR) and rotate every 2 minutes.
Is in the vicinity of an AED.	• Give five cycles of CPR before using the AED (in adults, an AED should be used as soon as it is available). • Apply child pads, if available.

index

image credits

Chapter 1
Opener Courtesy of Larry Newell; 1-1 From Vyrostek, S. B., Annest, J. L., Ryan, G. W. Surveillance for Fatal and Nonfatal Injuries–United States, 2001. *MMWR* 53 (SS07); 1-75 (September 3, 2004).

Chapter 2
Opener © Peter Steiner/Alamy Images; 2-1 © AbleStock.

Chapter 3
Opener © WizData, Inc./ShutterStock, Inc.

Chapter 4
Opener © Ingram Publishing/age fotostock; 4-2 © Jonathan Noden-Wilkinson/ShutterStock, Inc.; 4-3 Courtesy of the MedicAlert Foundation®. © 2006. All Rights Reserved. MedicAlert® is a federally registered trademark and service mark.

Chapter 5
Opener Courtesy of Larry Newell; 5-5 Photographed by Kimberly Potvin.

Chapter 6
Opener Courtesy of Larry Newell; 6-2 Source: American Heart Association; 6-8, 6-9 Courtesy of Philips Medical Systems. All rights reserved.

Chapter 7
Opener Photographed by Christine McKeen.

Chapter 8
Opener © Peter Morrison/AP Photos.

Chapter 9
Opener © Index Stock Imagery, Inc./Jupiterimages; 9-7, 9-10 © Howard Backer.

Chapter 10
Opener Photographed by Christine McKeen.

Chapter 11
11-1 © Suzanne Tucker/ShutterStock, Inc; 11-7 © Marilyn Barbone/ShutterStock, Inc.

Chapter 12
Opener © Joe Gough/ShutterStock, Inc.

Chapter 14
Opener Photographed by Christine McKeen.

Chapter 15
Opener © Christoph & Friends/Das Fotoarchiv/Alamy Images.

Chapter 16
Opener © Andres Rodriguez/ShutterStock, Inc.

Chapter 18
Opener © Stockbyte/Creatas; 18-4 © Doug Menuez/Photodisc/Getty Images; 18-5 Courtesy of DEA; 18-6 © Ben Smith/ShutterStock, Inc.; 18-7 Photographed by Kimberly Potvin; 18-8 © Thomas Photography LLC/Alamy Images; 18-9 © Thomas J. Peterson/Alamy Images; 18-10 Courtesy of U.S. Fish & Wildlife Service.

Chapter 19
Opener © Jonathan Plant/Alamy Images; 19-2 Courtesy of CDC; 19-5 © AbleStock; 19-6 Courtesy of Ray Rauch/U.S. Fish & Wildlife Services; 19-7 Courtesy of South Florida Water Management District; 19-8 Courtesy of Luther C. Goldman/U.S. Fish & Wildlife Services; 19-11 A: © Borut Gorenjak/ShutterStock, Inc., B: © Dwight Lyman/ShutterStock, Inc., C: © pixelman/ShutterStock, Inc., D: Heintje Joseph T. Lee/ShutterStock, Inc.; 19-14 © photobar/ShutterStock, Inc.; 19-15 Courtesy of Kenneth Cramer, Monmouth College; 19-16 © Nick Simon/ShutterStock, Inc.; 19-17 Kirubeshwaran/ShutterStock, Inc.; 19-21 Courtesy of Scott Bauer/USDA; 19-22 Courtesy of Daniel Wojcik/USDA; 19-23 © AbleStock; 19-24 Courtesy of NOAA; 19-25 © Nir Levy/ShutterStock, Inc.; 19-26 © Roger Dale Calger/ShutterStock, Inc.; 19-27 © AbleStock.

Chapter 20
Opener © Maxim Petrichuk/ShutterStock, Inc.; FYI box on page 316 Courtesy of the National Weather Service/NOAA.

Chapter 21
Opener © Laura Rauch/AP Photos.

Chapter 22
Opener © Craig Foster/ShutterStock, Inc.

Chapter 23
Opener © Dex Image/Jupiterimages; 23-1 Courtesy of Ron Dieckman, M.D.

Chapter 24

Opener © AbleStock; 24-7 © Riccardo Bastianello/ShutterStock, Inc.; 24-8 © AbleStock.

Chapter 25

25-4, 25-5 © U.S. Department of Transportation.

Chapter 26

Opener Courtesy of Dave Saville/FEMA; 26-1 Courtesy of D. Perkins/USGS; 26-2 Courtesy of Jocelyn Augustino/ FEMA; 26-4 © Photos.com; 26-5 Courtesy of the National Weather Service Forecast Office/NOAA; 26-6 Courtesy of John Hutmacher/USFS; 26-7 © Ron Frehm/AP Photos; 26-9 Courtesy of Andrea Booher/FEMA.

Appendix B

B-1 Courtesy of Dey, L.P.

Unless otherwise indicated, photographs are under copyright of Jones and Bartlett Publishers, courtesy of MIEMSS, or the American Academy of Orthopaedic Surgeons.